Pharmaceutical Applications of Analytical Chemistry

Pharmaceutical Applications of Analytical Chemistry

Edited by **Jessica Carol**

SYRAWOOD
PUBLISHING HOUSE

New York

Published by Syrawood Publishing House,
750 Third Avenue, 9ᵗʰ Floor,
New York, NY 10017, USA
www.syrawoodpublishinghouse.com

Pharmaceutical Applications of Analytical Chemistry
Edited by Jessica Carol

International Standard Book Number: 978-1-68286-127-1 (Hardback)

Contents

Preface

Analytical chemistry involves the identification and separation of chemical elements in both artificial and natural substances. This discipline has found its application in multiple fields like forensics, environmental and clinical analysis, etc. This book focuses on the experimental and analytical tools & methods utilized in the development and production of pharmaceutics. The researches included in this book provide new insights into the modern theories and applications of this field. It will serve as a valuable source of reference to students, academicians and professionals engaged in this area.

This book unites the global concepts and researches in an organized manner for a comprehensive understanding of the subject. It is a ripe text for all researchers, students, scientists or anyone else who is interested in acquiring a better knowledge of this dynamic field.

I extend my sincere thanks to the contributors for such eloquent research chapters. Finally, I thank my family for being a source of support and help.

Editor

Hafnium isotope analysis of mixed standard solutions by multi-collector inductively coupled plasma mass spectrometry: an evaluation of isobaric interference corrections

Min Seok Choi, Chang-Sik Cheong[*], Jeongmin Kim and Hyung Seon Shin

Abstract

Background: The Lu-Hf isotope system is widely used to decipher the crustal evolution and mantle differentiation of the Earth. The most critical point in obtaining accurate Hf isotope data is to correct the isobaric interferences of Yb and Lu imposed on the ^{176}Hf peak. In this study, we tested the validity of within-run correction protocol using MC-ICP-MS analysis of Hf standard solutions doped with Yb and Lu.

Findings: We found that the use of carefully selected Yb isotopic composition in the literature resulted in more reliable ^{176}Hf/^{177}Hf ratio. The ^{176}Hf/^{177}Hf ratios analyzed for a series of mixed Hf+Yb+Lu standard solutions could be quite accurately corrected for the mass bias and isobaric interferences. The systematic decreasing trend in the corrected ^{176}Hf/^{177}Hf ratios with increasing Yb/Hf ratios, however, indicates that the mass bias effect cannot be completely removed by the exponential law for samples high in Yb.

Conclusions: A close correlation of the calculated ^{176}Yb/^{177}Hf and ^{176}Lu/^{177}Hf ratios with the gravimetric values sheds light on the direct determination of inter-elemental isotope ratios without chemical purification.

Keywords: Lu-Hf, MC-ICP-MS, Isobaric interference, Mass bias

Introduction

Out of six naturally occurring isotopes of hafnium (^{174}Hf, ^{176}Hf, ^{177}Hf, ^{178}Hf, ^{179}Hf and ^{180}Hf), radiogenic ^{176}Hf is produced by the $^{\beta-}$ decay of ^{176}Lu with a half-life of 37.2 billion years in terrestrial samples (decay constant $\lambda = 1.865 \times 10^{-11}$ y^{-1}) (Scherer et al. 2001). Hafnium is more incompatible than lutetium during partial melting of mantle peridotite and thus long-term enrichment of the former relative to the latter in the continental crust has yielded unradiogenic ^{176}Hf/^{177}Hf ratios compared with those in the depleted mantle (Patchett et al. 1981). In this respect, the Lu-Hf system has been effectively used to trace crustal evolution and mantle differentiation of the Earth since the early 1980s (Patchett et al. 1981; Patchett & Tatsumoto 1980; Patchett

1983). Early Lu-Hf works were majorly undertaken by thermal ionization mass spectrometry but recent advances in multi-collector inductively coupled plasma mass spectrometry (MC-ICP-MS) have revolutionized the analysis of Lu-Hf isotopes, especially when combined with laser-ablation micro-sampling techniques (Thirlwall & Walder 1995; Griffin et al. 2000; Hawkesworth & Kemp 2006).

Accurate ^{176}Hf/^{177}Hf ratio is obtained only after the contribution of isobaric interferences by rare earth elements Yb and Lu on the ^{176}Hf signal is carefully corrected (Woodhead et al. 2004; Iizuka & Hirata 2005). This is particularly important where hafnium purification is unavailable prior to sample introduction to the ion source, as in the case of laser ablation analysis. The present study tests the validity of isobaric interference correction at mass 176 by using MC-ICP-MS analysis of Hf standard solutions doped with Yb and Lu. As the precise values of Yb isotope ratios selected for the

* Correspondence: ccs@kbsi.re.kr
Division of Earth and Environmental Sciences, Korea Basic Science Institute, Chungbuk 363-883, South Korea

correction of mass bias and isobaric contribution critically concern the reliability of corrected ^{176}Hf/^{177}Hf ratio, previous reports on Yb isotopic abundances will also be evaluated.

Instrumentation

In this study, Hf, Yb and Lu isotopic signals were measured by using a Neptune MC-ICP-MS installed at the Korea Basic Science Institute (KBSI) in Ochang. This instrument is a double focusing high-resolution ICP-MS equipped with eight motorized Faraday collectors and one fixed axial channel where ion beam intensities can be measured with either a Faraday collector or an ion counting electron multiplier. The gain calibration biases of the amplifiers are canceled out with the virtual amplifier design in which all Faraday collectors in a certain measurement are sequentially connected to all amplifiers. The Faraday collectors were statically set to simultaneously detect the required isotopes: ^{172}Yb (low 4), ^{173}Yb (low 3), ^{175}Lu (low 2), ^{176}(Yb+Lu+Hf) (low 1), ^{177}Hf (axial), ^{178}Hf (high 1), ^{179}Hf (high 2) and ^{180}Hf (high 3), respectively. The ion beam intensities were optimized by adjusting the torch position, gas flows and ion focus settings. The sensitivity on ^{180}Hf was typically around 25 V/Hf ppm (10^{+11} Ωresistors) in a low resolution (ca. 400) mode. Details of the other operational parameters are summarized in Table 1.

Measurement of standard solutions

The basic instrumental capability of the KBSI Neptune MC-ICP-MS was tested by using a JMC 475 Hf standard solution with a concentration of 200 ng ml^{-1}. The exponential law (Russel et al. 1978) was applied for mass bias

correction using ^{179}Hf/^{177}Hf = 0.7325 (Patchett et al. 1981). One run consists of 20 cycles, in which one cycle has an integration time of 4.194 s. The average ^{176}Hf/^{177}Hf ratio (0.282167±0.000005, n=5, 2σ S. E.) agrees well with previous recommended values (Blichert-Toft et al. 1997; Nowell et al. 1998; Vervoort & Blichert-Toft 1999) (Table 2). A range of shorter integration times (0.161, 0.262, 0.524 s) were tried with one block of 30 cycles (n=3). All results of ^{176}Hf/^{177}Hf ratio are quite reproducible and accurate (Figure 1) and thus it is concluded that the isotopic composition of a small quantity of hafnium (< 20 ng) could be analyzed with reasonable precision and accuracy in a short (< 1 minute) measurement time.

We also measured Hf isotope ratios of in-house standard solution JMC 14375, delivered from Alfa Aesar of Johnson Matthey Company (stock no. 14375, lot no. 83-084740F, plasma standard solution). The ^{176}Hf/^{177}Hf ratio of this standard solution (300 ng ml^{-1} Hf), measured with the same analytical design as that for the measurement of JMC 475 standard solution (20 cycles, 4.194 s integration) gave an average of 0.282228 ±0.000005 (n=10, 2σ S. E.) (Table 3).

Correction for isobaric interferences

Several analytical strategies were suggested to correct the isobaric interferences by Yb and Lu on ^{176}Hf: (1) Yb is doped with Hf isotope standard solution, and then use revised Yb isotopic compositions that give correct ^{176}Hf/^{177}Hf ratio (Thirlwall & Walder 1995; Griffin et al. 2000), (2) Determine the relationship between the Hf and Yb mass bias factors (Chu et al. 2002), (3) Yb mass bias factor is directly obtained from the Yb isotope ratios simultaneously measured with the Hf analysis (Woodhead et al. 2004; Iizuka & Hirata 2005). The last protocol would be the most effective unless Yb signal intensities are so low that precise isotope ratios are unavailable, considering that the mass bias factor is not a constant value during the MC-ICP-MS measurement (Woodhead et al. 2004; Iizuka & Hirata 2005). In this study, the isobaric interferences of ^{176}Lu and ^{176}Yb

Table 1 MC-ICP-MS instrumentation and operational parameters

RF forward power	1200 W
RF reflected power	< 2 W
Cooling gas	15 L/min.
Auxiliary gas	0.7 L/min.
Sample gas	1.018 L/min .
Extraction	−2 kV
Focus	−0.621 kV
Acceleration voltage	10 kV
Interface cones	Nickel
Spray chamber	Quartz dual cyclonic
Nebulizer	ESI PFA MicroFlow
Sample uptake rate	100 µL/min.
Instrumental resolution	ca. 400
Mass analyzer pressure	3.2 × 10^{-9} mbar

Table 2 Hf isotope ratios of JMC 475 standard solution

^{176}Hf/^{177}Hf	2σ S. E.	^{178}Hf/^{177}Hf	2σ S. E.
0.282171	0.000014	1.467249	0.000024
0.282153	0.000020	1.467270	0.000022
0.282167	0.000014	1.467247	0.000018
0.282174	0.000012	1.467248	0.000028
0.282173	0.000019	1.467256	0.000022
Average			
0.282167	0.000005	1.467254	0.000008

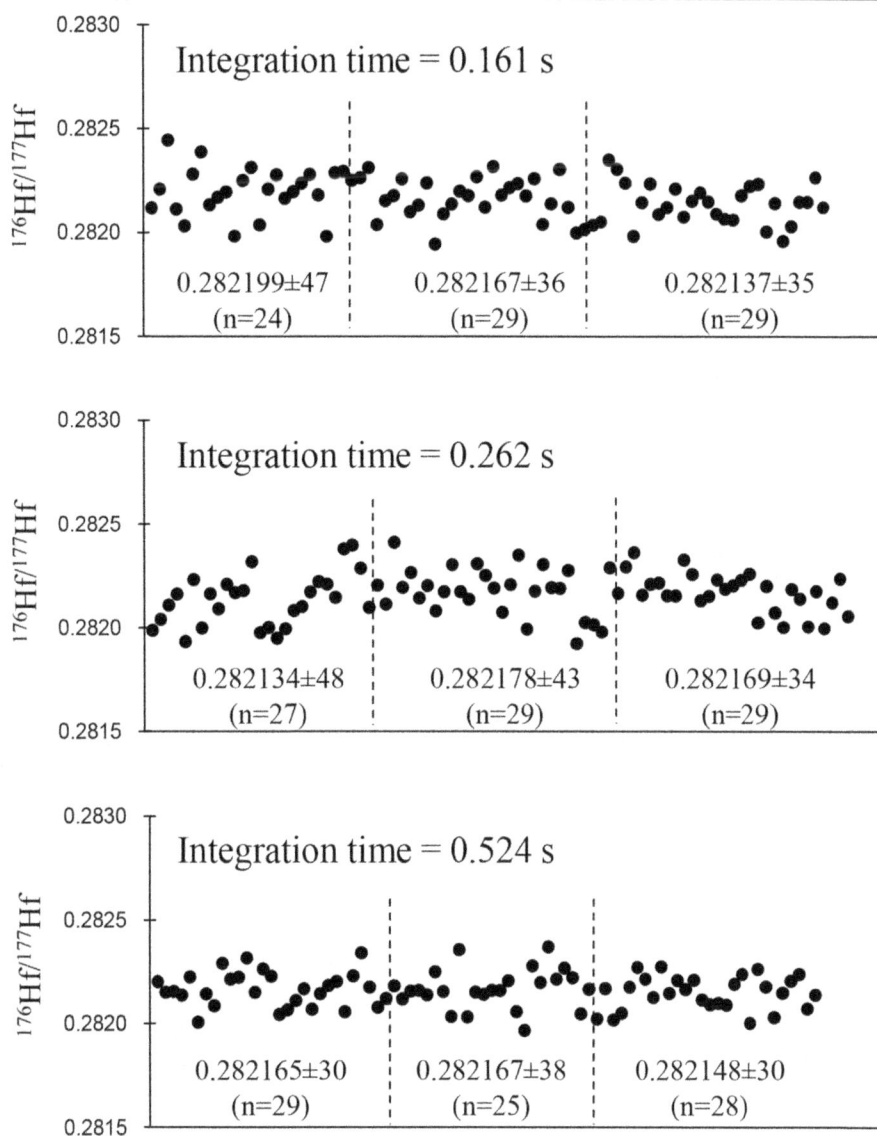

Figure 1 Hafnium isotope measurements of JMC 475 standard solution with integration times of 0.161, 0.262 and 0.524 s.

on ^{176}Hf were directly estimated by monitoring the intensities of interference-free Lu and Yb signals as the following:

$$^{176}\text{Hf}_{measured} = {}^{176}(\text{Hf} + \text{Lu} + \text{Yb})_{measured}$$
$$- \left[{}^{175}\text{Lu}_{measured} \times \left({}^{176}\text{Lu}/{}^{175}\text{Lu} \right)_{true} \times \left(M_{175}/M_{176(\text{Lu})} \right)^{\beta(\text{Lu})} \right]$$
$$- \left[{}^{173}\text{Yb}_{measured} \times \left({}^{176}\text{Yb}/{}^{173}\text{Yb} \right)_{true} \times \left(M_{173}/M_{176(\text{Yb})} \right)^{\beta(\text{Yb})} \right]$$

where $\beta(\text{Lu})$ and $\beta(\text{Yb})$ are respective exponential mass bias factors for Lu and Yb, and "M" denotes the mass of the isotope. The $\beta(\text{Hf})$ and $\beta(\text{Yb})$ values were measured by monitoring ^{179}Hf/^{177}Hf and ^{172}Yb/^{173}Yb ratios for a mixed standard solution of which concentrations were 298.7 ng ml^{-1} for JMC 14375 Hf, 30.4 ng ml^{-1} for

Table 3 Hf isotope ratios of JMC 14375 standard solution

^{176}Hf/^{177}Hf	2σ S. E.	^{178}Hf/^{177}Hf	2σ S. E.
0.282240	0.000014	1.467247	0.000022
0.282231	0.000012	1.467235	0.000030
0.282226	0.000011	1.467231	0.000028
0.282228	0.000011	1.467259	0.000036
0.282233	0.000010	1.467250	0.000038
0.282237	0.000012	1.467252	0.000024
0.282229	0.000015	1.467251	0.000028
0.282215	0.000009	1.467244	0.000028
0.282216	0.000015	1.467230	0.000032
0.282227	0.000010	1.467258	0.000028
Average			
0.282228	0.000005	1.467246	0.000006

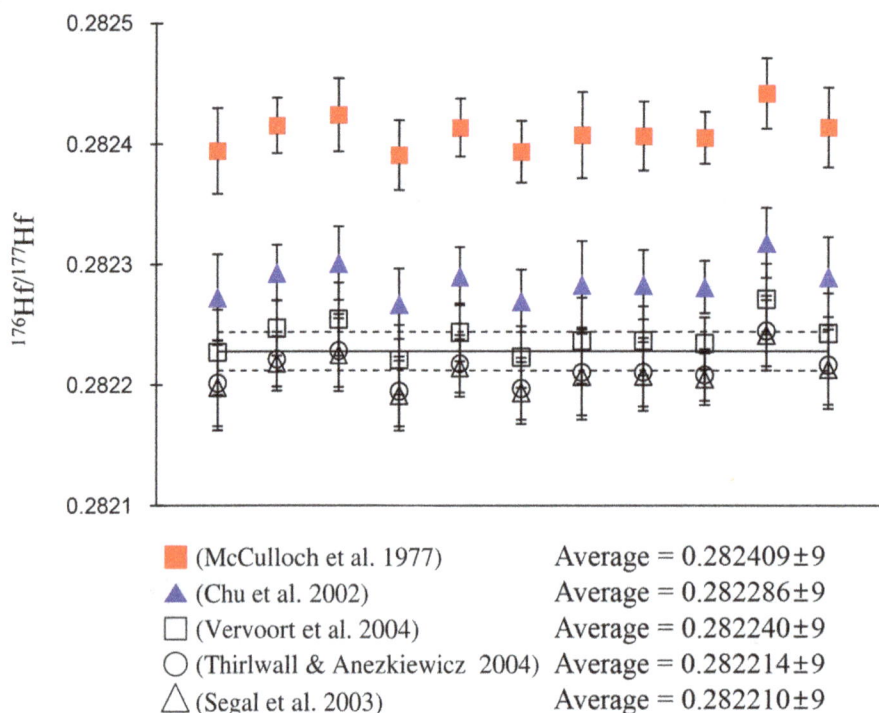

Figure 2 The ^{176}Hf/^{177}Hf isotopic measurements for a mixed standard solution of which concentrations were 298.7 ng ml^{-1} for JMC 14375 Hf, 30.4 ng ml^{-1} for Accu-Trace Yb and 3.0 ng ml^{-1} for Accu-Trace Lu. The isobaric interference corrections were made after previous reports on Yb isotopic composition (Chu et al. 2002; McCulloch et al. 1977; Segal et al. 2003; Thirlwall & Anczkiewicz 2004; Vervoort et al. 2004). Solid and dashed lines respectively represent the average ^{176}Hf/^{177}Hf of JMC 14375 and 2σ S. D. on the mean for the unspiked solution.

Accu-Trace Yb (lot no. B4035064-2B, reference standard) and 3.0 ng ml^{-1} for Accu-Trace Lu (lot no. B8045141, reference standard). For the calculation of β(Yb) and isobaric interference correction, an accurate Yb isotopic composition is needed but previous reports are not uniform (Chu et al. 2002; McCulloch et al. 1977; Segal et al. 2003; Thirlwall & Anczkiewicz 2004; Vervoort et al. 2004). The ^{176}Hf/^{177}Hf ratio of the

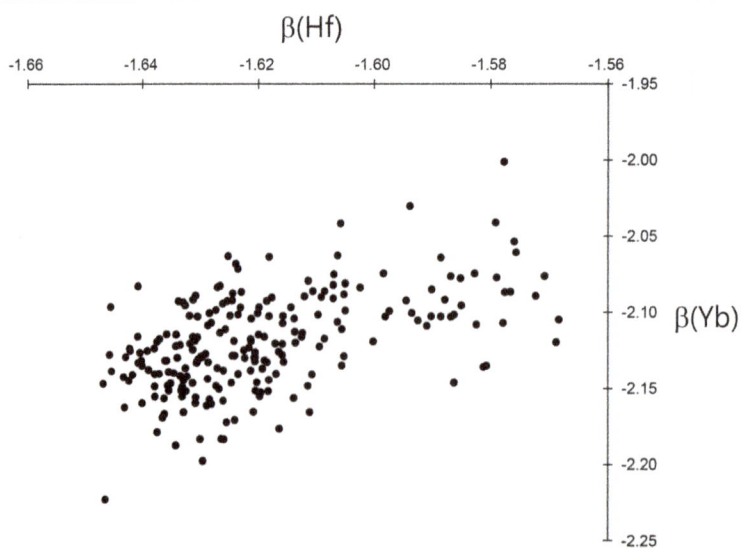

Figure 3 Relation between the Hf and Yb mass bias factors (β(Hf) and β(Yb)) for the same mixed standard solution as that described in Figure 2.

Table 4 Hf-Lu-Yb isotopic data for the mixed standard solutions

	$^{176}Hf/^{177}Hf$	2σ S. E.	$^{176}Lu/^{177}Hf$	2σ S. E.	$^{176}Yb/^{177}Hf$	2σ S. E.
Hf = 286.2 ng/ml, gravimetric $^{176}Lu/^{177}Hf$ =0.00072, $^{176}Yb/^{177}Hf$ = 0.03680						
	0.282214	0.000023	0.0009273	0.0000009	0.04969	0.00007
	0.282224	0.000024	0.0009419	0.0000004	0.05074	0.00003
	0.282228	0.000016	0.0009406	0.0000005	0.05068	0.00004
	0.282246	0.000025	0.0009408	0.0000014	0.05071	0.00011
	0.282218	0.000022	0.0009431	0.0000009	0.05087	0.00007
	0.282227	0.000020	0.0009428	0.0000005	0.05084	0.00004
	0.282237	0.000025	0.0009438	0.0000004	0.05093	0.00004
	0.282218	0.000024	0.0009348	0.0000003	0.05021	0.00002
	0.282217	0.000017	0.0009365	0.0000006	0.05037	0.00005
	0.282228	0.000014	0.0009397	0.0000004	0.05055	0.00004
Average	0.282226		0.0009391		0.05056	
2σ S. E.	0.000006		0.0000031		0.00024	
Hf = 298.7 ng/ml, gravimetric $^{176}Lu/^{177}Hf$ = 0.00142, $^{176}Yb/^{177}Hf$ = 0.07170						
	0.282201	0.000036	0.001851	0.000001	0.09813	0.00011
	0.282221	0.000023	0.001856	0.000001	0.09855	0.00012
	0.282229	0.000030	0.001866	0.000001	0.09932	0.00012
	0.282195	0.000029	0.001869	0.000002	0.09954	0.00011
	0.282218	0.000024	0.001867	0.000003	0.09942	0.00020
	0.282197	0.000026	0.001872	0.000002	0.09975	0.00016
	0.282210	0.000036	0.001874	0.000002	0.09992	0.00012
	0.282210	0.000029	0.001868	0.000001	0.09944	0.00009
	0.282208	0.000022	0.001873	0.000001	0.09983	0.00012
	0.282245	0.000029	0.001874	0.000002	0.09994	0.00012
	0.282217	0.000033	0.001874	0.000001	0.09995	0.00010
Average	0.282214		0.001868		0.09943	
2σ S. E.	0.000009		0.000004		0.00035	
Hf = 302.8 ng/ml, gravimetric $^{176}Lu/^{177}Hf$ = 0.00280, $^{176}Yb/^{177}Hf$ = 0.14151						
	0.282207	0.000033	0.003641	0.000003	0.19491	0.00025
	0.282216	0.000040	0.003662	0.000004	0.19654	0.00031
	0.282215	0.000045	0.003674	0.000004	0.19747	0.00029
	0.282185	0.000049	0.003674	0.000004	0.19748	0.00030
	0.282195	0.000030	0.003682	0.000002	0.19807	0.00013
	0.282206	0.000042	0.003681	0.000002	0.19788	0.00014
	0.282222	0.000033	0.003676	0.000003	0.19749	0.00021
	0.282196	0.000039	0.003675	0.000004	0.19732	0.00029
	0.282233	0.000031	0.003681	0.000003	0.19773	0.00025
	0.282184	0.000033	0.003671	0.000004	0.19685	0.00033
Average	0.282206		0.003672		0.19717	
2σ S. E.	0.000010		0.000008		0.00057	
Hf = 307.1 ng/ml, gravimetric $^{176}Lu/^{177}Hf$ = 0.00413, $^{176}Yb/^{177}Hf$ = 0.21282						
	0.282205	0.000030	0.005275	0.000003	0.28226	0.00022
	0.282176	0.000037	0.005289	0.000005	0.28333	0.00036

Table 4 Hf-Lu-Yb isotopic data for the mixed standard solutions *(Continued)*

0.282198	0.000028	0.005289	0.000003	0.28343	0.00026
0.282200	0.000045	0.005298	0.000004	0.28407	0.00029
0.282200	0.000036	0.005300	0.000003	0.28426	0.00021
0.282151	0.000035	0.005308	0.000007	0.28487	0.00051
0.282171	0.000047	0.005296	0.000007	0.28401	0.00051
0.282172	0.000041	0.005315	0.000004	0.28550	0.00030
0.282203	0.000038	0.005233	0.000007	0.27905	0.00052
0.282164	0.000037	0.005281	0.000004	0.28276	0.00026
Average 0.282184		0.005288		0.28335	
2σ S. E. 0.000012		0.000014		0.00111	

mixed standard solution was calculated using different sets of Yb isotope ratios as the followings.

^{172}Yb/^{173}Yb = 1.35260 (Chu et al. 2002),
     1.35704 (McCulloch et al. 1977),
     1.35428 (Segal et al. 2003),
     1.35823 (Thirlwall Anczkiewicz 2004),
     1.35272 (Vervoort et al. 2004)

^{176}Yb/^{173}Yb = 0.79618 (Chu et al. 2002),
     0.78759 (McCulloch et al. 1977),
     0.79381 (Segal et al. 2003),
     0.78696 (Thirlwall Anczkiewicz 2004),
     0.79631 (Vervoort et al. 2004)

As depicted in Figure 2, the results of 11 measurements (20 cycles, integration time=4.194 s) indicate that reports of Yb isotope ratios in (Chu et al. 2002; McCulloch et al. 1977) yielded incorrectly high ^{176}Hf/^{177}Hf ratios. Comparable ^{176}Hf/^{177}Hf ratios with that of unspiked JMC 14375 Hf (0.282228±0.000005) could be obtained by using Yb isotope ratios in (Segal et al. 2003; Thirlwall & Anczkiewicz 2004; Vervoort et al. 2004), and thus we hereafter give 1.35823 and 0.78696 as the (^{172}Yb/^{173}Yb)$_{true}$ and (^{176}Yb/^{173}Yb)$_{true}$ values, respectively (Thirlwall & Anczkiewicz 2004) for correcting mass fractionation of Yb and calculating its isobaric contribution to ^{176}Hf. Internal normalization of mass fractionation is not available for Lu, because it has only two natural isotopes (^{175}Lu and ^{176}Lu). In this study, the β(Lu) is assumed to be identical to the β(Hf), and (^{176}Lu/^{175}Lu)$_{true}$ of 0.026549 (Chu et al. 2002) is employed to calculate the signal intensities of ^{176}Lu. Possible difference between the β(Lu) and β(Hf) values does not affect the corrected Hf isotope ratio significantly because the contribution of ^{176}Lu to ^{176}Hf is typically very small in the crustal materials (*ca.* 1%, (Rudnick & Fountain 1995)). The β(Yb) value of each cycle is plotted against the β(Hf) value in Figure 3. This diagram confirms that the two values are not identical,

and should be measured independently during the run. They are positively correlated with each other but a distinct regression line is not identified.

We further tested the validity of isobaric interference correction described above by using Hf+Yb+Lu solutions mixed with different elemental proportions (Hf = 300 ng ml^{-1} JMC 14375, Hf:Yb:Lu ≈ 200:10:1, 100:10:1, 50:10:1, 30:9:1). The results with 10 blocks of 20 cycles (integration time = 4.194 s) (Table 4) show that the correction protocol works pretty well. There is, however, a systematic decreasing trend in the corrected ^{176}Hf/^{177}Hf ratio with increasing Yb/Hf ratios, indicating that mass bias is not perfectly corrected by the exponential law for samples high in Yb. The ^{176}Yb/^{177}Hf and ^{176}Lu/^{177}Hf ratios are calculated as the followings (Iizuka & Hirata 2005):

$$\left(^{176}\text{Lu}/^{177}\text{Hf}\right)_{corrected} = \left(^{176}\text{Lu}/^{175}\text{Lu}\right)_{true} \times \left(^{175}\text{Lu}/^{177}\text{Hf}\right)_{measured}$$
$$\times \left(M_{177}/M_{175}\right)^{\beta(Hf)}$$

$$\left(^{176}\text{Yb}/^{177}\text{Hf}\right)_{corrected} = \left(^{176}\text{Yb}/^{173}\text{Yb}\right)_{true} \times \left(^{173}\text{Yb}/^{177}\text{Hf}\right)_{measured}$$
$$\times \left(M_{176(Yb)}/M_{173}\right)^{\beta(Yb)} / \left(M_{176(Yb)}/M_{177}\right)^{\beta(Hf)}$$

The calculated ratios are not identical to the gravimetric values (Table 4) due to differences in elemental sensitivity but the two values are quite perfectly correlated with each other ((^{176}Lu/^{177}Hf)$_{calculated}$ = 1.277 × (^{176}Lu/^{177}Hf)$_{gravimetric}$; (^{176}Yb/^{177}Hf)$_{calculated}$ = 1.327 × (^{176}Yb/^{177}Hf)$_{gravimetric}$, R^2 > 0.98), leaving a possibility that these inter-elemental isotope ratios can be accurately measured directly from the sample solution without chemical purification.

Conclusions

We tested the capability of a Neptune MC-ICP-MS in obtaining accurate Hf isotope ratios of the mixed Hf+Yb+Lu standard solution. Careful selection of Yb isotope compositions was essential for the correction of mass bias and isobaric interferences from Yb and Lu on the ^{176}Hf peak. The validity of within-run correction protocol described here was confirmed by analyzing a series of mixed standard solutions, although the systematic decreasing trend in the corrected ^{176}Hf/^{177}Hf ratio with increasing Yb/Hf ratios indicated that mass bias was not completely corrected by the exponential law for samples high in Yb. A quite perfect correlation of the calculated ^{176}Yb/^{177}Hf and ^{176}Lu/^{177}Hf ratios with the gravimetric values leaves a probability to determine the inter-elemental isotope ratios directly from the sample solution without chemical separation.

Competing interests
The authors declare that they have no competing interest.

Authors' contributions
CSC, JK and HSS designed the study. MSC prepared the sample solutions and carried out isotope measurements. CSC drafted the manuscript. All authors read and approved the final manuscript.

Acknowledgements
This study was supported by Korea Basic Science Institute grants (G32221, G32210 and C32710). Valuable comments of two anonymous reviewers are acknowledged.

References
Blichert-Toft J, Chauvel C, Albarede F (1997) Separation of Hf and Lu for high-precision isotope analysis of rock samples by magnetic sector-multiple collector ICP-MS. Contrib. Mineral. Petrol. 127:248–260

Chu NC, Taylor RN, Chavagnac V, Nesbitt RW, Boella M, Milton JA (2002) Hf isotope ratio analysis using multi-collector inductively coupled plasma mass spectrometry: an evaluation of isobaric interference corrections. J. Anal. At. Spectrom. 17:1567–1574

Griffin WL, Pearson NJ, Belousova EA, Jackson SE, O'Reily SY, van Achterberg E, Shee SR (2000) The Hf-isotopic composition of cratonic mantle: LAM-MC-ICPMS analysis of zircon megacrysts in kimberlites. Geochim. Cosmochim. Acta. 64:133–147

Hawkesworth CJ, Kemp AIS (2006) Using hafnium and oxygen isotopes in zircons to unravel the record of crustal evolution. Chem. Geol. 226:144–162

Iizuka T, Hirata T (2005) Improvements of precision and accuracy in in situ Hf isotope microanalysis of zircon using the laser ablation-MC-ICPMS technique. Chem. Geol. 220:121–137

McCulloch MT, Rosman KJR, De Laeter JR (1977) The isotopic and elemental abundance of ytterbium in meteorites and terrestrial samples. Geochim. Cosmochim. Acta. 41:1703–1707

Nowell GM, Kempton PD, Noble SR, Fitton JG, Saunders AD, Mahoney JJ, Taylor RN (1998) High precision Hf isotope measurements of MORB and OIB by thermal ionization mass spectrometry: insights into the depleted mantle. Chem. Geol. 149:211–233

Patchett PJ (1983) Importance of the Lu-Hf isotopic system in studies of planetary chronology and chemical evolution. Geochim. Cosmochim. Acta. 47:81–91

Patchett PJ, Tatsumoto M (1980) Hafnium isotope variations in oceanic basalts. Geophy. Res. Lett. 7:1077–1080

Patchett PJ, Kouvo O, Hedge CE, Tatsumoto M (1981) Evolution of continental crust and mantle heterogeneity: evidence from Hf isotopes. Contrib. Mineral. Petrol. 78:279–297

Rudnick RL, Fountain DM (1995) Nature and composition of the continental crust: A lower crustal perspective. Rev. Geophys. 33:267–309

Russel WA, Papanastassiou DA, Tombrello TA (1978) Ca isotope fractionation on the earth and other solar system materials. Geochim. Cosmochim. Acta. 42:1075–1090

Scherer E, Münker C, Mezger K (2001) Calibration of the lutetium-hafnium clock. Science. 293:683–687

Segal I, Halicz L, Platzner IT (2003) Accurate isotope ratio measurements of ytterbium by multi-collector inductively coupled plasma mass spectrometry applying erbium and hafnium in an improved double external normalization procedure. J. Anal. At. Spectrom. 18:1217–1223

Thirlwall MF, Anczkiewicz R (2004) Multidynamic isotope ratio analysis using MC-ICP-MS and the causes of secular drift in Hf, Nd and Pb isotope ratios. Int. J. Mass Spectrom. 235:59–81

Thirlwall MF, Walder AJ (1995) In-situ hafnium isotope ratio analysis of zircon by inductively coupled plasma multiple collector mass spectrometry. Chem. Geol. 122:241–247

Vervoort JD, Blichert-Toft J (1999) Evolution of the depleted mantle: Hf isotope evidence from juvenile rocks through time. Geochim. Cosmochim. Acta. 63:533–556

Vervoort JD, Patchett PJ, Söderlund U, Baker M (2004) Isotopic composition of Yb and the determination of Lu concentrations and Lu/Hf ratios by isotope dilution using MC-ICPMS. Geochem. Geophys. Geosystem. 5, Q11002. doi:10.1029/2004GC000721

Woodhead J, Hergt J, Shelley M, Eggins S, Kemp R (2004) Zircon Hf-isotope analysis with an excimer laser, depth profiling, ablation of complex geometries, and concomitant age estimation. Chem. Geol. 209:121–135

2

Spectrofluorimetric determination of certain antidepressant drugs in human plasma

Mahmoud A Omar[1*], Osama H Abdelmageed[2], Sayed M Derayea[1], Tadayuki Uno[3] and Tamer Z Atia[1,3]

Abstract

Background: Certain antidepressant drugs namely Sertraline hydrochloride, Fluoxetine hydrochloride, Paroxetine hydrochloride, Thioridazine hydrochloride and Amineptine hydrochloride were studied throughout this work using spectrofluorimetric method.

Methods: The spectrofluorimetric method is based on the charge-transfer reaction of these drugs as n-electron donors with 7,7,8,8-tetracyanoquinodimethane (TCNQ) as π-electron acceptor. The drug-TCNQ complexes showed excitation maxima ranged from 290-301 nm and emission maxima ranged from 443-460 nm.

Results and discussion: The different experimental parameters affecting the formation and stability of the complexes were carefully studied and optimized. The calibration plots were constructed over the range of 50-450 ng mL-1 for Fluoxetine and Sertraline, 50-550 ng mL-1 for Paroxetine, 50-650 ng mL-1 for Thioridazine and 50-750 ng mL-1 for Amineptine. The proposed method was validated according to ICH and USP guidelines with respect to specificity, linearity, accuracy, precision and robustness.

Conclusion: A simple, reliable, sensitive and selective spectrofluorimetric method has been developed for determination of certain antidepressant. The proposed method was successfully applied to the analysis of the cited drugs in dosage forms. The high sensitivity of the proposed method allows determination of investigated drugs in spiked and real human plasma.

Keywords: Antidepressant drugs,7,7,8,8-tetracyanoquinodimethane (TCNQ), Dosage forms, Human plasma, Spectrofluorimetric determination

Background

Depression: a common mental disorder is a chronic or recurrent illness that affects both economic and social functions of patients and can eventually lead to suicidal behaviors. Antidepressant medications have been used to treat all forms of major depressive disorders (Parfitt & Martindale 2002). In the last years prescription of antidepressants has increased dramatically in Egypt. Sertraline, paroxetine, fluoxetine and amineptine are extensively used as antidepressant drugs in Egypt while thioridazine is a potent antipsychotic agent which is used in treatment of depression accompanied with anxiety. The chemical structures of the studied drugs in this work are shown in Table 1. Several methods have been published for determination of these drugs in bulk or in different pharmaceutical formulations as well as in biological fluids. These methods include Volumetric methods (Bueno et al. 2000; Delazzeri 2005; Basavaiah et al. 1999), Spectroscopic methods (Onal et al. 2005; Darwish & Refaat 2006; Patel et al. 2009; Darwish 2005; Mohamed et al. 2005; Mohamed et al. 2007), Electrochemical methods (Nouws et al. 2006; Atta-Politou et al. 2001), Chromatographic methods (Zainaghi et al. 2003; Nevado et al. 2006; Meiling et al. 2002; Sbarra et al. 1979, 1981; Tsaconas et al. 1989) and Capillary electrophoretic methods (Labat et al. 2002; Mandrioli et al. 2002).

The wide use of these drugs necessitates the development of simple, accurate, sensitive, applicable and cheaper method for their determination in pure forms, pharmaceutical formulations, spiked and real

* Correspondence: momar1971g@yahoo.com
[1]Analytical Chemistry Department, Faculty of pharmacy, Minia University, Minia 61519, Egypt
Full list of author information is available at the end of the article

Table 1 Structural formula of the studied drugs

Name	Chemical name	Structure
Sertraline Hydrochloride	(1S,4S)-4 [3,4-dichlorophenyl]- 1,2,3,4 tetrahydro-N-methyl-1-naphthylamine	
Paroxetine Hydrochloride	(3S, 4R)-3-[(1,3-Benzodioxol-5-yloxy)methyl]- 4-(4-fluorophenyl) piperidine hydrochloride	
Fluoxetine Hydrochloride	(3RS)-N-methyl-3-phenyl-3-[4-(trifluoromethyl) phenoxy] propane-1-amine hydrochloride	
Thioridazine Hydrochloride	10-[2-(1-methylpiperidin-2-yl) ethyl] -2-methylsulfanyl-phenothiazine hydrochloride.	
Amineptine Hydrochloride	dihydro-IO,1 I-dibenzo[a,&ycloheptenyl-5-amino-7-heptanoic acid	

human plasma. So this study describes a simple and very sensitive spectrofluorimetric method for determination of these drugs depending on the formation of charge-transfer complexes.

Experimental and Methods
Apparatus

- A perkin Elmer LS 45 Luminescence spectrometer (United Kingdom) connected to an IBM PC computer loaded with FL WINLABTM software.
- SpectronicTM GenesysTM 2PC. Ultraviolet/Visible spectrophotometer (Milton Roy Co, USA) with

matched 1 cm quartz cell connected to IBM computer loaded with winspecTM application software.
- Milwakee SM 101 pH meter (Portugal).
- Digital analytical balance (AG 29, Meltter Toledo, Glattbrugg, Switzerland).
- Laboratory centrifuge 4000 rpm (Bremsen ECCO, Germany).

Materials and reagents
All materials were of analytical reagent grades and the solutions were prepared with double distilled water. Samples of investigated drugs were generously supplied by their

respective manufacturers and were used without further purification; Sertraline hydrochloride was kindly provided by Pfizer Egypt, S.A.E., Cairo, Egypt. Fluoxetine hydrochloride was kindly provided by EIPICO, El Asher Ramadan City, Cairo, Egypt. Paroxetine hydrochloride was kindly provided by Pharaonia Pharmaceuticals Pharo Pharma, Alexandria, Egypt. Amineptine hydrochloride was kindly provided by Servier Egypt Industries Limited, 6th October City, Giza, Egypt and thioridazine hydrochloride was supplied by Delta Pharm, S.A.E, El Asher Ramadan City, Cairo, Egypt.

7,7,8,8-tetracyanoquinodimethane (TCNQ) (Sigma Chemical Co., USA) was prepared as 1×10^{-3} M in acetonitrile. Solution was found to be stable for at least one week at 4°C. Acetonitrile, diethyl ether and methanol (Riendel-De-Haen AG, Germany). Chloroform, 1, 2 Dichloromethane, Ethanol and 33% W/V ammonia solution (El Nasr chemical Co., Abu Zabbal, Egypt).

Plasma was kindly provided by EL-Minia Hospital of Psychiatric medicine and kept frozen until assay.

Pharmaceutical formulations

The following available commercial preparations were analyzed; Lustral® tablets (Pfizer Egypt, S.A.E., Cairo, Egypt) labeled to contain 50 mg sertraline per tablet. Flutin® capsules (EIPICO, El Asher Ramadan City, Cairo, Egypt) labeled to contain 20 mg Fluoxetine per capsule. Paxetin® tablets (Pharaonia Pharmaceuticals Pharo Pharma, Alexandria, Egypt) labeled to contain 20.0 mg of paroxetine per tablet. Survector® tablets (Servier Egypt Industrial Limited, 6th October City, Giza, Egypt) labeled to contain 100.0 mg of Amineptine hydrochloride per tablet. Thiozine® tablets (Delta Pharm, S.A.E, El Asher Ramadan City, Cairo, Egypt) labeled to contain 100 mg of Thioridazine hydrochloride per tablet.

Preparation of standard solutions

An accurately weighed 20.0 mg salt of each investigated drugs, was transferred into 125-mL separating funnel containing about 20 mL of distilled water. The resultant solution was rendered distinctly alkaline with dropwise addition of 33% w/v aqueous ammonia solution. The librated free base was extracted with three potions of 5 mL chloroform. The combined chloroformic extracts were filtered through anhydrous sodium sulfate supported on Whitman filter paper. The filter paper was washed thoroughly with two portions of 5 mL chloroform. The combined extracts and washings were diluted to volume with chloroform to provide a stock standard solution containing 200.0 μg mL^{-1}. This solution was further diluted with the same solvent to prepare working standard solutions containing 0.50 - 4.50 μg mL^{-1} of fluoxetine and sertraline, 0.50- 5.5 μg mL^{-1} of paroxetine, 1.0-6.5 μg mL^{-1} of thioridazine and 1.0-7.5 μg mL^{-1} of

amineptine. The standard solutions were stable for seven days when kept in the refrigerator.

General analytical procedure

Into a series of 10 mL volumetric flasks, 1.0 mL of working standard solution of each drug was transferred over the cited concentration. One mL of 1×10^{-3} M TCNQ solution was added and mixed well. The reaction mixture was allowed to stand at room temperature (25.0 ± 5°C) for 40 min for fluoxetine, sertraline and paroxetine; 35 min for thioridazine and 45 min for amineptine then completed to the mark with chloroform. The fluorescence intensity of the complexes was measured at 443, 447, 447, 450 and 458 nm after excitation at 290, 291, 291, 295 and 301 nm for fluoxetine, sertraline, paroxetine, amineptine and thioridazine respectively. Blank experiment was carried out simultaneously. The relative fluorescence intensity of each sample solution for each investigated drugs was accurately measured and plotted against the final drug concentration (ng mL^{-1}) to get the calibration graphs.

Procedure for pharmaceutical formulations (tablets and capsules)

A quantity of finely powdered twenty tablets or mixed capsules contents equivalent to 100.0 mg of active component was transferred to 50-mL volumetric flask, sonicated for about 10 minute with about 30 mL double distilled water. The volume was made up with distilled water, mixed well and filtered. The first portion of the filtrate was discarded; twenty mL of the clear solution was transferred quantitatively to a 125 mL separating funnel. The contents of the funnel were rendered alkaline with dropwise addition 33% w/v aqueous ammonia solution, and the procedure was completed as described under preparation of the standard solutions.

Procedure for spiked human plasma

5.0 mL of drug free human blood sample was taken from three healthy volunteers into a heparinized tubes, centrifuged at 3000 rpm for 30 minutes then 1.0 mL of the drug free plasma (supernatant) was spiked with 1.0 mL of investigated drugs containing 5.0-45.0 μg mL^{-1} of fluoxetine and sertraline, 5.0- 55.0 μg mL^{-1} of paroxeine, 10.0- 65.0 μg mL^{-1} of thioridazine and 10.0-75.0 μg mL^{-1} of amineptine. 2.0 mL of acetonitrile was added as precipitating agent for protein then centrifuged at 4000 rpm for about 20 min. The supernatant was rendered alkaline by adding 1.0 mL of 33% w/v aqueous ammonia and then extract the librated free base three times with 3×3 mL of chloroform. The combined chloroformic extracts were filtered through anhydrous sodium sulfate supported on Whitman filter paper. The filter paper was washed thoroughly with two portions of

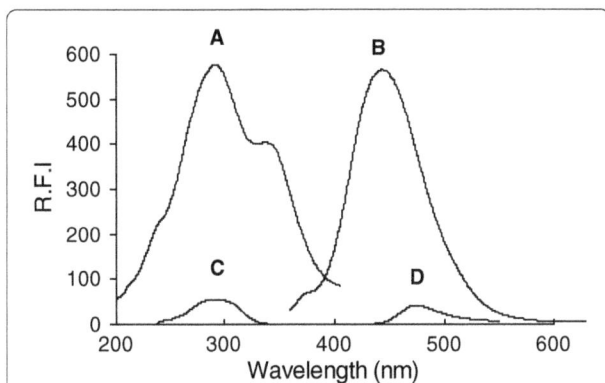

Figure 1 Fluorescence spectra of the produced CT-complex of fluoxetine (450 ngml^{-1}) with 1×10^{-3} M TCNQ where; A) Excitation spectrum B) Emission spectrum, C) Excitation spectrum of blank and D) Emission spectrum of blank.

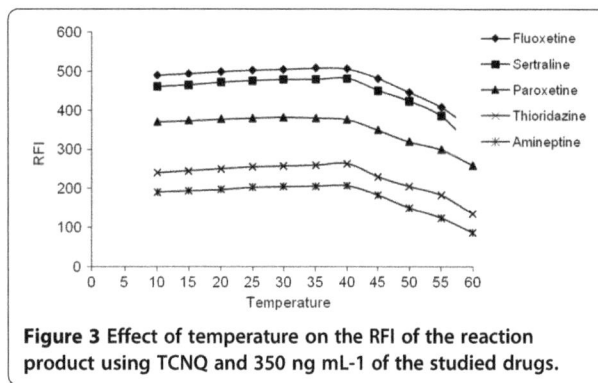

Figure 3 Effect of temperature on the RFI of the reaction product using TCNQ and 350 ng mL-1 of the studied drugs.

5 mL chloroform. The combined extracts and washings were diluted to volume with chloroform. Aliquotes covering the working concentration range was transferred into 10-mL volumetric flasks; then the general procedure was followed. A blank value was determined by treating the drug free blood sample in the same manner.

Procedure for real human plasma

For fluoxetine, 20.0 mg was taken orally once daily by three healthy human volanteers for 4 weeks. 5.0 mL of human blood sample was taken by using heperanized tube after an average of 6 hrs following the last oral administration and centrifuged at 3000 rpm for 30 minute. 3.0 mL of plasma obtained was treated with 2.0 mL of acetonitrile as precipitating agent for protein then centrifuged at 4500 rpm for about 20 minute. The supernatant was rendered alkaline by adding 1.0 mL of 33% w/v aqueous ammonia followed by extraction with 3×3 mL of chloroform. The combined extracts were diluted to volume with chloroform; then the general procedure was followed.

For paroxetine, 40.0 mg was taken orally once daily by three healthy human volanteers for 14 days. 10.0 mL

of human blood sample was taken by using heperanized tube after an average of 12 hrs following the last oral administration and centrifuged at 3000 rpm for 30 minute. 6.0 mL of plasma obtained was treated with 4.0 mL of acetonitrile as precipitating agent for protein then centrifuged at 4500 rpm for about 20 minute; then the procedure was followed as described for fluoxetine starting from "The supernatant was rendered alkaline by...".

For bupropion, 150.0 mg was taken orally every 12 hrs by three healthy human volanteers for 14 days. 5.0 mL of human blood sample was taken by using heperanized tube after an average of 6 hrs following the last oral administration; then the procedure was followed as described for fluoxetine.

For sertraline, 50.0 mg was taken orally once daily by three healthy human volanteers for 14 days. 5.0 mL of human blood sample was taken by using heperanized tube after an average of 12 hrs following the last oral administration; then the procedure was followed as described for fluoxetine.

For thioridazine, 100.0 mg was taken orally four times daily by three healthy human volunteers for 7 days. 5.0 mL of human blood sample was taken by using heperanized tube at 8 th day, 3 hrs after the last morning oral administration; then the procedure was followed as described for fluoxetine.

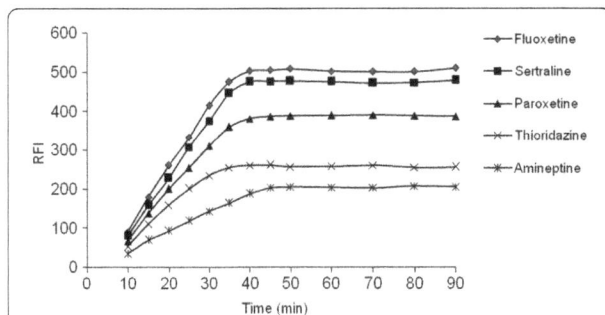

Figure 2 Effect of reaction time on the RFI of the reaction product using TCNQ and 350 ng mL-1 of the studied drugs.

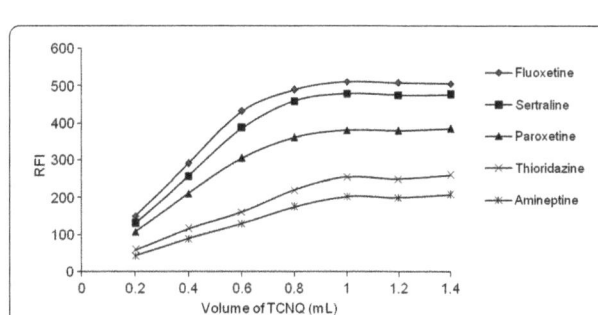

Figure 4 Effect of $1 \times 10\text{-}3$ M TCNQ volume on its reaction with 350 ng mL-1 of the studied drugs.

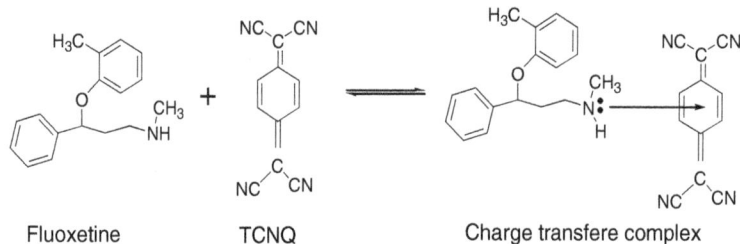

Figure 5 The suggested reaction pathway between fluoxetine as representative example of the studied drugs with TCNQ.

Results and discussion

The aim of this work is to establish a simple, sensitive, reliable, selective and cheap spectrofluorimetric method for the analysis of investigated drugs in pure forms, pharmaceutical formulations, spiked and real human plasma. The developed method was based on reaction of investigated drugs with 7,7,8,8-tetracyanoquinodimethane (TCNQ) to form highly fluorescent product, measured fluorometrically.

Fluorescence spectrum

Solutions of the studied drugs have very weak native fluorescence intensity, however in presence of TCNQ, the fluorescence intensity increases substantially. The formed CT complexes between the investigated drugs and TCNQ were probably through the lone pair of electron donated by the N atom in investigated drugs (n-donor) to TCNQ (π-acceptor). The fluorescence intensity of the reaction product was measured at 443, 447, 447, 450 and 458 nm after excitation at 290, 291, 291, 295 and 301 nm for fluoxetine, sertraline, paroxetine, amineptine and thioridazine respectively. Figure 1 shows the fluorescence spectra of the reaction product of fluoxetine as a representative example of investigated drugs TCNQ.

Optimization of variables

The spectrofluorimetric properties of the fluorescent product as well as the different experimental parameters affecting the development and stability of the CT-complex were carefully studied and optimized. Each factor was changed individually while the others were kept constant.

The studied factors include diluting solvent, reaction time, temperature and concentration of the reagent.

In order to select the suitable solvent for CT-complex formation, the reaction of TCNQ with studied drugs was carried out in different solvents. The studied solvents are chloroform, acetonitrile, ethanol, methanol and 1,2-dichloroethane. It was found that chloroform was considered to be the best solvent for the fluorescence development proved by the highest RFI observed relative to other solvents.

The fluorescence intensity of the formed CT-complex was monitored at different time intervals. It was found that complete fluorescence developments were attained after 40 minutes for fluoxetine, sertraline and paroxetine; after 35 min for thioridazine and after 45 min for amineptine (Figure 2). The fluorescence intensity remained stable for at least 2 hours.

The effect of temperature on the formed charge transfer complexes was studied in the range of 10 - 60°C. All the formed complexes were stable up to 40°C. At temperature higher than 40°C, the RFI decreases probably due to dissociation of the complex. Thus, the determinations of studied drugs were carried out at 25 ± 5°C (Figure 3).

Different volumes of 1×10^{-3} M of TCNQ reagent were used ranging from 0.2 to 1.4 mL. It was observed that the relative fluorescence intensity (RFI) increases by increasing volume of TCNQ and reaches its maximum values at 1 mL of 1×10^{-3} M of TCNQ after which no further increase in RFI was observed. So 1 mL of 1×10^{-3} M of TCNQ was chosen as an optimum concentration for further investigation (Figure 4).

Table 2 Analytical parameters of spectrofluorimetric determination of investigated drugs with TCNQ

Investigated drugs	Linear range ng mL^{-1}	Intercept (a)	Standard deviation of intercept (Sa)	Slope (b)	Correlation coefficient (r)	LOD ng mL^{-1}	LOQ ng mL^{-1}
Fluoxetine	50-450	−0.20	2.58	1.45	0.9995	5.35	17.85
Sertraline	50-450	−2.18	2.82	1.36	0.9998	6.23	20.77
Paroxetine	50-550	0.63	2.45	1.10	0.9997	6.68	22.26
Thioridazine	100-650	−1.47	2.68	0.71	0.9992	11.37	37.90
Amineptine	100-750	−0.43	2.37	0.57	0.9990	12.48	41.61

Table 3 Evaluation of accuracy of the investigated analytical procedure at three concentration levels within the specified range

Drug	50.0 ng mL^{-1}	Recovery %[a] 250.0 ng mL^{-1}	450.0 ng mL^{-1}
Fluoxetine	100.94 ± 1.29	99.80 ± 0.51	100.41 ± 0.28
Sertraline	99.84 ± 1.69	98.91 ± 0.55	100.14 ± 0.30
	50.0 ng mL^{-1}	**Recovery %[a] 250.0 ngmL^{-1}**	**550.0 ngmL^{-1}**
Paroxetine	100.92 ± 1.28	100.09 ± 0.67	100.06 ± 0.31
	100.0 ngmL^{-1}	**Recovery %[a] 350.0 ngmL^{-1}**	**650.0 ngmL^{-1}**
Thioridazine	100.44 ± 1.57	101.31 ± 0.95	100.48 ± 0.41
	100.0 ngmL^{-1}	**Recovery %[a] 450.0 ngmL^{-1}**	**750.0 ngmL^{-1}**
Amineptine	100.14 ± 1.87	98.81 ± 0.72	100.47 ± 0.44

[a] Mean of Six replicate measurements.

Stoichiometry and Mechanism of the reaction

The stoichiometric of the reaction mechanism was studied adopting the job's method (Job 1964) of continuous variation. The molar ratio of TCNQ to each of investigated drugs was 1:1. The reaction pathway proposed in Figure 5 is presented.

Validation of the proposed method

Concentration range (Topic Q2A 1994) was established by confirming that the analytical procedure provided a suitable degree of precision, accuracy and linearity when applied to the sample containing amount of analyte within or at the extreme of the specified range of the analytical procedure (Topic Q2B 1996; The United States Pharmacopoeia XXV and NF XX 2002). In this work, concentration ranging from 50 to 450 ng mL^{-1} (for fluoxetine and sertraline), 50 to 550 ng mL^{-1} (for paroxetine), 100 to 650 ng mL^{-1} (for thioridazine) and 100 to 750 ng mL^{-1} (for amineptine) were studied. The whole set of experiments were carried out within this range to ensure the validation of the proposed procedure. Linear calibration graphs were obtained for all the studied drugs by plotting the RFI of the studied drugs versus the drug concentration (ng mL^{-1}) within the specified range.

Linearity was indicated by high correlation coefficient obtained. The correlation coefficients (r) of the formed products were in the range 0.9990 to 0.9998 indicating good linearity, as shown in Table 2.

Accuracy (The United States Pharmacopoeia XXV and NF XX 2002) was checked at three concentration levels within the specified range. Six replicate measurements were recorded at each concentration level. The results were expressed as percent recovery ± standard deviation (Table 3). The obtained results show the close agreement between the measured and true values. Meanwhile, comparison of the obtained results from the analysis of the drug products by the proposed procedure with those obtained from the reported methods (Darwish 2005; Mohamed et al. 2005, 2007) revealed that their is no significant difference between them with respect to accuracy as indicated by t- and F- tests (Table 4).

Precision (The United States Pharmacopoeia XXV and NF XX 2002) was checked at three concentration levels, eight replicate measurements were recorded at each concentration level; the results are summarized in Table 5. The calculated relative standard deviations were below 2.2% indicating excellent precision of the proposed procedure at both levels of repeatability and intermediate precision.

Limit of detection (Topic Q2A 1994) was calculated based on standard deviation of response and the slope of calibration curve (Topic Q2B 1996). The limit

Table 4 Statistical analysis of the results obtained using the proposed procedures and reference method for spectrofluorimetric analysis of authentic samples using TCNQ

Drug	% Recovery ± SD		t-value[b]	F-value[b]
	Proposed methods	Reported method[#]		
Fluoxetine	100.34 ± 0.89	99.95 ± 1.08	0.62	1.44
Sertraline	99.61 ± 1.57	99.67 ± 1.61	0.06	1.05
Paroxetine	99.29 ± 1.02	99.38 ± 1.20	0.13	1.40
Thiridazine	100.32 ± 1.24	100.39 ± 1.30	0.09	1.09
Amineptine	100.37 ± 1.04	100.57 ± 1.69	0.23	2.63

[b]Tabulated value at 95% confidence limit; F = 6.338 and t = 2.306.
[#]References (Darwish 2005; Mohamed et al. 2005, 2007).

Table 5 Evaluation of precision of the proposed spectrofluorimetric method for the determination of the investigated drugs

Drug	Conc. µg/ml	Mean[c]	S.D	RSD
Fluoxetine	50	100.84	1.33	1.32
	250	98.81	0.62	0.63
	450	100.47	0.41	0.41
Sertraline	50	99.77	1.50	1.50
	250	98.87	0.50	0.51
	450	100.17	0.28	0.27
Paroxetine	50	100.71	1.32	1.31
	250	100.14	0.69	0.69
	550	100.08	0.28	0.28
Thioridazine	100	100.86	1.58	1.57
	350	101.31	0.76	0.75
	650	100.46	0.37	0.37
Amineptine	100	100.10	1.84	1.84
	450	98.77	0.65	0.66
	750	100.53	0.39	0.39

[c]mean is average of eight determinations.

of detection was expressed as (The United States Pharmacopoeia XXV and NF XX 2002):

$$LOD = 3\sigma/S \tag{1}$$

Where σ is the standard deviation of intercept. S is the slope of calibration curve.

The results are summarized in Table 2. The calculated detection limits for all the studied drugs were less than 12.48 ng mL^{-1} indicating good sensitivity of the proposed method.

Limit of quantitation (Topic Q2A 1994) was calculated based on standard deviation of intercept and slope of calibration curve. In this method, the limit of quantitation is expressed as (The United States Pharmacopoeia XXV and NF XX 2002):

$$LOQ = 10\sigma/S \tag{2}$$

The calculated quantitation limits for all the studied drugs were all less than 41.61 ngmL^{-1}, as shown in Table 2, indicating good sensitivity of the proposed method. So it can be applied for analysis of drug in biological fluids.

Specificity and interference
The specificity of the method was investigated by observation of any interference encountered from the common tablet excipients, such as talc, starch, gum acacia, lactose and magnesium stearate. This study indicates that the presence of these excipients did not interfere with the proposed method as proved by the excellent recoveries obtained, as shown in Table 6.

Application to pharmaceutical dosage forms
The proposed method was applied for determination of investigated drugs in commercial pharmaceutical dosage forms. The results were statistically compared with those of reported methods (Darwish 2005; Mohamed et al. 2005, 2007), in respect to accuracy and precision. The obtained mean recovery values were 100.62-101.01 ± 0.66-1.39%, as shown in Table 7. According to t- and F- tests, no significant difference was found between the proposed and reported methods at 95% confidence level. This indicates good level of precision and accuracy.

Application to spiked human plasma
The high sensitivity attained by the proposed method allowed the determination of the studied drugs in spiked human plasma. The concentrations of investigated CNS drugs were computed from their corresponding regression equations. The obtained mean recovery values of the obtained amount were 99.76-100.39 ± 1.33 - 1.99% (Table 8).

Analysis of cited drugs in real human plasma
Fluoxetine is metabolized into its active metabolite norfluoxetine (Lemberger et al. 1985). Norfluoxetine concentrations are approximately equal to those of the parent drug during chronic therapy (Brunswick et al. 2002a). After a fixed daily dose of fluoxetine (20.0 mg day^{-1}), the

Table 6 Analysis of the investigated drugs (100.0 ng mL^{-1}) in presence of some common excipients using the proposed spectrofluorimetric method

Excipients	Amount Added µgmL^{-1}	% Recovery [d] ± SD				
		Fluoxetine	Sertraline	Paroxetine	Thioridazine	Amineptine
Starch	50	100.07 ± 0.61	99.19 ± 0.72	99.85 ± 0.87	100.80 ± 0.78	101.29 ± 0.79
Lactose	50	98.21 ± 0.91	99.83 ± 0.63	98.78 ± 0.61	100.73 ± 0.71	98.12 ± 0.45
Mg stearate	50	101.25 ± 0.54	98.24 ± 1.25	101.58 ± 1.61	99.86 ± 0.33	101.62 ± 1.07
Gum acacia	50	99.25 ± 0.59	99.76 ± 1.01	98.82 ± 0.86	100.28 ± 0.89	101.98 ± 0.49
Talc	50	100.38 ± 1.58	100.18 ± 0.25	98.21 ± 0.67	99.70 ± 0.51	99.81 ± 0.34

[d]Average of three determinations.

Table 7 Statistical analysis of the results obtained using the proposed spectrofluorimetric and reported methods for analysis of the investigated drugs in pharmaceutical dosage forms

Drug	Pharmaceutical dosage forms	Proposed method ± SD (n = 5)	Reported methods [8-10] ± SD (n = 5)
Fluoxetine	Neurazine® tablets	100.94 ± 1.390	100.53 ± 1.46
		t = 0.45 [e] F = 1.09 [e]	
Sertraline	Thiozine® tablets	100.18 ± 1.15	100.13 ± 1.68
		t = 0.06 F = 2.13	
Paroxetine	Stellasil® tablets	100.01 ± 1.196	99.98 ± 0.95
		t = 0.04 F = 1.59	
Thioridazine	Tryptizol® tablets	100.62 ± 0.663	100.22 ± 1.07
		t = 0.71 F = 2.59	
Amineptine	Survector® capsules	100.14 ± 1.26	99.88 ± 1.59
		t = 0.29 F = 1.59	

[e]Tabulated value at 95% confidence limit; F = 6.338 and t = 2.306.

Table 9 % Recoveries after application of the proposed method for determination of investigated CNS drugs in real human plasma sample

Drug	Intraday assay % Recovery$_{invivo}$	Interday assay % Recovery$_{invivo}$
Fluoxetine		
Mean ± SD	91.53 ± 5.11	86.28 ± 5.27
Sertraline		
Mean ± SD	88.83 ± 5.38	85.50 ± 5.947
Paroxetine		
Mean ± SD	76.76 ± 4.82	75.28 ± 7.94
Thioridazine		
Mean ± SD	91.53 ± 5.11	92.26 ± 2.73
Amineptine		
Mean ± SD	86.29 ± 6.44	87.41 ± 3.87

concentration of the drug and its active metabolite in the blood continued to grow through the first few weeks of treatment, and their steady concentration in the blood is achieved only after four weeks (Pérez et al. 2001; Brunswick et al. 2002b). Paroxetine is completely absorbed after oral administration and metabolized in the liver forming three main metabolites: the two isomers (3S,4R)-4-(4-fluorophenyl)- 3-[(4-hydroxy-3-methoxyphenoxy)methyl]-piperidine (M1), (3S,4R)-4-(4-fluorophenyl)-3-[(3-hydroxy-4-methoxyphenoxy)methyl]-piperidine(M2) and (3S,4R)-3-hydroxymethyl- 4-(4-fluorophenyl) piperidine (M3) (Hiemke & Hartter 2000). Steady-state plasma paroxetine concentrations were achieved after approximately 10 days following 40-mg once daily dose (Mandrioli et al. 2007). Thioridazine is mainly metabolized into mesoridazine and sulphoridazine. Steady-state

plasma thioridazine concentrations were achieved after approximately 7 days following four 100-mg doses per day (Vanderheeren & Muusze 1977). Sertraline is mainly metabolized into N-desmethylsertraline. Steady state plasma concentration level for sertraline and its metabolite were achieved after approximately one week of a 50-mg once-daily dosing (Package Insert, Zolofi@, Pfizer Inc 1992; Mandrioli et al. 2006). Amineptine is mainly metabolized by beta-oxidation of the side chain, its principle metabolites has the same structure as the parent compound except that its side chain is reduced to five carbon atom (Lachatre et al. 1989). Steady state plasma level is achieved at 8 th day following two 100.0 mg doses per day (Rop Pok et al. 1990).

According to the reported metabolic pathway of all the cited drugs; the proposed method can be used specifically for determination of fluoxetine and sertraline only in presence of their metabolites in plasma because the metabolic products are considered as compounds containing primary

Table 8 Application of the proposed method to the determination of studied drugs in spiked human plasma

Concentration (ngmL^{-1})	% Recovery [f]				
	Fluoxetine	Sertraline	Paroxetine	Thioridazine	Amineptine
50	97.79	100.12	102.40	99.01	100.84
100	98.62	97.68	99.20	99.36	101.64
150	103.03	103.22	97.54	100.05	102.39
250	99.11	98.56	99.46	97.21	98.84
350	98.42	100.76	98.22	101.64	99.31
450	101.10	99.85	101.55	99.40	99.56
550	-	-	99.72	99.25	101.61
650	-	-	-	102.19	98.76
750	-	-	-	-	100.61
Mean ± SD	99.68 ± 1.99	100.03 ± 1.92	99.73 ± 1.73	99.76 ± 1.565	100.39 ± 1.33

[f]Mean of three replicate measurements.

amino group (as norfluoxetine and norsertraline); which should not interfere upon application of the suggested procedure, while for thioridazine, paroxetine and amineptine, their metabolites can interfere with the determination of the parent drugs because they contain the same function group (secondary or tertiary amine moiety) as well.

So % recovery of fluoxetine and sertraline in plasma were calculated by using the following equation

$$\%Recovery_{in\ vivo} = (concentration_{found}/concentration_{taken}) \times 100 \tag{3}$$

Where,

% Recovery $_{in\ vivo}$ is % recovery for drug in real human sample.
Concentration $_{found}$ is concentration of the drug founded in real human sample.
Concentration $_{taken}$ is concentration of the drug reported in real human sample.
While % recovery of thioridazine, paroxetine and amineptine and their metabolites in plasma were calculated by using the same equation

Where,

% Recovery $_{in\ vivo}$ is % recovery for drug and their metabolites in real human sample.
Concentration $_{found}$ is concentration of the drug and their metabolites founded in real human sample.
Concentration $_{taken}$ is reported concentration of the drug and their metabolites in real human sample.
% Recoveries after application of the proposed method for determination of investigated CNS drugs in real human plasma sample by intra and inter day assay are shown in Table 9.

Conclusion

The proposed spectrofluorimetric method has the advantage of being simple, highly sensitive and low cost method for determination of the investigated antidepressant drugs in pure forms, pharmaceutical formulations, without any interference from common excipients present and with minimum detection limits. Furthermore the proposed method was successfully applied for analysis of the cited drugs in spiked and real human plasma. Therefore, the developed method can be considered as suitable for routine analysis of investigated antidepressant drugs in quality control and clinical laboratories. Also it is suitable for selective determination of fluoxetine and sertraline only without their metabolites in human plasma.

Competing interests

All authors declare that there is no competing of interest.

Authors' contributions

Dr Mahmoud M. Omar and Dr. Sayed M. Derayea proposed the idea and design the experimental section. Dr Tamer Z. Attia, Dr. Sayed M. Derayea and Dr Mahmoud M. Omar carried out the experimental parts and participated in sequence alignment and drafted the manuscript. All authors participated in preparation of the discussion and result section. Dr Osama H. Abdelmageed and Dr. Tadayuki Uno revised the final manuscript. Finally all authors read and approved the final manuscript.

Acknowledgements

The authors express their gratitude to Egyptian government for providing financial support to achieve this paper. Also, the authors express their gratitude to Dr. Monsef Mahfuz a consultant psychiatrist and manager of Minia hospital for psychiatric medicine (Minia, Egypt) for providing the plasma samples.

Author details

[1]Analytical Chemistry Department, Faculty of pharmacy, Minia University, Minia 61519, Egypt. [2]Pharmaceutical Chemistry Department, Faculty of Pharmacy, King Abdulaziz University, Jeddah, Kingdom of Saudi Arabia. [3]Graduate School of Pharmaceutical Sciences, Osaka University, 1-6 Yamadaoka, Suita, Osaka 565-0871, Japan.

References

Atta-Politou J, Skopelitis I, Apatsidis I, Koupparis M (2001) Eur J Pharmaceut Sci 12:311
Basavaiah K, Manjunatha Swamy L, Krishnamurthy G (1999) Chem Pharm Bull 47:1351
Brunswick DJ, Amsterdam JD, Fawcett J, Quitkin FM, Reimherr JF, Beasley CM (2002a) J Affect Disord 68:243
Brunswick DJ, Amsterdam JD, Fawcett J, Quitkin FM, Reimherr FW, Rosenbaum JF, Beasley CM (2002b) J Affect Disord 68:243
Bueno F, Bergold AM, Fröehlich PE (2000) Boll Chim Farm 139:256
Darwish IA (2005) J AOAC INTERNATIONAL 88:38
Darwish IA, Refaat IH (2006) J AOAC INTERNATIONAL 89:326
Delazzeri L (2005) Caderno de Farmácia 21:37
Hiemke C, Hartter S (2000) Pharmacol Ther 85:11
Job P (1964) Advanced Physicochemical Experiments, 2nd edition. Oliner and Boyd, Edinburgh, p 54. Ann. Chem. 1936, 16, 97
Labat L, Deveaux M, Dallet P, Dubost JP (2002) J Chromatogr B773:17
Lachatre G, Piva C, Riche C, Dumont D, Defrance R, Mocaer EV (1989) V Nicot Fundam Clin Pharmacol 3:19
Lemberger L, Bergstrom RF, Wolen RL, Farid NA, Enas GG, Aronoff GR (1985) J Clin Psychiatry 46:14
Mandrioli R, Pucci V, Visini D, Varani G, Raggi MAJ (2002) Pharm Biomed Anal 29:1127
Mandrioli R, Saracino MA, Ferrari S, Berardi D, Kenndler E, Raggi MA (2006) J Chromatogr B836:116
Mandrioli R, Mercolini L, Ferranti A, Furlanetto S, Boncompagni G, Roggi MA (2007) Anal Chim Acta 591:141
Meiling Q, Peng W, Yingshu G, Junling G, Ruonong FJ (2002) Clin Pharmaceut Sci 11:16
Mohamed FA, Mohamed HA, Hussein SA, Ahmed SA (2005) Pharm Biol Anal 39:139
Mohamed GG, Nour El-Dien FAF, Mohamed NA (2007) Spectrochim Acta A68:1244
Nevado JJB, Llerena MJV, Cabanillas CG, Robledo VR, Buitrago S (2006) J Separ Sci 29:103
Nouws HPA, Delerue-Matos C, Barros AA, Rodrigues JA (2006) J Pharm Biomed Anal 42:341
Onal A, Kepekçi SE, Oztunç A (2005) J AOAC INTERNATIONAL 88:490

Package Insert, Zolofi@, Pfizer Inc (1992). Jan. through analytical profile of drug substances, vol 25, p 443

Parfitt K, Martindale E (2002) The Complete Drug Reference, 33rd edition. Pharmaceutical Press, London, UK

Patel KN, Patel JK, Rathod IS (2009) J Pharm Res 2:1525

Pérez V, Puiigdemont D, Gilaberte I, Alvarez E, Artigas F (2001) J Clin Psychopharmacol 21:36

Rop Pok P, Spinazzola J, Bresson M (1990) J Chromatogr B532:351

Sbarra C, Negnm P, Fanelh R (1979) J Chromatogr 162:31

Sbarra C, Castelh MG, Noseda A, Fanelh R (1981) Eur J Drug Metab Pharmarmacokin 6:123

The United States Pharmacopoeia XXV and NF XX (2002). American Pharmaceutical Association, Washington, DC

Topic Q2A (1994) Text on validation of analytical procedure. International Conference on Harmonization (ICH)

Topic Q2B (1996) Validation of analytical procedure. Methodology, International Conference on Harmonization (ICH)

Tsaconas C, Padteu P, d'Athts P, Mocaer E, Bromet N (1989) J Chromatogr 487:313

Vanderheeren FHJ, Muusze RG (1977) Eur J Clin Pharmacol 11:135

Zainaghi IA, Lanchote VL, Queiroz RHC (2003) Pharmacol Res 48:217

3

Development and validation of RP-HPLC-PDA method for the quantification of eugenol in developed nanoemulsion gel and nanoparticles

Kannissery Pramod[1], Ura Kottil Ilyas[2], Yoonuskunju Thajudeenkoya Kamal[2], Sayeed Ahmad[2], Shahid Hussain Ansari[2] and Javed Ali[1*]

Abstract

Background: Eugenol is a potent phytochemical, and a plethora of delivery systems for this bioactive agent is being developed. Reversed-phase high-pressure liquid chromatography equipped with photodiode array detector (RP-HPLC-PDA) method is very useful in the quantification of the phytochemicals.

Methods: The RP-HPLC-PDA system with C18 reversed-phase column (250 × 4.6 mm, particle size 5 μm) was used in this study. Acetonitrile and water in 1:1 (v/v) ratio was chosen as the mobile phase under a column temperature of 25°C. The detection wavelength was set at 280 nm with a flow rate of 1 mL/min. Method validation was performed according to the International Conference on Harmonization guidelines.

Results: HPLC method for the quantification of eugenol was successfully developed and validated. The method was validated in terms of linearity and range, accuracy, precision, specificity, robustness, detection limit, and quantitation limit.

Conclusions: The developed RP-HPLC-PDA could be successfully employed for the quantification of eugenol in nanoemulsion gel and nanoparticles.

Keywords: Accuracy; Precision; Specificity; Robustness; ICH guidelines

Background

A good number of novel delivery systems of eugenol (Chen et al. 2009; Gomes et al. 2011; Jadhav et al. 2004; Kriegel et al. 2010; Pokharkar et al. 2011) have been reported owing to its potent bioacitivity. Anti-inflammatory and anti-microbial actions are among other major pharmacological actions of eugenol (Pramod et al. 2010). Development of a suitable analytical method will be needed when eugenol is formulated in nanocarriers for targeted delivery.

Quantification of the pharmacologically active component in a dosage form is indispensable to the quality control of these systems. Quality control checks the suitability of a drug delivery system for the intended application. It serves as a marker for the consistency and predictability of the performance of dosage forms (Levi et al. 1964). High-pressure liquid chromatography (HPLC) methods are widely reported for the quantitative estimation of bioactive phytochemicals, but to this day, no reports are available on reversed-phase HPLC equipped with photodiode array detector (RP-HPLC-PDA) methods for the quantification of eugenol in nano-structured delivery systems such as nanoemulsion gel and nanoparticles. Besides this, none of the methods are available for eugenol quantification from formulations where a high specificity is required to overcome the probable interference of the excipients.

Nanoemulsion gel and nanoparticles have been developed as novel drug delivery systems of eugenol (Pramod et al. 2012, 2013). The major aim of the present work was to develop a RP-HPLC-PDA method for the quantitative estimation of eugenol in these drug delivery systems for anti-inflammation and periodontal infection.

* Correspondence: javedaali@yahoo.com
[1]Department of Pharmaceutics, Faculty of Pharmacy, Jamia Hamdard, Hamdard Nagar, New Delhi – 110 062, India
Full list of author information is available at the end of the article

Methods

Chemicals and reagents

Eugenol (pure) was purchased from Central Drug House (Delhi, India). Poly-ε-caprolactone (MW 14,000), chitosan, sodium alginate and Pluronic F-68 were purchased from Sigma-Aldrich Co. (MO, USA). Tween 80 and polyvinyl alcohol were purchased from Central Drug House (New Delhi, India). Carbopol 940 was a gift sample from Noveon Corporation (Cleveland, OH, USA). Tween 80 and triethanolamine were purchased from S D Fine-Chem Ltd. (Mumbai, India). Ethanol (99.9%) was purchased from Jiangsu Huax Co., Ltd. (Jiangsu, China). HPLC-grade water and acetonitrile were purchased from Merck (Mumbai, India).

Preparation of eugenol-loaded nanoemulsion gel and nanoparticles

Aqueous titration method was employed for the preparation of eugenol-loaded nanoemulsion. The formulated eugenol-loaded nanoemulsion was converted to nanoemulsion gel by dispersing 1% (w/w) Carbopol 940 in it. Tween 80 and ethanol were used as surfactant and co-surfactant, respectively. For S_{mix}, a specific volume ratio of 4:1 (Tween 80/ethanol) was used (Pramod et al. 2012). For the preparation of the sample solution of nanoemulsion gel, an accurately weighed gel sample was taken in methanol, sonicated (Altrasonics, Mumbai, India) for 20 min, and filtered using a 0.2-μm syringe filter (Axiva Sichem Biotech, New Delhi, India).

Solvent displacement method was employed for the preparation of eugenol-loaded nanoparticles (Reis et al. 2006). Polycaprolactone (encapsulating polymer) and eugenol were dissolved in acetone (organic solvent phase) by mild heating. The solution of eugenol and polymer was injected dropwise into aqueous Pluronic F-68 (stabilizer) solution under magnetic stirring, and stirring was continued until complete evaporation of acetone occurred. Centrifugation of the suspension of nanoparticles thus obtained was carried out at 15,000 rpm for 1 h. The obtained nanoparticles were washed twice with distilled water and then freeze-dried (Pramod et al. 2013). For the preparation of the sample solution from nanoparticles, accurately weighed sample of dried nanoparticles was dissolved in 1 mL of acetone and then was added to 5 mL of methanol. Acetone was then evaporated. The sample was sonicated (Altrasonics, Mumbai, India) for 20 min, then was made up to 10 mL with methanol, and was filtered using a 0.2-μm syringe filter (Axiva Sichem Biotech, New Delhi, India) (Pramod et al. 2013).

HPLC instrumentation and chromatographic conditions

The HPLC method for the determination of eugenol was carried out on a Waters Alliance e2695 separating module (Waters Co., MA, USA) using a photodiode array detector (Waters 2998) with autosampler and column oven. The instrument was controlled by Empower 2 software (Europa Science, Ltd., Cambridge, UK) installed with equipment for data collection and acquisition. Compounds were separated on a C18 reversed-phase column (250 × 4.6 mm, particle size 5 μm; Merck, Darmstadt, Germany) maintained at room temperature.

Mobile phase

Acetonitrile and water in the ratio of 1:1 (v/v) was chosen as the mobile phase.

Chromatographic system

The chromatographic system is composed of the following (Table 1): Chromatographic conditions.

Preparation of the mobile phase

HPLC-grade water was mixed with HPLC-grade acetonitrile in the volume ratio of 1:1. The prepared mobile phase was then filtered through a 0.45-μm nylon filter and sonicated in an ultrasonic bath for 15 min.

Method validation

Linearity and range

A stock solution of eugenol (10 mg mL^{-1}) was prepared in methanol. Standard calibration solutions (5 to 1,000 μg mL^{-1}) for the assessment of linearity were prepared from this stock solution using the mobile phase. The solutions were filtered through a 0.45-μm nylon filter. The filtered solution was then injected into the HPLC system. The data of peak area versus drug concentration were treated by linear least square regression.

Accuracy as recovery

Accuracy was determined by recovery studies using standard addition method. The pre-analyzed samples were spiked with extra 50%, 100%, and 150% of the standard

Table 1 Chromatographic conditions

Composition	Value
Column	C18 reverse phase column (250 × 4.6 mm, particle size 5 μm; Merck, Darmstadt, Germany)
Flow rate	1 mL min^{-1}
Retention time	7.968 ± 0.042 min
Detector	PDA detector (Waters 2998)
Detection wavelength	280 nm
Injection volume	20 μL
Temperature	25°C
Elution type	Isocratic
Run time	20 min

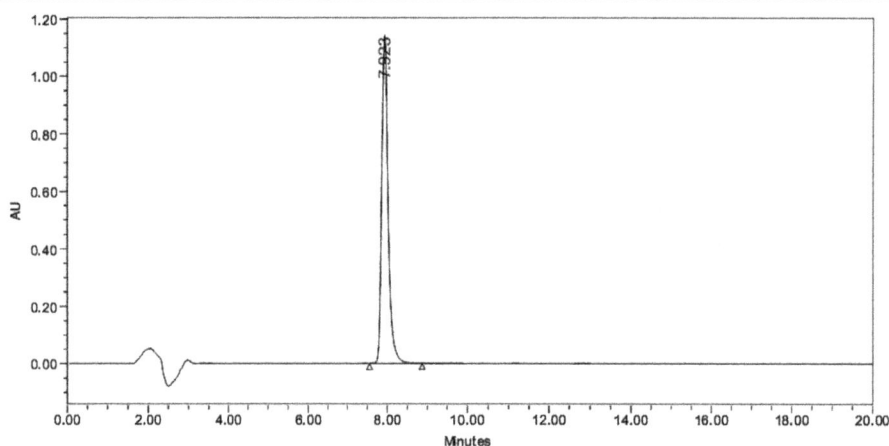

Figure 1 HPLC chromatogram of eugenol.

eugenol, and the mixtures were analyzed by the proposed method. The experiment was conducted in triplicate.

Precision

The intraday (repeatability) and interday (intermediate precision) variations for the determination of eugenol was carried out at three concentration levels of 20, 100, and 600 µg mL^{-1}. The determinations were carried out in triplicate.

Specificity

The specificity of the method was ascertained by analyzing the standard drug and sample. The band for eugenol in nanoemulsion gel and nanoparticle samples was confirmed by comparing the R_f values and spectra of the band with that of the standard. The peak purity of eugenol was assessed by comparing the spectra at three different levels, that is, peak start, peak apex, and peak end positions of the spectrum.

Robustness

Robustness of the method was carried out by introducing very small changes in the analytical methodology at

a single concentration level (100 µg mL^{-1}). Robustness of the proposed method was determined in two different ways, i.e., by making deliberate changes in the mobile phase ratio, flow rate, and detection wavelength of analysis. The percentage of relative standard deviation (%RSD) of the experiment was calculated to assess the robustness of the method.

Detection and quantitation limits

The detection limit (DL) is the lowest amount of analyte in a sample, which can be detected but not necessarily quantitated. The quantitation limit (QL) is the lowest amount of analyte in a sample, which can be quantitatively determined with suitable precision and accuracy. The limit of quantification and limit of detection were determined based on the technique of signal-to-noise ratio (ICH Guidelines Q2(R1) 2005) using Equations 1 and 2:

$$QL = 10\,\sigma/S \tag{1}$$

$$DL = 3.3\,\sigma/S \tag{2}$$

where σ is the standard deviation of the intercept of the calibration plot and S is the slope of the calibration curve.

Results and discussion

Although limited HPLC methods for the determination of eugenol have been reported (Dighe et al. 2005; Li

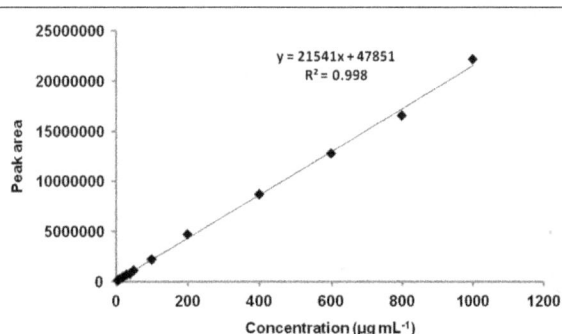

Figure 2 Calibration curve of eugenol by HPLC method.

Table 2 Linear regression data for the calibration curve ($n = 3$)

Parameter	Mean ± SD	%RSD
Linearity range (µg mL^{-1})	5 to 1,000	-
Correlation coefficient (R^2)	0.9984 ± 0.0001	0.02
Slope	215,40.54 ± 63.93	0.30
Intercept	47,851.22 ± 2,880.31	6.02

Table 3 Recovery data for the accuracy of the HPLC method

Excess of eugenol added (%)	Concentration of sample (µg mL^{-1})	Theoretical concentration of spiked sample (µg mL^{-1})	Concentration of spiked sample ± SD (µg mL^{-1}) (n = 3)	Recovery ± SD (%)	%RSD
50	100	150	149.41 ± 1.87	99.60 ± 1.24	1.25
100	100	200	202.15 ± 1.36	101.07 ± 0.68	0.67
150	100	250	252.01 ± 1.82	100.80 ± 0.73	0.72

et al. 2004), none of them reported their specificity in quantifying eugenol in nanostructured delivery systems. Moreover, the application of PDA detector is an added advantage for the developed method. Detection of an entire spectrum simultaneously is possible with PDA detector. While UV–vis detectors visualize the obtained result in two dimensions (light intensity and time), only PDA adds the third dimension (wavelength). This is convenient to determine the most suitable wavelength without repeating analyses. No methods are available for eugenol quantification from formulations where a high specificity is required to overcome the probable interference of the excipients.

Calibration curve

A representative chromatogram of eugenol in the developed HPLC method is shown in Figure 1. A retention time of 7.923 min can be observed from the HPLC chromatogram in Figure 1. The calibration curve for eugenol by the developed HPLC method is shown in Figure 2. The linear regression data for the calibration curve demonstrated a good linear relationship over the concentration range of 5 to 1,000 µg mL^{-1}. A good linearity was established by a correlation coefficient (R^2) value of 0.9984 ± 0.0001 (Table 2). Correlation coefficient is a statistical tool used to measure the degree or strength of this type of relationship, and here, a high correlation coefficient value (a value very close to 1.0) indicates a high level of linear relationship between the concentration of eugenol and peak area. No significant differences were observed in the slopes of standard curves as indicated by the low %RSD of 0.30. Table 2 displays the linear regression data for the calibration curve of eugenol.

Accuracy as recovery

Accuracy was investigated by analyzing three concentrations of the standard drug solution previously analyzed using standard addition technique. The recovery studies were carried out to check the sensitivity of the method to estimate eugenol. The standard addition technique was carried out by adding 50%, 100%, and 150% of eugenol concentration in the sample. The percentage recoveries of the three concentrations were found to be 99.60% to 101.07%, which is indicative of high accuracy. The values of percentage recovery and %RSD are displayed in Table 3. The mean percentage recovery values, close to 100%, and their low %RSD values indicated high accuracy of the analytical method.

Precision

The repeatability of developed HPLC method, by intraday assay, is expressed in the terms of %RSD, and the results (Table 4) demonstrated the repeatability of the method. The interday variation of eugenol at three different concentration levels of 20, 100, and 600 µg mL^{-1} establishes the intermediate precision of the method. The low values of %RSD for repeatability and intermediate precision suggested an excellent precision of the developed HPLC method.

Specificity

The specificity of the developed method for the analysis of eugenol in the nanoemulsion gel and nanoparticle samples was confirmed by comparing the spectra obtained in the standard and sample analyses (Figure 3). The peak start, peak apex, and peak end positions of these spectra were matching.

Robustness

Robustness was studied by introducing small changes in the mobile phase ratio, flow rate, and detection wavelength of analysis. The standard deviation and %RSD of peak area and retention time (R_t) was calculated and

Table 4 Repeatability and intermediate precision of HPLC method

Concentration (µg mL^{-1})	Repeatability (n = 3)		Intermediate precision (n = 3)	
	Mean peak area ± SD	%RSD	Mean peak area ± SD	%RSD
20	468283.0 ± 3410.6	0.73	467144.7 ± 3398.0	0.73
100	2213959.7 ± 11480.9	0.52	2213539.0 ± 8008.9	0.36
600	12800060.3 ± 45178.8	0.35	12778185.3 ± 40768.0	0.32

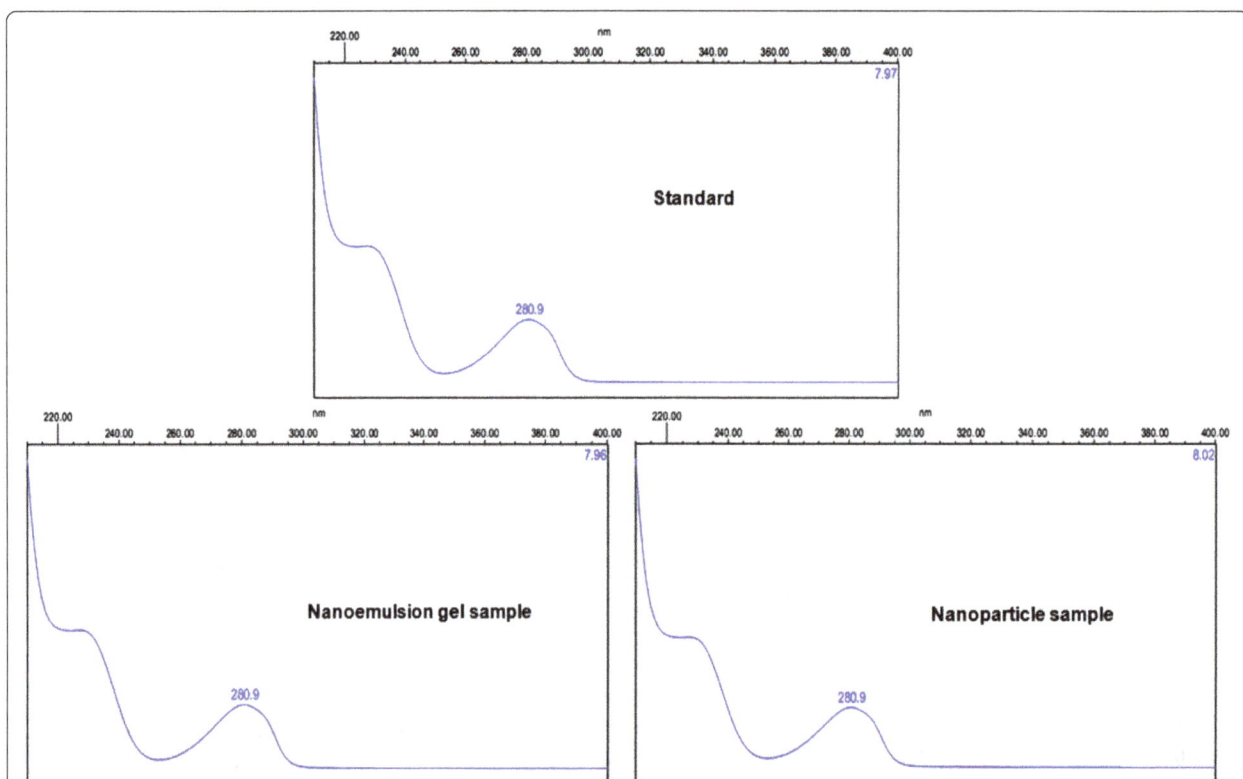

Figure 3 UV absorption spectra of eugenol in standard, nanoemulsion gel sample, and nanoparticle sample.

listed in Table 5. The low values of %RSD show the robustness of the method.

Detection and quantitation limits

The DL and QL were determined as per the ICH Guidelines Q2(R1) (2005) and were found to be 0.44 and 1.34 µg mL^{-1}, respectively.

Conclusions

The RP-HPLC-PDA system with C18 reversed-phase column (250 × 4.6 mm, particle size 5 µm) was used in this study. Acetonitrile and water in the ratio of 1:1 (v/v) was chosen as the mobile phase, and a detection wavelength of 280 nm was used with a flow rate of 1 mL min^{-1}. The method validation was performed according to the guidelines of the

Table 5 Robustness data of the HPLC method

Parameter	Study condition			Mean area ± SD	%RSD of area	R_t ± SD	% RSD of R_t
	Original	Used	Level				
Mobile phase ratio (ACN/water)	50:50	48:52	−1	2218634.9 ± 6686.7	0.30	7.968 ± 0.024	0.30
		50:50	0				
		52:48	+1				
Flow rate (mL min^{-1})	1.0	0.9	−1	2216384.3 ± 8147.4	0.37	7.958 ± 0.068	0.85
		1.0	0				
		1.1	+1				
Detection wavelength (nm)	280	278	−1	2214941.3 ± 13356.9	0.60	7.967 ± 0.030	0.38
		280	0				
		282	+1				

$n = 3$ at each level. Concentration = 100 µg mL^{-1}.

International Conference on Harmonization (ICH). HPLC method for the quantification of eugenol was successfully developed and validated. The method was validated in terms of linearity and range, accuracy, precision, specificity, robustness, detection limit, and quantitation limit. The DL and QL were determined as per the ICH guidelines and were found to be 0.44 and 1.34 μg mL^{-1}, respectively. The developed RP-HPLC-PDA could be successfully employed for the quantification of eugenol in its nanoemulsion gel and nanoparticles.

Competing interests
The authors declared that they have no competing interests.

Authors' contributions
KP, SHA and JA proposed the idea and design the experiment. KP and JA carried out the preparation of nanoemulsion and nanoparticles. UKI assisted in framing the experiments. UKI prepared standards and samples for analysis. YTK and SA carried out the HPLC analysis of the samples and standard. All authors participated in the preparation of the manuscript. All authors read and approved the final manuscript.

Acknowledgements
Pramod K gratefully acknowledges Indian Council of Medical Research (ICMR), New Delhi, India, for providing Senior Research Fellowship (No. 35/3/10/NAN/BMS).

Author details
[1]Department of Pharmaceutics, Faculty of Pharmacy, Jamia Hamdard, Hamdard Nagar, New Delhi – 110 062, India. [2]Department of Pharmacognosy & Phytochemistry, Faculty of Pharmacy, Jamia Hamdard, Hamdard Nagar, New Delhi – 110 062, India.

References
Chen F, Shi Z, Neoh KG, Kang ET (2009) Antioxidant and antibacterial activities of eugenol and carvacrol-grafted chitosan nanoparticles. Biotechnol Bioeng 104(1):30–39
Dighe W, Gursale AA, Sane RT, Menon S, Patel PH (2005) Quantitative determination of eugenol from Cinnamomum tamala Nees and Eberm: leaf powder and polyherbal formulation using reverse phase liquid chromatography. Chromatographia 61:443–446
Gomes C, Moreira RG, Castell-Perez E (2011) Poly (DL-lactide-co-glycolide) (PLGA) nanoparticles with entrapped trans-cinnamaldehyde and eugenol for antimicrobial delivery applications. J Food Sci 76(2):N16–N24
ICH Guidelines Q2(R1) (2005) Validation of analytical procedures: text and methodology, http://www.ich.org/fileadmin/Public_Web_Site/ICH_Products/Guidelines/Quality/Q2_R1/Step4/Q2_R1__Guideline.pdf. Accessed 10 Mar 2011
Jadhav BK, Khandelwal KR, Ketkar AR, Pisal SS (2004) Formulation and evaluation of mucoadhesive nanocapsules containing eugenol for the treatment of periodontal diseases. Drug Dev Ind Pharm 30:195–203
Kriegel C, Kit KM, McClements DJ, Weiss J (2010) Nanofibers as carrier systems for antimicrobial microemulsions: II: release characteristics and antimicrobial activity. J Appl Polym Sci 118:2859–2868
Levi L, Walker GC, Pugsley LI (1964) Quality control of pharmaceuticals. Can Med Assoc J 91(15):781–785
Li Y, Sun Z, Zheng P (2004) Determination of vanillin, eugenol and isoeugenol by RP-HPLC. Chromatographia 60:709–713
Pokharkar VB, Shekhawat PB, Dhapte W, Mandpe LP (2011) Development and optimization of eugenol loaded nanostructured lipid carriers for periodontal delivery. Int J Pharm Pharm Sci 3:138–143
Pramod K, Ansari SH, Ali J (2010) Eugenol: a natural compound with versatile pharmacological actions. Nat Prod Commun 5(12):1999–2006
Pramod K, Shanavas S, Ansari SH, Ali J (2012) Eugenol nanodroplet gel as novel biomaterial in nanomedicine. Adv Sci Lett 10:1–13
Pramod K, Ansari SH, Ali J (2013) Fabrication and tailoring of eugenol loaded polycaprolactone nanoparticles using response surface methodology. Adv Sci Eng Med 5(11):1166-1175
Reis CP, Neufeld RJ, Ribeiro AJ, Veiga F (2006) Nanoencapsulation I: methods for preparation of drug-loaded polymeric nanoparticles. Nanomedicine 2:8–21

4

Simultaneous determination of methaqaulone, saccharin, paracetamol, and phenacetin in illicit drug samples by hplc

Mohd Idris[1*], Cijo John[1], Priyankar Ghosh[1], Sudhir Kumar Shukla[2] and Tulsidas Ramachandra Rao Baggi[3]

Abstract

Background: Saccharin, a low calorie artificial sweetener was found as a new diluent / adulterant present along with paracetamol and phenacetin in an illicit methaqualone sample.

Methods: All these components were simultaneously analyzed by the proposed reverse phase high performance liquid chromatography method using C_{18} column using acetonitrile: water (90:10 v/v) as mobile phase with a flow rate of 1 mL/min.

Results: The percentages of saccharin, phenacetin, paracetamol and methaqualone in illicit drug sample were found to be 15.0, 45.6, 25.1 and 12.0 respectively. The method was validated for limit of detection, limit of quantification, linearity, accuracy, precision and reproducibility with the help of the exhibit and simulated samples.

Conclusions: The proposed method is simple, accurate and fast. It can be applied to the routine analysis of illicit methaqualone samples as well as for their impurity profiles for tracing the origin.

Keywords: Saccharin, Methaqualone, Diluents, Illicit drug samples, HPLC, Drug profiling

Background

The ever-growing problem of drug abuse is of great concern to the society. The drugs of abuse may be encountered in forensic practice in either pure form, diluted and/or adulterated forms. The reasons for the presence of many substances as impurities, diluents or adulterants in illicit drugs are often varied. Sometimes it may be unintentional because of the imperfect and bad manufacturing and laboratory practices. Most of the time these diluents and adulterants could be added as cutting agents to increase the bulk, dilute, complement or enhance the effects of the drugs and to mimic the taste of a genuine drug. The evidence suggests that illicit drugs are more commonly adulterated with either neutraceuticals such as sucrose, lactose, dextrose, mannitol and vitamins or pharmaceuticals that will mimic the taste of illicit drugs such as quinine, caffeine, paracetamol and aspirin or some innocuous substances such as talc, starch, chalk and magnesium stearate (Behrman 2008) etc. On one hand the identification as well as determination of a controlled substance is important for forensic science laboratories for prosecutorial purposes and on the other hand profiling of decomposition products, side reaction products, precursors, impurities, solvents, adulterants and diluents are of prime importance to trace the geographical origin of the illicit sample.

Paracetamol or acetaminophen, (Figure 1) is a widely used over-the-counter analgesic (pain reliever) and antipyretic (fever reducer). It is commonly used for the relief of headaches, other minor aches and pains, and is a major ingredient in numerous cold and flu remedies. In combination with opioid analgesics, paracetamol can also be used in the management of more severe pain such as post surgical pain and providing palliative care in advanced cancer patients. It was found as adulterant in illicit heroin, methaqualone, phenobarbitone, cocaine, methamphetamine (Atasoy et al. 1988; Battisti et al. 2006; Brunt et al. 2009).

Phenacetin (Figure 2) is an analgesic, once widely used but nowadays its use has been declined because of its adverse effects. It was reported as adulterant in illicit cocaine, methaqualone and heroin samples (Fucci 2004; Fucci & Giovanni 1998; Furst 2000).

* Correspondence: md_idris3@yahoo.com
[1]Chemistry Division, Central Forensic Science Laboratory, Hyderabad, India
Full list of author information is available at the end of the article

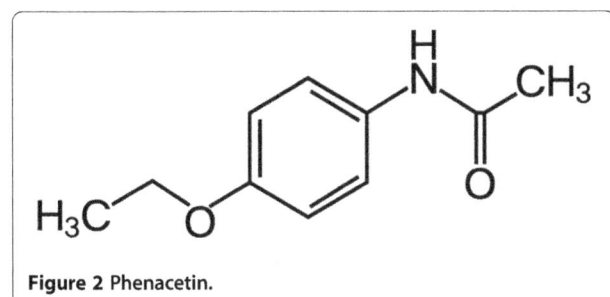

Figure 1 Paracetamol.

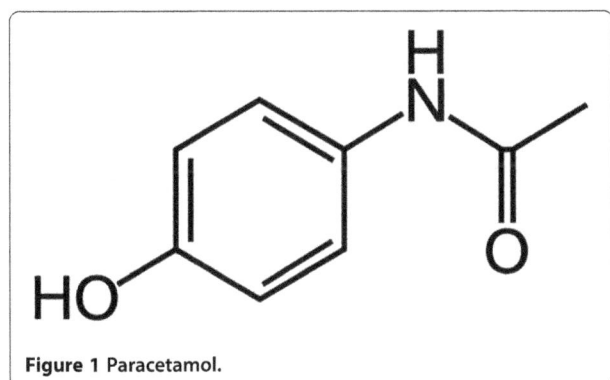

Figure 3 Methaqualone.

Methaqualone (Figure 3) is a sedative-hypnotic drug that is similar in effect to barbiturates, a general central nervous system depressant. It was widely used in the 1960s and 1970s as a hypnotic, for the treatment of insomnia, and as a sedative and muscle relaxant. It has also been used illegally as a recreational drug, commonly known as Mandrax. The drug was used during sexual activity because of heightened sensitivity and lowered inhibition coupled with relaxation and euphoria (Kacker & Zaheer 1951; Smyth et al. 1973).

Saccharin (1, 2-benzisothiazol-3(2H)-one-1, 1-dioxide), (Figure 4) is a non-glucose, low-calorie sugar substitute. It is found to be new cutting agent added in bulk or as diluent in illicit drugs because of its easy availability and low cost. Earlier in a study it was reported as diluent in illicit cocaine samples (Fucci & De Giovanni 1998). But in some recent cases saccharin was found in illicit methaqualone samples along with paracetamol and phenacetin.

Saccharin was determined individually in soft drinks, dietetic food samples (Filho & Nobrega 1994; Fo et al. 1993), determined simultaneously along with preservatives and flavoring agents in drinks (Ikai et al. 1988; Terada & Sakade 1985), also along with other non-nutritive sweeteners in dietetic samples (Chen et al. 1997; Biemer 1989; Zhu et al. 2005; Sastry et al. 1995; Valley et al. 2007). It was also determined individually in faces sample (Tibbels & Smith 1988). Limited references are available on the occurrence and determination of saccharin as diluent/adulterant in illicit drug samples

(Fucci & De Giovanni 1998). Most of the methods of analysis of drugs and other compounds were designed for their determination in routine pharmaceutical analysis and not for illicit drugs which might contain a variety of drugs and chemicals as diluents and adulterants, which are not present in official preparations. When the standard pharmaceutical procedures are applied to the illicit drugs they are fraught with interferences, difficulties in separation, identification and quantification. Therefore, there is always a need to develop new methods and procedures for the analysis of illicit drug samples where we can separate the adulterants, diluents and other impurities encountered in the forensic samples.

In this presentation a simple liquid chromatographic method has been described for the simultaneous determination of saccharin, paracetamol, phenacetin and

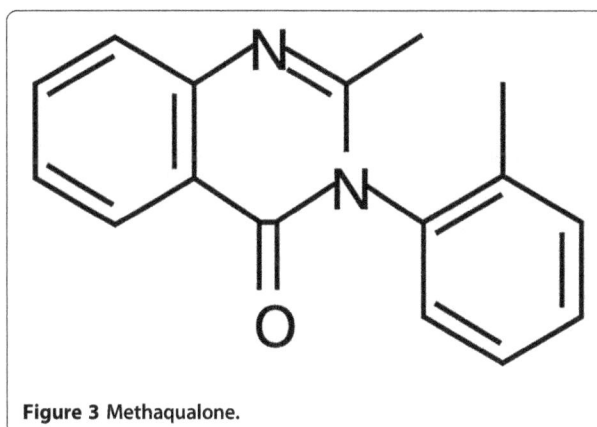

Figure 4 Saccharin.

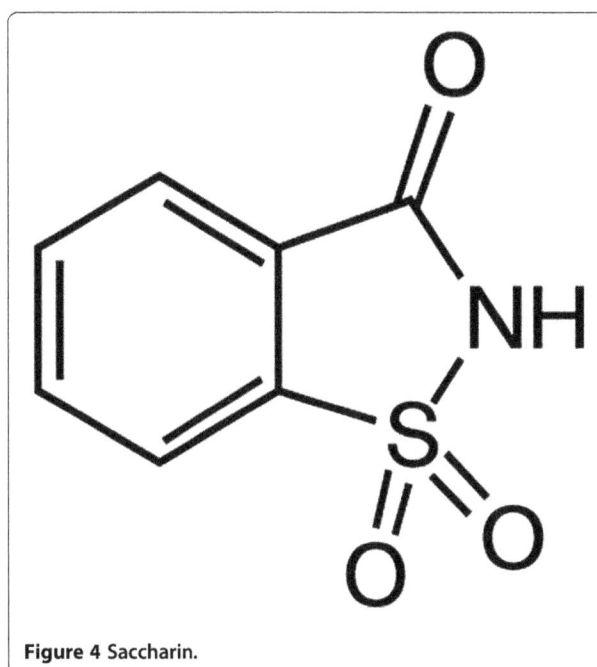

Figure 2 Phenacetin.

methaqualone in an illicit methaqualone samples. To demonstrate the usefulness of this method samples were also analyzed by employing Clarke's HPLC methods (Anthony et al. 2003) for determination of paracetamol, phenacetin and methaqualone where as Tibbels and Smith method (Tibbels & Smith 1988) was used for analysis of saccharin.

Experimental

Chemicals and reagents

Saccharin was supllied by Kare Labs (India), paracetamol; phenacetin and methaqualone were purchased from Sigma-Aldrich (India). HPLC grade acetonitrile and water were purchased from Qualigens (India).

Apparatus

High Performance Liquid Chromatography (HPLC) System (Waters) consisting of a 600E controller pump, a 717 plus auto sampler, 2996 PDA detector and an inline-degasser. Millinium32 software for data processing and C_{18} (Waters, Spherisorb 5 um ODS2, 4.6 × 250 mm) analytical column was used for separation.

Standard preparation

A standard stock solution containing a mixture of saccharin, phenacetin, paracetamol, and methaqualone having a concentration of 2 mg/mL of each of these substances was prepared in the mobile phase. The stock solution was further diluted with mobile phase to give the five different concentrations (containing saccharin, paracetamol, phenacetin and methaqualone in the range of 0.2 μg/10 μL to 1.8 μg/10 μL, 0.4 μg/10 μL to 2 μg/10 μL, 0.4 μg/10 μL to 2 μg/10 μL and 0.2 μg/10 μL to 1 μg/10 μL, respectively). Five replicates of each of these five solutions were injected for plotting the calibration curve.

For limit of detection and limit of quantification a standard solution containing each of saccharin, phenacetin, paracetamol and methaqualone (1 mg/mL each) was diluted to give the different concentrations (0.05 μg/10 μL to 2 μg/10 μL). Recovery studies were carried out by standard addition method where three different concentrations of above said components were prepared with in the calibration range of corresponding components.

Sample preparation

A homogenized representative sample (10 mg) was transferred to a 10 mL volumetric flask and made up to the mark with mobile phase with intermittent shaking. Simulated samples were simultaneously prepared by mixing methaqualone, phenacetin, paracetamol and saccharin in different proportions. The simulated samples were analyzed by the proposed method for validation studies.

Standards and samples were ultrasonicated for 15 min and filtered through a Whatmann No.1 (Cellulose,

Particle retention of 11μm) filter paper prior to injection into the HPLC system.

Chromatography

Chromatography was carried out at ambient temperature. The mobile phase consisted of acetonitrile and water (90:10). The flow-rate of the mobile phase was 1mL/min. 10 μL of each of the standard solutions of the four compounds were injected in the HPLC to prepare a calibration graph. Then ten micro liters of sample solution was injected and concentration of each component was determined through the calibration graphs of the respective standards.

Method validation

Preliminary validation of the method was performed by checking the linearity, precision, recovery, detection and quantification limits, and repeatability.

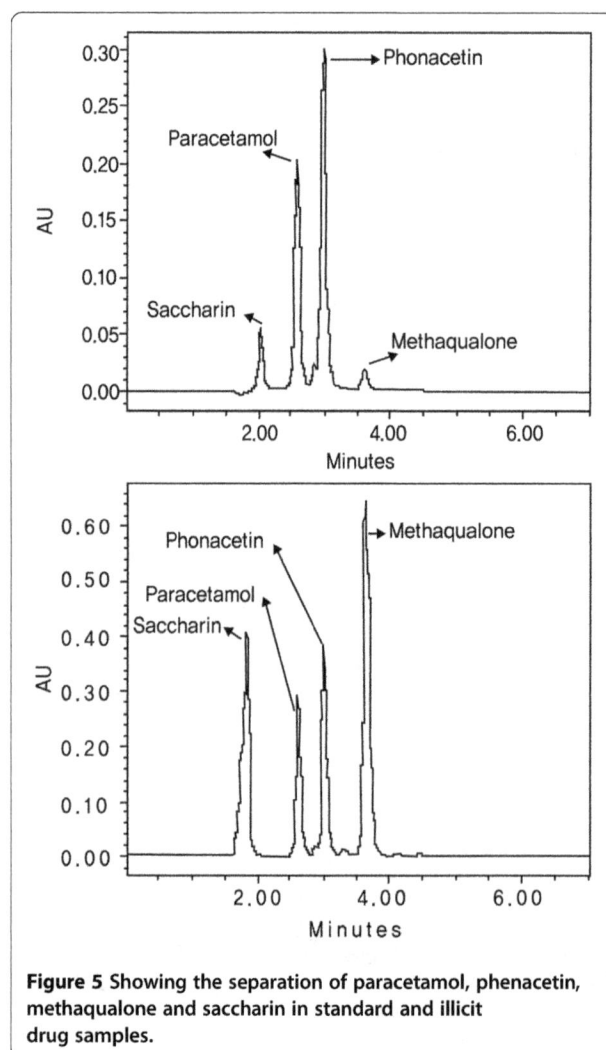

Figure 5 Showing the separation of paracetamol, phenacetin, methaqualone and saccharin in standard and illicit drug samples.

Limits of detection and determination

The detection and quantification limit were determined based on signal (S) to noise (N) ratio by injecting diluted solutions (made from stock solution (2 mg/mL)) into the HPLC system. Limit of detection (LOD) was calculated as S/N × 3 where as limit of quantification (LOQ) was calculated as S/N × 10.

Linearity

For linearity checking Stock solution (2 mg/mL) containing a mixture of saccharin, phenacetin, paracetamol and methaqualone was further diluted with mobile phase to give the final concentration of 0.1 µg/mL. And these solutions were injected into the HPLC system and the resultants peak areas of each component were recorded.

Precision

The precision of the method was evaluated on the basis of analyzing the three different concentrations of each component in the linearity range for repeating three times.

Recovery/accuracy

The accuracy of the method was expressed as the percentage recovery of each component. Recovery studies were carried out by standard addition method where three different concentrations of above said components were prepared with in the calibration range of corresponding components. And also recovery study was carried out by using simulated samples.

Repeatability

The consistency of the results for the same analytes samples were checked by repeating the experiment for 6 times per day (intraday) and consecutive for 3 days (interday). And standard deviation of the repeated recovery values was calculated.

Robustness

Robustness is a measure of a method's immunity to small but deliberate variations in the conditions used. Acetonitrile, water ratio (± 10%) and flow rate (± 10%) were deliberately changed and effects were monitored.

Table 1 Showing the data of limit of detection, limit of quantification and linearity range

Compound	Limit of detection (LOD)	Limit of quantification (LOQ)	Linearity range
Saccharin	15 ng	48 ng	200 ng – 1800 ng
Phenacetin	10 ng	33 ng	200 ng – 2000 ng
Paracetamol	6 ng	19 ng	100 ng – 2200 ng
Methaqualone	5 ng	16 ng	100 ng – 1400 ng

Table 2 Showing the regression equation, slope and intercept value of calibration curve obtained for different analytes

Analytes	Regression equation $y = mx + c$	Regression value (R^2)
Saccharin	Y = 1007.5x + 790110	0..9991
Phenacetin	Y = 1348.5x + 139111	0..9996
Paracetamol	Y = 2420.6x + 37789	0..9993
Methaqualone	Y = 5011.3x - 77962	0.9982

Results and discussion

In the analysis of illicit drugs like methaqualone, in addition to its identity and quantization, it is very important to give the complete profile of the sample with respect to the presence of active component, its decomposition products, side reaction products, impurities, adulterants and diluents so that this data can be compared and correlated with samples of known origin. Many methods are available for the analysis of individual components present in the samples. Analyzing individual components in different unknown samples is a time consuming and costly process. Under these circumstances methods which can determine the individual components simultaneously, accurately and quickly are desirable. The proposed method has been developed by keeping in view these factors. By the proposed method, which needs minimum sample preparation, it was possible to separate and determine saccharin, paracetamol, phenacetin and methaqualone simultaneously in illicit methaqualone samples.

The present HPLC method shows the well resolved peaks with a short analysis time of only 6 minutes. Saccharin, paracetamol, phenacetin and methaqualone were eluted at 2.0, 2.5, 3.0 and 3.6 minutes respectively

Table 3 Showing the recovery and precision data

Compound	Expected amount	Amount recovered in ng	% Recovery	±SD [% n=3]
Saccharin	600	600.16	100.02	4
	1000	1005.83	100.58	2.51
	1400	1408	100.57	3.51
Phenacetin	500	499.5	99.99	2.38
	1000	1015.33	101.53	2.73
	1500	1507.5	100.5	2.59
Paracetamol	500	507.16	101.43	2.27
	1000	1004.83	100.48	4.14
	1500	1500.66	100.04	4.66
Methaqualone	400	402.16	100.54	2.07
	600	598.33	99.72	3.28
	800	797.66	99.70	2.83

Table 4 Showing intraday and interday reproducibility data

Compound	Intraday recovery value (n=6)	± S.D	Interday recovery value (3 days)	± S.D
Saccharin	100.02, 101.31, 100.98, 99.99, 104.53, 101.54	1.66	100.02, 104.34, 102.54	2.16
Phenacetin	99.99, 99.87, 101.72, 103.64, 101.73, 100.11	1.47	98.99, 101.76, 102.70	1.92
Paracetamol	101.43, 102.70, 101.11, 100.68, 101.99, 99.76	1.02	101.43, 104.37, 104.01	1.60
Methaqualone	100.54, 100.96, 102.73, 101.13, 100.02, 99.99	1.05	100.54, 98.67, 103.54	2.45

(Figure 2) under the experimental conditions used. The samples were analyzed in the wavelength ranges from 210 nm to 350 nm by using PDA detector. For detection of saccharin, paracetamol, phenacetin and methaqualone an optimized wavelength of 238 nm was chosen. The mobile phase was optimized by varying mobile phase compositions and flow rate. It was found that mobile phase (acetonitrile: water, 90:10 v/v) with a flow rate of 1mL/min was found to be optimum for efficient resolution of the peaks (Figure 5).

The method was validated accordingly ICH guideline. The limit of detection (LOD), limit of quantification (LOQ), and linearity range and coefficient correlation data is presented in Table 1. The recovery of this method was found to be better than 99% (Table 2). And the standard deviation (+ SD) of this method was found to be in the range from 2 to 5 (Table 3). Intraday and interday studies also shows good reproducibility in respect of recovery (Table 4), and it was found to be precise and accurate. The method remained unaffected, by small but deliberate variations, in the LC flow rate (± 10%) and mobile phase ratio (± 10%). The quantification of the components was studied on simulated samples. The percentage of methaqualone, phenacetin, paracetamol and saccharin in a typical illicit drug sample as well as simulated samples in Table 5.

Conclusion

The proposed method is simple, accurate, reproducible and fast. It can determine the methaqualone, the adulterants/diluents including saccharin simultaneously. The present method can be routinely used for the analysis of these components in illicit methaqualone samples and it will be a valuable method for drug profiling.

Table 5 Percentage of amount found in different samples & comparative correlation of new method with reference methods

Sample	Compounds	% Amount expected	% Amount found by new method	% Amount found by reference methods	± SD (n=3)
Sample 1 (Unknown)	Methaqualone Phenacetin Paracetamol Saccharin	-	12.04	12.45	0.28
		-	45.60	45.09	0.36
		-	25.08	26.18	0.77
		-	15.01	14.31	0.49
Sample 2 (Mixed different proportion of four compounds)	Methaqualone Phenacetin Paracetamol Saccharin	25	26.15	24.68	1.03
		25	24.49	24.10	0.27
		25	23.98	25.35	0.96
		25	27.05	26.78	0.19
Sample 3 (Mixed different proportion of four compounds)	Methaqualone Phenacetin Paracetamol Saccharin	20	18.92	21.35	1.71
		20	21.05	21.69	0.45
		30	28.19	30.70	1.77
		30	32.11	29.85	1.59
Sample 4 (Mixed different proportion of four compounds)	Methaqualone Phenacetin Paracetamol Saccharin	30	31.98	30.51	1.03
		30	28.70	31.59	2.04
		20	19.25	18.75	0.35
		20	22.70	20.96	1.23
Sample 5 (Mixed different proportion of four compounds)	Methaqualone Phenacetin Paracetamol Saccharin	35	33.69	36.68	2.11
		30	28.18	31.32	2.22
		20	21.83	18.96	2.02
		15	13.76	14.13	0.26

Competing interests
The authors declare that they have no competing interests.

Authors' contributions
MI design the experiment, carried out the experiment, and contributed in framing the article. CJ assisted in the analysis using HPLC. PG collected the samples, assisted in the framing of experiment. SKS and TRB contributed in designing the experiment and framing the article. All authors read and approved the final manuscript.

Acknowledgement
Two of the authors (MI and CJ) are grateful to Dr C. N. Bhattacharya, Chief Forensic Scientist I/C, Directorate of Forensic Science, Government of India, New Delhi, for providing them research fellowships. The authors would like to thank Mr. A.K.Ganjoo, Director, CFSL, Hyderabad for extending necessary facilities and giving constant encouragement during the course of this work. Our thanks are due to Mr. S.N. Rasool, JSO, CFSL, Hyderabad, India, for technical help. Authors also thanks to M/s Kare Labs (Goa, India) for providing Reference standard of Saccharin.

Author details
[1]Chemistry Division, Central Forensic Science Laboratory, Hyderabad, India.
[2]Chemistry Division, Central Forensic Science Laboratory, Chandigarh, India.
[3]Forensic Science Institute, Osmania University, Hyderabad, India.

References
Anthony CM, Osselton MD, Widdop B (2003) Clarke's Analysis of Drugs and Poisons, vol 1 & 2, 3rd edn. Pharmaceutical Pharmaceutical, London

Atasoy S, Bicer F, Acikkol M, Bilgic Z (1988) Illicit drug abuse in the Marmara region of Turkey. J Forensic Sci Int 38(1–2):75–81

Battisti MC, Noto AR, Nappo S, De A, Carlini E (2006) A profile of ecstasy (MDMA) use in Sao Paulo, Brazil: An ethnographic study. J Psycho Drugs 38(1):13–18

Behrman AD (2008) Luck of the Draw: Common Adulterants found in illicit Drugs. J Emer Nursing 34:80–82

Biemer TA (1989) Analysis of Saccharin, Acesulfame-K and Sodium Cyclamate by high performance ion chromatography. J Chromatogr A 463:463–468

Brunt TM, Rigter S, Hoek J, Vogels N, Van Dijk P, Niesink RJM (2009) An analysis of cocaine powder in the Netherlands: Content and health hazards due to adulterants. Addiction 104(5):798–805

Chen Q, Mou S, Liu K, Ni Z (1997) Simultaneous determination of four artificial sweeteners and citric acid by High-Performance Anion Exchange Chromatography. J Chromatogr A 771:135–143

Filho OF, Nobrega JA (1994) Flow injection potentiometric determination of Saccharin in dietary products with relocation of filtration unit. Talanta 41:731–734

Fo OF, Moraes AJ, Santos GD (1993) Potentiometric determination of Saccharin in dietary products using mercurous nitrate as titrant. Talanta 40:737–740

Fucci N (2004) Phenacetin and cocaine in a body packer. J Forensic Sci Int 141 (1):59–61

Fucci N, De Giovanni N (1998) Adulterants encountered in the illicit Cocaine market. J Forensic Sci Int 95:247–252

Fucci N, Giovanni ND (1998) Adulterants encountered in the illicit cocaine market. J Forensic Sci Int 95:247–252

Furst RT (2000) The re-engineering of heroin: An emerging heroin "cutting" trend in New York City. Addict Resear Theory 8(4):357–379

Ikai Y, Oka H, Kawamura N, Yamada M (1988) Simultaneous determination of nine food additives using High Performance Liquid Chromatography. J Chromatogr A 457:333–343

Kacker IK, Zaheer SH (1951) Potential Analgesics. Part I. Synthesis of substituted 4 Quinazolones. J Ind Chem Soc 28:344–346

Sastry CSP, Srinivas KR, Prasad KMMK, Krishnamacharyulu AG (1995) Rapid, routine method for the analysis of non-nutritive sweeteners in food stuffs. Analyst 120:1793–2012

Smyth RD, Lee JK, Polk A, Chemburkar PB, Savacool AM (1973) Bioavailability of methaqualone. J Clin Pharmacol 13(10):391–400

Terada H, Sakade Y (1985) Studies on the analysis of food additives by High Performance Liquid Chromatography: V. Simultaneous determination of preservatives and Saccharin in foods by ion-pair Chromatography. J Chromatogr A 346:333–340

Tibbels TS, Smith RA (1988) Determination of saccharin in diet and biological materials. J Chromatogr A 441:448–453

Valley LFC, Jimenez JFG, Valencia MC (2007) Simultaneous determination of antioxidants, preservatives and sweetener additives in food and cosmetics by flow injection analysis coupled to a monolithic column. J Anal Chim Acta 594:226–233

Zhu Y, Guo Y, Ye M (2005) Separation and simultaneous determination of four artificial sweeteners in food and beverages by ion chromatography. J Chromatogr A 1085:143–146

5

Novel radiochemical and biological characterization of ^{99m}Tc-histamine as a model for brain imaging

M H Sanad

Abstract

Background: Histamine was successfully labeled with technetium-99 m (^{99m}Tc). The studied reaction parameters included substrate concentration, reducing agent concentration, pH of the reaction mixture, reaction time, in vitro stability of the ^{99m}Tc-histamine, and biodistribution in experimental animals.

Method: Accurately weighed 3 mg histamine was dissolved and transferred to an evacuated penicillin vial. Exactly 50 µg SnCl$_2$ dihydrate was added and the pH of the mixture was adjusted to 4 using 0.1N HCl, then the volume of the mixture was adjusted to one ml by N$_2$-purged distilled water. One ml of freshly eluted ^{99m}TcO4- (~ 400MBq) was added to the above mixture. The reaction mixture was vigorously shaken and allowed to react at room temperature for sufficient time to complete the reaction

Result: The complex gives a maximum labeling yield of 98.0% ± 0.34%, and maintained stability throughout the working period (6 h). Biodistribution investigation showed that the maximum uptake of the ^{99m}Tc-histamine in the brain was 7.1% ± 0.12% of the injected activity/g tissue organ, at 5 min post-injection. The clearance from the mice appeared to proceed via the circulation mainly through the kidneys and urine (approximately 37.8% of the injected dose at 2 h after injection of the tracer).

Conclusions: Brain uptake of ^{99m}Tc-histamine is higher than that of (^{99m}Tc-ECD and ^{99m}Tc-HMPAO) therefore ^{99m}Tc-histamine could be used for brain single-photon emission computed tomography (SPECT). Furthermore, ^{99m}Tc-histamine could be considered as a novel radiopharmaceutical for brain imaging.

Keywords: Histamine; Hexamethylpropyleneamine oxime and ethyl cysteinate dimer; Technetium-99 m; Labeling; Biodistribution; Brain; Imaging

Background

Several recent reviews describe the use of single-photon emission computed tomography (SPECT) alone or in combination with PET and/or functional magnetic resonance imaging (fMRI) in studies of human cognition, imaging of neuroreceptor systems, aiding diagnosis or assessment of progression or treatment response in various psychiatric and neurologic disorders, neuropharmacologic challenge studies and in the new field of molecular imaging, including imaging of transgene expression (Devous 2002; Catafau 2001; Mazziotta and Toga 2002; Lee and Newberg 2005; Bonte and Devous 2003; Devous Sr 1998;

Brooks 2005; Heinz et al. 2000; Dickerson and Sperling 2005; Bammer et al. 2005; Eckert and Eidelberg 2005; Kuzniecky 2005). Brain SPECT is now commonly used in the diagnosis, prognosis assessment, evaluation of response to therapy, risk stratification, detection of benign or malignant viable tissue, and choice of medical or surgical therapy, especially in head injury, malignant brain tumors, cerebrovascular disease, movement disorders, dementia, and epilepsy (Lee and Newberg 2005; Bonte and Devous 2003; Devous Sr 1998; Brooks 2005; Heinz et al. 2000; Dickerson and Sperling 2005; Bammer et al. 2005; and Kuzniecky 2005). The selection of the proper isotope to be used in labeling and in imaging is important because it should have a suitable short half-life to avoid unwarranted harmful exposure to radiation and suitable photon energy

Correspondence: msanad74@yahoo.com
Labeled Compounds Department, Radioisotopes Production and Radioactive Sources Division, Hot Laboratories Center, Atomic Energy Authority, P.O. Box 13759, Cairo, Egypt

within the range of gamma camera. The two most proper isotopes that fulfill these two precautions are ^{123}I and ^{99m}Tc. Brain imaging in humans is currently achieved by using ^{99m}Tc-ethyl cysteinate dimer (^{99m}Tc-ECD), ^{99m}Tc-hexamethylpropyleneamine oxime (^{99m}Tc-HMPAO), ^{125}I-sibutramine, and ^{125}I-fluoxetine (Ogasawara et al. 2001; Chang et al. 2002; Bonte et al. 2010; and El-Ghany et al. 2007). The major disadvantage of these compounds is their poor brain uptake in experimental animals (4.7% for ^{99m}Tc-ECD and 2.25% for ^{99m}Tc-HMPAO) (Walovitch et al. 1989; Neirinckx et al. 1987). Such low uptake enforces us to try to find novel radiopharmaceuticals that can overcome this limitation and can be used as more efficient brain imaging agents. Histamine [2-(1H-imidazol-4-yl)] ethanamine is an organic nitrogen compound involved in local immune responses as well as regulating physiological function in the gut and acting as a neurotransmitter (Marieb 2001). Histamine increases the permeability of the capillaries to white blood cells and some proteins to allow them to engage pathogens in the infected tissues (Di Giuseppe et al. 2003). Histamine is known to be involved in so many physiological functions because of its chemical properties that allow it to be so versatile in binding (Noszal et al. 2004). In this paper, histamine was labeled with the most widely used imaging radionuclide, ^{99m}Tc. Factors affecting the labeling yield of ^{99m}Tc-histamine complex and biological distribution in Swiss Albino mice (25 to 30 g) were studied in detail (Motaleb and Sanad 2012). The radiochemical yield of the product was determined by paper chromatography, paper electrophoresis, and high-performance liquid chromatography (HPLC).

Methods

Drugs and chemicals

Histamine was purchased from Sigma-Aldrich Chemical Company, St. Louis, MO, USA, and all other chemicals were purchased from Merck (Whitehouse Station, NJ, USA) and they were reactive grade. The water used is purged deoxygenated bidistilled water.

Labeling of histamine

Accurately weighed 3 mg histamine was dissolved and transferred to an evacuated penicillin vial. Exactly 50 μg SnCl$_2$ dihydrate was added and the pH of the mixture was adjusted to 4 using 0.1 N HCl, then the volume of the mixture was adjusted to 1 ml by N$_2$-purged distilled water. One milliliter of freshly eluted ^{99m}TcO$_4^-$ (approximately 400 MBq) was added to the above mixture. The reaction mixture was vigorously shaken and allowed to react at room temperature for sufficient time to complete the reaction (Boyd 1986). The proposed structure of the ^{99m}Tc-histamine via reaction of histamine with ^{99m}TcO$_4^-$ in the presence of stannous chloride dihydrate at pH 4 at room temperature is shown in Figure 1b, where the oxidation state of ^{99m}Tc changed from +7 into +5 to form a complex with two

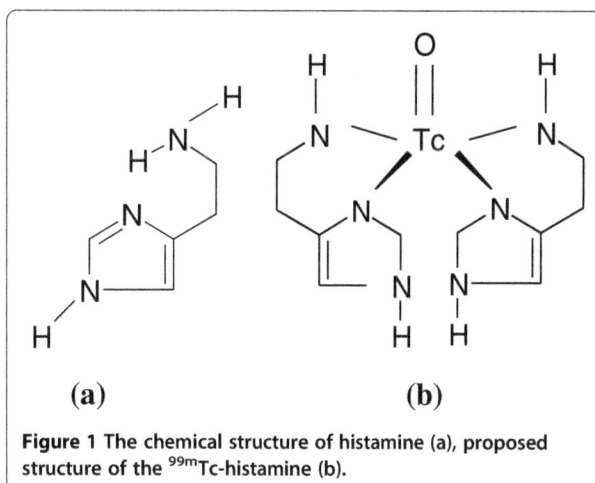

Figure 1 The chemical structure of histamine (a), proposed structure of the ^{99m}Tc-histamine (b).

molecules of histamine. ^{99m}Tc-histamine complex coordinated as a Tc (V) oxocore, leading to complexes in which a TcO^{3+} core exists (Jurisson et al. 1986; Abrams et al. 1991).

Factors affecting % labeling yield

This experiment was conducted to study the different factors that affect labeling yield such as tin content as (SnCl$_2$ · 2H$_2$O), substrate content, pH of the reaction, and reaction time. In the process of labeling, trials and errors were performed for each factor under investigations till obtains the optimum value. The experiment was repeated with all factors kept at optimum changing except the factor under study, till the optimal conditions are achieved (Robbins 1984).

Quality control
Paper chromatography

Radiochemical yield of ^{99m}Tc-histamine was checked by paper chromatography method in which, the reaction product was spotted on ascending paper chromatography strips (10 × 1.5 cm). Free ^{99m}TcO$_4^-$ in the preparation was determined using acetone as the mobile phase. Reduced hydrolyzed technetium was determined by using an ethanol/water/ammonium hydroxide mixture (2:5:1) or 5 N NaOH as the mobile phase. After complete development, the strips were dried then cut into 0.5-cm pieces and counted in a well-type γ-scintillation counter.

HPLC analysis

An HPLC analysis of histamine solution was done by an injection of 10 μl from the reaction mixture into the column (RP-18-250 × 4.6 mm^2, 5 μm, Lischrosorb) built in an HPLC Shimadzu model (Kyoto, Japan) which consists of pumps LC-9A, Rheohydron injector and UV spectrophotometer detector (SPD-6A) adjusted to the 256-nm wavelength. The column was eluted with mobile phase methanol/H$_2$O (50:50) and the flow rate was adjusted to 1 ml/min. Then fractions of 1 ml were collected separately using a fraction collector up to 20 ml and counted in a well-type γ-scintillation counter.

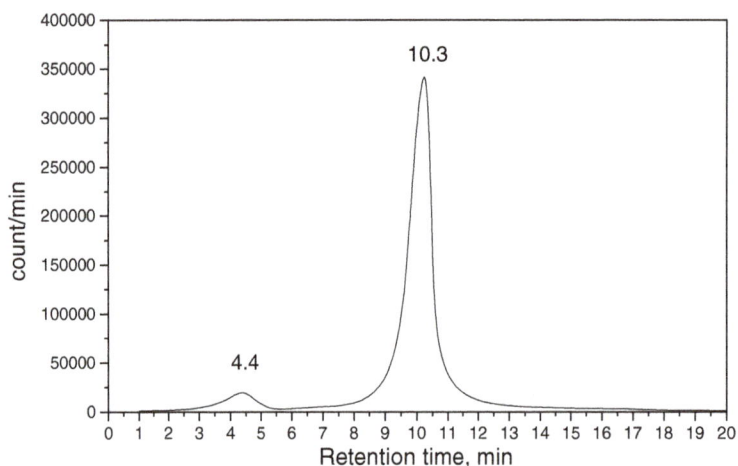

Figure 2 HPLC radiochromatogram of ^{99m}Tc-histamine complex.

Stability of ^{99m}Tc-histamine in human serum

The stability of ^{99m}Tc-histamine was studied in vitro by mixing 1.8 ml of normal human serum and 0.2 ml of ^{99m}Tc-histamine and incubated at 37°C for (24 h). Exactly 0.2 ml aliquots were withdrawn during the incubation at different time intervals up to 6 h and subjected to paper chromatography for determination of the percent of ^{99m}Tc-histamine, reduced hydrolyzed technetium and free pertechnetate

Animal studies

The study was approved by the animal ethics committee, Labeled Compound Department, and was in accordance with the guidelines set out by the Egyptian Atomic Energy Authority. Swiss Albino mice (25 to 30 g) were intravenously injected with 100 μl (100 to 150 MBq) of sterile ^{99m}Tc-histamine adjusted to physiological pH via the tail vein and kept alive in metabolic cage for different intervals of time under normal conditions. For quantitative determination of organ distribution, five mice were used for each experiment and the mice were sacrificed at different times post-injection. Samples of fresh blood, bone, and muscle were collected in pre-weighed vials and counted. The different organs were removed, counted, and compared to a standard solution of the labeled histamine. The average percent values of the administered dose/organ were calculated. Blood, bone, and muscles were assumed to be 7%, 10%, and 40%, respectively, of the total body weight (Motaleb 2001). Corrections were made for background radiation and physical decay during experiment. Differences in the data were evaluated with the Student's t test. Results for P using the two-tailed test are reported and all the results are given as mean ± SEM. The level of significance was set at $P < 0.05$.

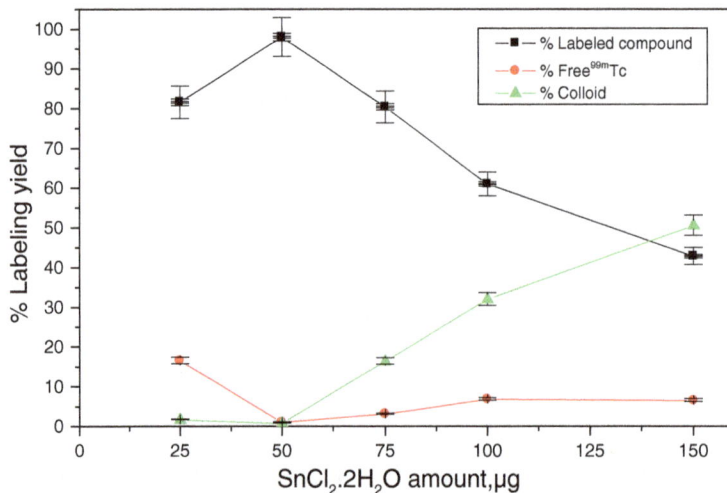

Figure 3 Effect of Sn (II) amount on the labeling yield of ^{99m}Tc-histamine, complex. Conditions: 3 mg histamine, 25-150 μg Sn (II), pH 4 and 30 min. reaction time, n=3.

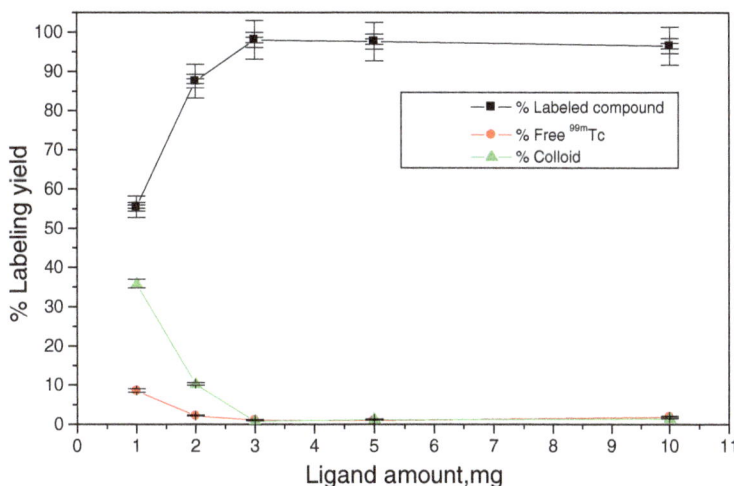

Figure 4 Effect of histamine amount on the labeling yield of ^{99m}Tc-histamine complex. Conditions: 1-10 mg of histamine, 50 µg Sn (II), pH 4 and 30 min. reaction time, n=3.

Determination of the partition coefficient of ^{99m}Tc-histamine

The partition coefficient was determined by mixing ^{99m}Tc-histamine with equal volumes of 1-octanol and phosphate buffer (0.025 M at pH 7.4) in a centrifuge tube.

The mixture was vortexed at room temperature for 1 min and then centrifuged at 5,000 rpm for 5 min. Subsequently, 100 µl samples from the 1-octanol and aqueous layers were pipetted into other test tubes and counted in a gamma counter. The measurement was repeated five times. The partition coefficient value was expressed as log p (Motaleb et al. 2011).

$$P = \frac{\text{Counts per min in octanole} - \text{Counts per min back ground}}{\text{Counts per min in buffer} - \text{Counts per min back ground}}$$

Results and discussion
Separation of ^{99m}Tc-histamine complex

In the case of the ascending paper chromatographic method, acetone was used as the developing solvent; free ^{99m}TcO$_4^-$ moved with the solvent front ($R_f = 1$), while ^{99m}Tc-histamine and reduced hydrolyzed technetium remained at the point of spotting. In the case of the ascending paper chromatographic method, mixture was used as the developing solvent; reduced hydrolyzed technetium remains at the origin ($R_f = 0$), while other species migrate with the solvent front ($R_f = 1$). The radiochemical purity was determined by subtracting the sum of the percent of reduced hydrolyzed technetium and free pertechnetate from 100%. The radiochemical yield is the mean value of five experiments.

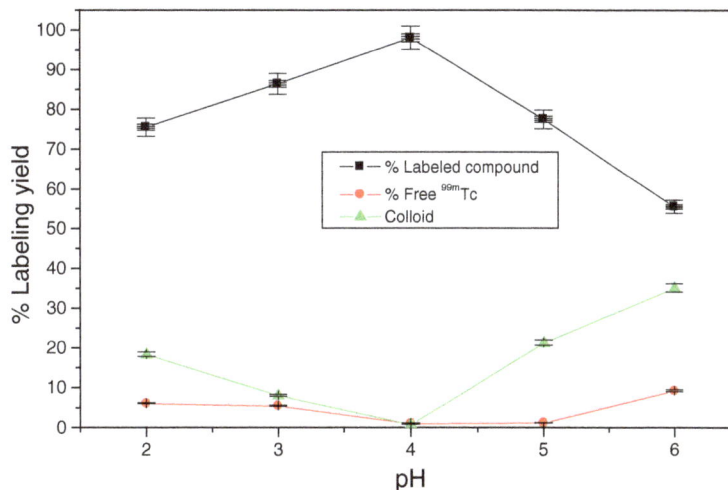

Figure 5 Effect of pH of the reaction mixture of ^{99m}Tc-histamine complex. Conditions: 3 mg histamine, 50 µg Sn (II), pH 2-6 and 30 min. reaction time, n=3.

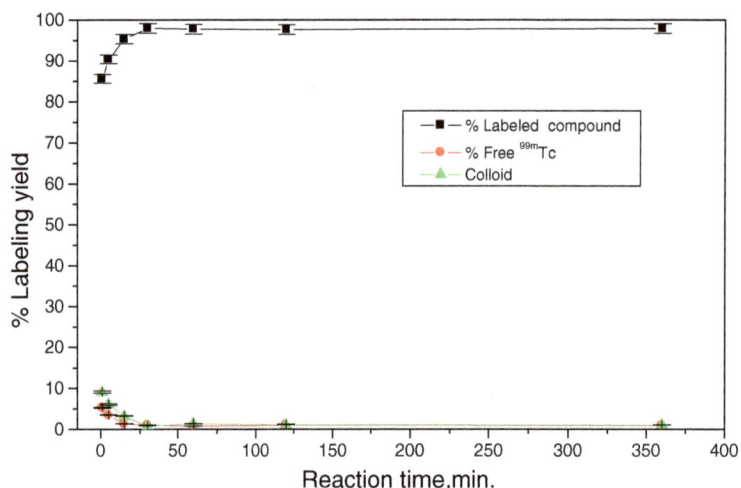

Figure 6 Effect of reaction time on the labeling yield of ^{99m}Tc-histamine complex. Conditions: 1-360 min. at optimum conditions, reaction time, n=3.

HPLC chromatogram was presented in Figure 2 and shows two peaks, one at fraction No. 4.4, which corresponds to ^{99m}TcO$_4^-$, while the second peak was collected at fraction No. 10.3 for ^{99m}Tc-histamine, which was found to coincide with the UV signal.

Factors affecting labeling yield
Effect of SnCl$_2 \cdot$ 2H$_2$O amount
As shown in Figure 3, the radiochemical yield was dependent on the amount of SnCl$_2 \cdot$ 2H$_2$O present in the reaction mixture. At 25 μg SnCl$_2 \cdot$ 2H$_2$O, the labeling yield of ^{99m}Tc-histamine was 81.6% due to the fact that SnCl$_2 \cdot$ 2H$_2$O amount was insufficient to reduce all

pertechnetate so the percentage of ^{99m}TcO$_4^-$ was relatively high (16.6%). The labeling yield significantly increased by increasing the amount of SnCl$_2 \cdot$ 2H$_2$O from 25 to 50 μg (optimum amount), at which a maximum labeling yield of 98% was obtained. By increasing the amount of SnCl$_2 \cdot$ 2H$_2$O above the optimum concentration value, the labeling yield decreased again because the excess SnCl$_2 \cdot$ 2H$_2$O was converted to colloid (50.6% at 150 μg SnCl$_2 \cdot$ 2H$_2$O) (Liu et al. 2004).

Effect of histamine amount
The labeling yield of ^{99m}Tc-histamine complex was 55.5% at 1 mg histamine and increased with increasing the

Table 1 Biodistribution of ^{99m}Tc-histamine in normal mice

Organs and body fluid	% I.D./organ and body fluid at different post-injection times				
	5 min	15 min	30 min	120 min	240 min
Liver	8.11 ± 0.3	6.2 ± 0.1	5.2 ± 0.2	3.2 ± 0.1	1.3 ± 0.02
Urine	5.10 ± 0.2	8.60 ± 0.11	18.1 ± 1.1	23.0 ± 2.3	31.5 ± 2.3
Kidneys	10.5 ± 0.1	12.25 ± 0.3	16.8 ± 1.2	15.2 ± 0.3	6.30 ± 22
Blood	28.4 ± 0.5	24.8 ± 0.9	6.1 ± 0.12	3.50 ± 0.1	1.2 ± 0.05
Heart	1.3 ± 0.01	1.40 ± 0.02	1.6 ± 0.01	0.9 ± 0.03	0.70 ± 0.02
Lung	30.5 ± 0.2	12.8 ± 0.3	11.30 ± 0.2	5.40 ± 0.10	3.25 ± 0.6
Intestine	3.50 ± 0.1	2.80 ± 0.2	1.4 ± 0.02	1.2 ± 0.03	0.9 ± 0.02
Stomach	1.6 ± 0.06	1.20 ± 0.02	2.2 ± 0.05	3.3 ± 0.13	3.70 ± 0.2
Spleen	1.6 ± 0.03	4.52 ± 0.21	6.20 ± 0.2	5.3 ± 0.32	3.80 ± 0.16
Bone	1.90 ± 0.1	1.6 ± 0.3	2.0 ± 0.11	1.80 ± 0.30	1.70 ± 0.13
Muscle	1.8 ± 0.01	1.6 ± 0.03	1.5 ± 0.01	1.2 ± 0.06	1.10 ± 0.02
Brain	7.1 ± 0.12	4.85 ± 0.6	1.4 ± 0.02	0.83 ± 0.06	0.62 ± 0.03
Thyroid	1.3 ± 0.05	0.9 ± 0.02	0.7 ± 0.03	0.55 ± 0.01	0.32 ± 0.01
Brain/blood	0.25	0.2	0.23	0.24	0.52

amount of histamine till reaching the maximum value of 98% at 3 mg (Figure 4). The formed complex remained stable with increasing the amount of histamine up to 10 mg. So the optimum amount of histamine was 3 mg (Liu et al. 2004; Sanad 2007).

Effect of pH of the reaction mixture

As shown in Figure 5, at pH 2, the labeling yield of ^{99m}Tc-histamine complex was small and equal to 75.5% and this yield increased with increasing the pH of the reaction mixture where pH 4 gave the maximum labeling yield of 98%. By increasing the pH greater than 4, the labeling yield decreased again till it became 55.5% at pH 6 where colloid was the main impurity (35.2% at pH 6) after pH 6 more colloidal solutions are formed (Liu et al. 2004).

Effect of reaction time

Figure 6 describes the effect of incubation time on the radiochemical purity of ^{99m}Tc-histamine complex. At 1 min post labeling, the yield was small and equal to 85.6% which increased with time till reaching its maximum value of 98% at 30 min. The yield remains stable at 97.9% for a time up to 6 h (Liu et al. 2004).

Stability test

In vitro stability of ^{99m}Tc- histamine was studied in order to determine the suitable time for injection to avoid the formation of the undesired products that result from the radiolysis of complex. These undesired radioactive products might be accumulated in non-target organs. The results of stability showed that the ^{99m}Tc-histamine is stable up to 24 h and that at 37°C, resulted in no release of radioactivity (n = five experiments) from the ^{99m}Tc-histamine, as determined by paper chromatography (Motaleb et al. 2011).

Partition coefficient for ^{99m}Tc- histamine

The partition coefficient values were 1.48 ± 0.02, showing that the ^{99m}Tc-histamines are lipophilic and can cross the blood–brain barrier.

Biodistribution of ^{99m}Tc-histamine

The biodistribution patterns of ^{99m}Tc-histamine is shown in Table 1, the ^{99m}Tc-histamine was injected in normal mice via intravenous route and was distributed all over the body organs and fluids. All radioactivity levels are expressed as average percent-injected dose per gram (%ID/g ± SD). ^{99m}Tc-histamine was removed from the circulation mainly through the kidneys and urine (approximately 37.8% injected dose at 2 h after injection of the tracer). The liver uptake decreased markedly with time for ^{99m}Tc-histamine from 8.11 ± 0.3, at 5 min till reaching 1.3 ± 0.02 at 4 h (Sanad 2013; Motaleb et al. 2012).

The high accumulation of ^{99m}Tc-histamine in lungs is decreased markedly with time from 30.5 ± 0.2, at 5 min till reaching 3.5 ± 0.6 at 4 h (Suhara et al. 1998; Sanad and Ibrahim 2013; Ibrahim and Sanad 2013; Sanad and El-Tawoosy 2013). The biodistribution data showed substantial uptake of 7.1 ± 0.12 (%ID/g ± SD) in the brain at 5 min post-injection. After this time point, radioactivity dropped to 4.85 ± 0.6 at 15 min post-injection. The maximum brain uptake of ^{99m}Tc-histamine (7.1 ± 0.12) is higher than that of currently used radiopharmaceuticals for brain imaging, ^{99m}Tc-ethyl cysteinate dimer (^{99m}Tc-ECD) and ^{99m}Tc- hexamethylpropyleneamine oxime (^{99m}Tc-HMPAO) which have maximum brain uptake of 4.7% and 2.25%, respectively (Walovitch et al. 1989; Neirinckx et al. 1987); therefore, ^{99m}Tc-histamine could be successfully used for brain SPECT.

Conclusion

Histamine can be labeled easily with ^{99m}Tc using 50 µg stannous chloride dihydrate ($SnCl_2 \cdot 2H_2O$) as a reducing agent and 3 mg histamine at pH 4 for 30 min at room temperature to give ^{99m}Tc-histamine complex with a radiochemical yield of 98%, which is higher than that of the commercially available kit. Biodistribution studies showed that the uptake of ^{99m}Tc-histamine in the brain (7.1% ± 0.12) is higher than that of currently used radiopharmaceuticals for brain imaging, ^{99m}Tc-ethyl cysteinate dimer (^{99m}Tc-ECD) and ^{99m}Tc-hexamethylpropyleneamine oxime (^{99m}Tc-HMPAO), respectively. ^{99m}Tc-histamine could be used for brain SPECT. Furthermore, ^{99m}Tc histamine could be considered as a novel radiopharmaceutical for brain imaging.

Competing interests

The author declares that he has no competing interests.

References

Abrams MJ, Larsen S, Zubieta J (1991) Fluoride as a terminal bridging ligand for copper: isolation and X-ray crystallographic characterization of monomeric and dimeric forms of a copper (II)-fluoride complex. Inorg Chem 30:2031–2035

Bammer R, Skare S, Newbould R, Liu C, Thijs V, Ropele S, Clayton DB, Krueger G, Moseley ME, Glover GH (2005) Foundations of advanced magnetic resonance imaging. NeuroRx 2:167–196

Bonte FJ, Devous MD (2003) SPECT brain imaging. In: Sandler MP, Coleman RE, Patton JA, Wackers FJTH, Gottschalk A (eds) Diagnostic nuclear medicine 4th edn. Lippincott Williams and Wilkins, Philadelphia, pp 757–782

Bonte FJ, Hynan L, Harris TS, White CL (2010) ^{99m}T-HMPAO brain blood flow imaging in the dementias with histopathologic correlation in 73 patients. J Mol Imaging 2011:409101

Boyd RE (1986) Technetium generators: status and prospects. Nucl Spectrum 2:18–25

Brooks DJ (2005) Positron emission tomography and single-photon emission computed tomography in central nervous system drug development. NeuroRx 2(2):226–236

Catafau AM (2001) Brain SPECT in clinical practice. part I: Perfusion. J Nucl Med 42:259–271

Chang C, Shiau Y, Wang J, Ho S, Kao A (2002) Abnormal regional cerebral blood flow on ^{99m}Tc ECD brain SPECT in patients with primary Sjögren's syndrome and normal findings on brain magnetic resonance imaging. Ann Rheum Dis 61:774–778

Devous MD, Sr (1998) SPECT brain imaging in cerebrovascular disease. In "Nuclear Medicine in Clinical Diagnosis and Treatment." 2nd edn Murray IPC, Ell PJ (ed). McGraw- Hill, New York, pp 631–649

Devous MD, Sr (2002) Functional brain imaging in the dementias: role in early detection, differential diagnosis, and longitudinal studies. Eur J Nucl Med Mol Imaging 29(12):1685

Di Giuseppe M, Sergienko AV, Saleh BEA, et al. (2003) Nelson biology 12. Thomson Canada Ltd, Toronto, p 473. ISBN 0-17-625987-2

Dickerson BC, Sperling RA (2005) Neuroimaging biomarkers for clinical trials of disease-modifying therapies in Alzheimer's disease. NeuroRx 2(2):348–360

Eckert T, Eidelberg D (2005) Neuroimaging and therapeutics in movement disorders. NeuroRx 2(2):361–371

El-Ghany EA, Amine AM, El-Kawy OA, Magdy A (2007) Technetium-99 m labeling and freeze-dried kit formulation of levofloxacin (L-Flox): a novel agent for detecting sites of infection. J Label Compd Radiopharm 50(1):25–31

Heinz A, Jones DW, Raedler T, Coppola R, Knable MB, Weinberger DR (2000) Neuropharmacological studies with SPECT in neuropsychiatric disorders. Nucl Med Biol 27(7):677–682

Ibrahim IT, Sanad MH (2013) Radiolabeling and biological evaluation of losartan as a possible cardiac imaging agent. J Radiochemistry 55(3):336–340

Jurisson S, Schlemper EO, Troutner DE, Canning LR, Nowotnik DP, Neirinckx RD (1986) Synthesis characterization and X-ray structural determination of Tc (V)-oxo-tetradenatate amine oxime complex. Inorg Chem 25:543-549

Kuzniecky RI (2005) Neuroimaging of epilepsy: therapeutic implications. NeuroRx 2(2):384–393

Lee B, Newberg A (2005) Imaging in traumatic brain imaging. NeuroRx 2(2):372–383

Liu FEI, Youfeng HE, Luo Z (2004) Technical Report Series No 426. IAEA, Austria, p 37

Marieb E (2001) Human anatomy & physiology. Benjamin Cummings, San Francisco, p 414. ISBN 0-8053-4989-8

Mazziotta JC, Toga AW (2002) Brain mapping: the methods, 2nd edition. Academic, San Diego, USA, p 513

Motaleb MA (2001) Synthesis and evaluation of some 99mTc- Complexes; applied in nuclear medicine, Ph.D. Thesis, Faculty of Science, Ain-Shams University, Cairo, Egypt

Motaleb MA, Sanad MH (2012) Preparation and quality control of 99mTc-6-[[2-amino- 2-(4-hydroxyphenyl)-acetyl]amino]-3,3-dimethyl- 7-oxo- 4-thia- 1-azabicyclo-heptane- 2-carboxylic acid complex as a model for detecting sites of infection. Arab J Nucl Sci and Appli 45(3):71–78

Motaleb MA, Moustapha ME, Ibrahim IT (2011) Synthesis and biological evaluation of 125I-nebivolol as a potential cardioselective agent for imaging β1-adrenoceptors. J Radioanal Nucl Chem 289(1):239–245

Motaleb MA, Abdallah HEM, Atef M (2012) Synthesis and evaluation of 99mTc-NIDA and 99mTc-DMIDA complexes for hepatobiliary imaging. J Radiochmestry 54(5):501–505

Neirinckx RD, Canning LR, Piper IM, Nowotnik DP, Pickett RD, Holmes RA, Volkert WA, Forster AM, Weisner PS, Marriott JA, Chaplin SB (1987) 99mT–D, L HMPAO a new radiopharmaceutical for SPECT imaging of regional cerebral blood flow. J Nucl Med 28:191–202

Noszal B, Kraszni M, Racz A (2004) Histamine: fundamentals of biological chemistry. In: Falus A, Grosman N, Darvas Z (ed) Histamine: Biology and Medical Aspects. SpringMed Publishing Ltd, Budapest, p 15

Ogasawara K, Ogawa A, Ezura M, Konno H, Suzuki M, Yoshimoto T (2001) Brain single-photon emission CT studies using 99mTc-HMPAO and 99mTc-ECD early after recanalization by local intraarterial thrombolysis in patients with acute embolic middle cerebral artery occlusion. Am J Neuroradiol 22:48–53

Rbbins PJ (1984) Chromatography of technetium-99 m radiopharmaceuticals, a practical guide. Society of Nuclear Medicine, New York, NY, USA

Sanad MH (2007) Synthesis and labeling of some organic compounds with one of the most radioactive isotope; Ph.D. Thesis, Chemistry Department, Faculty of Science, Ain-Shams University, Cairo, Egypt

Sanad MH (2013) Labeling of omeprazole with technetium-99 m for diagnosis of stomach. J Radiochemistry 55(6):605–609

Sanad MH, El-Tawoosy M (2013) Labeling of ursodeoxycholic acid with technetium-99 m for hepatobiliary imaging. J Radioanal Nucl Chem 298(2):1105–1109

Sanad MH, Ibrahim IT (2013) Radiodiagnosis of peptic ulcer with technetium-99 m pantoprazole. J Radiochemistry 55(3):341–345

Suhara T, Sudo Y, Yoshida K, Okubo Y, Fukuda H, Obata T, Yoshikawa K, Suzuki K, Sasaki Y (1998) Novel radioiodinated sibutramine and fluoxetine. Lancet 351:332–335

Walovitch RC, Hill TC, Garrity ST, Cheesman EH, Burgess BA, O'Leary DH, Watson AD, Ganey MV, Morgan RA, Williams SJ (1989) Characterization of technetium-99 m-L, L-ECD for brain perfusion imaging, Part 1: Pharmacology of technetium-99 m ECD in nonhuman primates. J Nucl Med 30(11):1892–1901

6

Method development for simultaneous detection of ferulic acid and vanillin using high-performance thin layer chromatography

Swarali S Hingse, Shraddha B Digole and Uday S Annapure[*]

Abstract

Background: A simple, accurate, and reliable high-performance thin-layer chromatography (HPTLC) method was developed for separation and detection of ferulic acid and vanillin.

Methods: Separation of ferulic acid and vanillin was carried out on 20 × 10 cm thin layer chromatography (TLC) plates using mobile phase containing toluene/1, 4-dioxan/acetic acid in the ratio 9:2.5:0.4 (v/v). The FA and vanillin were scanned at 320 and 312 nm, respectively. Method was validated for linearity, accuracy, precision, robustness, limit of detection, limit of quantification, and specificity.

Results: Retention factor (Rf) obtained for ferulic acid and vanillin was 0.48 and 0.56, respectively. The correlation coefficients, 0.9975 and 0.9991 with an average recovery of 98.77% and 98.45% obtained for ferulic acid and vanillin respectively by this method were satisfactory.

Conclusion: The optimized method was found to be efficient, precise, accurate, specific, and economic. Therefore, the method would be useful for both qualitative and quantitative routine analysis in pharmaceutical, food industry, and research laboratories.

Keywords: Ferulic acid; Vanillin; High-performance thin layer chromatography (HPTLC); Simultaneous detection

Background

Aromatic compounds are present in natural sources with substantial combinations which are directly responsible for its odor and sensitivity. They can be categorized as volatile organic compounds like aldehydes, alcohols, ketones, esters, lactones, and terpenes (Raisi et al. 2008). They are known to be precursors for the production of numerous products employed in the food, pharmaceutical, and chemical industries and are present at very low concentrations in natural sources. According to US and European legislations, synthetic flavor production is not considered as natural. Alternatively, biotechnology offers microorganisms as production hosts for different types of aromatic compounds in industrial fermentative processes (Lomascolo et al. 1999). The most intensively studied biotransformation using microorganisms is the bio conversion of ferulic acid (FA) to produce natural vanillin (Priefert et al. 2001).

FA is an important precursor of vanillin that is available in abundance in plant cell walls linked to polysaccharide by an ester or ether bonds (Xu et al. 2005). FA is a potent antioxidant because it effectively scavenges free radicals and even possesses antimicrobial properties by preventing the lipid peroxidation caused by microbes (Graf 1992). Moreover, it is used in cosmetics for the photo protection of skin and in protection against various inflammatory diseases.

Vanillin is widely used in food industry as a flavoring agent but also has applications in some fragrances and pharmaceuticals (Priefert et al. 2001). It is also known to possess anti-metastatic, anticancer (Ho et al. 2009) and anti-inflammatory (Wu et al. 2009) activities. It exhibits antimicrobial properties due to its phenolic nature and hence used to develop antimicrobial films used in packaging of bakery products (Rakchoy et al. 2009).

FA and vanillin are generally determined by various chromatographic methods. Different approaches such as UV spectrophotometry (Mabry et al. 1970; Macheix et al. 1990)

* Correspondence: udayannapure@gmail.com
Food Engineering and Technology Department, Institute of Chemical Technology, Nathalal Parekh Marg, Matunga, Mumbai - 400019, India

gas chromatography (GC), capillary electrophoresis (CE), high-pressure liquid chromatography (HPLC), thin layer chromatography (TLC), and high-performance thin layer chromatography (HPTLC) are some of the frequently used methods for the detection, qualitative analysis, and quantification (Sharma et al. 2007).

Spectrophotometric methods are used for identification of phenolic acids and are generally carried between a range of 220 to 320 nm (Mabry et al. 1970; Macheix et al. 1990); however, methods such as the Folin Ciocalteu spectrophotometric method results in nonspecific detection of the phenolic compounds and the interference of components such as ascorbic acid in food samples, that behave as reducing agents. Absorption of phenolic compounds is affected by pH, solvents used in the method and the interference of proteins and amino acids (Constantine et al. 2007).

Volatile compounds are directly analyzed by gas chromatography, a technique of unsurpassed separation capacity (Sostaric et al. 2000). GC is a major chromatographic technique employed for the analysis of essential phenolic acids in plants. It deals with high sensitivity and selectivity (Chiou et al. 2007) but requires derivatization step of hydroxyl groups in phenolic compounds. They are modified by various reagents to make more volatile compounds by a process such as methylation, conversion into trimethylsilyl (TMS) derivatives. However, problems such as poor separation and low stability after derivatization state are some of the shortcomings of this method. CE is too employed for analysis of phenolic compounds (Huck et al. 2005; Butehorn et al. 1996). Mostly, the method falls in the field of natural product research, including the analysis of plants, vegetables, herbs, and other plant- or fruit-derived products. It results in oxidation of phenolic compounds by dissolved oxygen and increase in migration time of flavonoids due to the increase in buffer concentrations (Constantine et al. 2007).

TLC methods have the ability to screen phenolic compounds easily (Tilay et al. 2008). The results obtained by TLC method are generally quantified using more multifaceted techniques like HPTLC (Mabinya et al. 2006). However detection of vanillin by spraying with 2, 4-dinitrophenylhydrazine (2, 4-DNPH) is not significant as the peaks are not detected properly. Currently, the main qualitative and quantitative techniques for phenolic compound detection are HPLC (Rao et al. 1999; Zheng et al. 2007). The European pharmacopoeia suggests the development of such analytical method which demands the adequate amount of reagents, solvents, and material (European Pharmacopoeia 2008). HPTLC allows for the simultaneous analysis of large sample size using small quantities of solvents, thus reducing time and cost of the analysis. The sensitivity for phenolic compounds performed by HPTLC is more as compared to HPLC (Prinjaporn et al. 2013). Mobile phase having pH 8 and above can be employed. Sample with turbidity and

different combinations of solvent can be directly applied. It facilitates automated application and repeated scanning of the chromatogram with the same or different parameters (Bakshi et al. 2002). Therefore, this technique should be taken into consideration as an alternative to HPLC.

HPTLC is a sophisticated instrumental technique which allows a fast and inexpensive method for analysis. Special advantage of HPTLC includes high sample throughput and low cost per analysis. HPTLC offers a great variety of stationary phases with unique selectivity for mixture components and their separation simultaneously. Processing of standards and samples identically on the same plate directs to better accuracy and precision of method for assessment. HPTLC development is extensive as the mobile phases are fully evaporated before the detection step thus preventing solvent interference in analysis. It minimizes exposure risks and significantly discarding toxic organic effluent problems were reduced thereby reducing possibilities of environment pollution. In response to this, HPTLC-based methods could be considered as a good alternative as they are being explored as an important tool in routine analysis. The HPTLC-developed method is actively used in application of qualitative and quantitative analyses of a wide range of compounds, such as herbal and botanical dietary supplements and nutraceuticals. It helps in identifying compounds present in a given substance; to check starting raw materials (plant extracts, extracts of animal origin, fermentation mixtures) identification of drugs and their metabolites in biological media such as urine, plasma, or gastric fluid (pharmacological, toxicological, pharmacokinetic) (Renger 1993; 1998).

The aim of the present study is to develop rapid, economic, selective HPTLC method for analysis and simultaneous determination of FA and vanillin with proper peak separation and hence can be used for routine high-throughput detection and determination of phenolic compounds. It is a one-step biotransformation process using culture *Pycnoporus cinnabarinus* which undergoes propenoic acid chain degradation of FA to vanillin (Tilay et al. 2008).

Methods
Chemicals/Reagents
Standard FA and vanillin (99% purity), maltose, diammonium tartarate, yeast extract, malt extract, potassium dihydrogen orthophosphate, magnesium sulfate, calcium chloride, thiamine hydrochloride, sodium hydroxide, and agar powder were procured from Hi-Media Laboratory (Mumbai, India). HPLC grade toluene, 1, 4-dioxan, acetic acid, ethyl acetate, and methanol were procured from Hi-Media (Mumbai, India).

Instrumentation
CAMAG TLC system consist of a CAMAG Linomat V (Muttenz, Switzerland) sample applicator and CAMAG

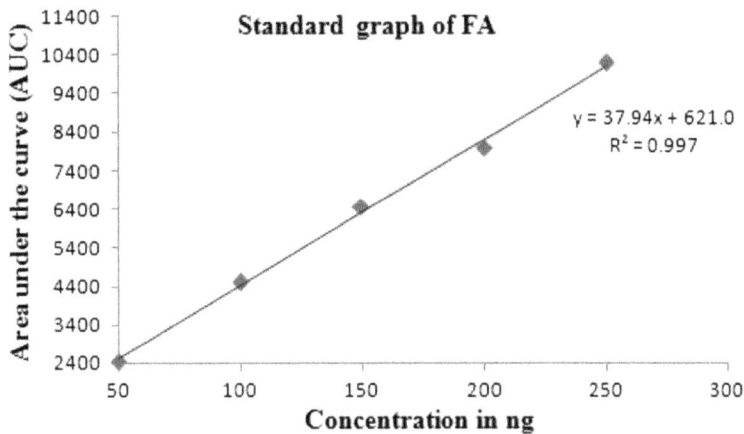

Figure 1 Standard graph of FA by HPTLC method.

TLC Scanner 3 controlled by WinCats software (1.4.3.6336); CAMAG glass twin-trough chambers ($20 \times 10 \times 4$ cm^3); 100-μl Hamilton syringe; Silica gel plates (G60F$_{254}$, 20×10 cm) were procured from E-Merck Pvt. Ltd., Mumbai, India. For extraction of vanillin, Buchi evaporator system was used consisting of Buchi evaporator R-124, Buchi water bath B-480, and Buchi vacuum controller B-721.

Preparation of stock solution
Standard stock solutions were prepared by dissolving 25 mg of vanillin and 25 mg of FA in 25 ml of methanol. Working standard solution was diluted (1:200) from stock solution of FA and vanillin to attain concentration of 5 μg/ml.

Microorganism
Pycnoporus cinnabarinus NCIM 1181 was procured from National Centre for Industrial Microorganism (NCIM), National Chemical Laboratory (NCL), Pune, India. Culture was maintained on potato dextrose agar slants at 4°C.

Media for vanillin production
A production media consisting of maltose 20 g/l, diammonium tartarate 1.8415 g/l, KH$_2$PO$_4$ 0.2 g/l, CaCl$_2$ 2H$_2$O 0.0132 g/l, MgSO$_4$·7H$_2$O 0.5 g/l, yeast extract 0.5 g/l, and thiamine hydrochloride 2.5 mg/l was adjusted to pH 7 and inoculated using mycelium fragments of *P. cinnabarinus* (Gross et al. 1993). This was further incubated on an incubator shaker (150 rpm) at 37°C for 6 days. After 3 days of growth, sterile solution of FA (0.03 g/100 ml) was added to the media prepared by dissolving FA in 0.1 N NaOH in the form of sodium ferulate.

Extraction of FA and vanillin from the culture media
The broth obtained after fermentation was filtered and the filtrate was acidified to obtain a pH of 1 to 2.80 ml of the above acidified solution was extracted thrice with equal volume of ethyl acetate. The extracts and the residue were redissolved in 50% (*v/v*), respectively. The organic phase containing FA and vanillin was concentrated (up to 2 to 3 ml) using a rotary vacuum

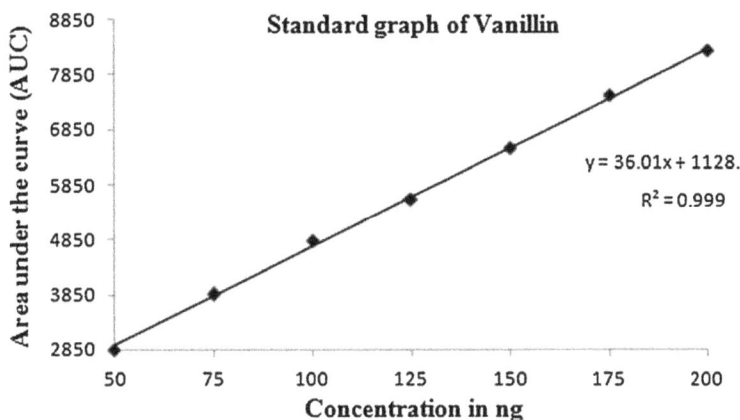

Figure 2 Standard graph of vanillin by HPTLC method.

Table 1 Intra- and inter-day precision (n = 5)

Compound	Std amount (ng/band)	Intra-day precision		Inter-day precision	
		SD[a]	%RSD[b]	SD[a]	%RSD[b]
Ferulic acid	100	4.52	0.021	1.64	0.053
	150	2.93	0.015	4.66	0.091
	200	4.51	0.001	4.57	0.050
Vanillin	100	2.09	0.044	2.21	0.040
	150	2.97	0.048	2.77	0.042
	200	1.93	0.022	2.02	0.023

SD, standard deviation (n = 5); RSD, percent relative standard deviation (n = 5).

evaporator with conditions (55°C, 150 rpm, <80 mbar) followed by reconstitution in 2 ml of methanol 50% (v/v) (Tilay et al. 2010). This solution was used for quantification of FA and vanillin by HPTLC.

Instrumentation and chromatographic parameters

HPTLC was executed using silica gel 60F$_{254}$ plates. A 10 µl of standard working solutions of FA and vanillin were applied to the plates of size 20 × 10 cm with a 5-mm band length. Ascending chromatography silica gel plate development traveled to a distance of 85 mm at temperature of 25°C with toluene/1, 4-dioxan/acetic acid (9:2.5:0.4; v/v) as mobile phase. After development, the plates were dried and chromatograms were recorded at 320 and 312 nm, respectively using CAMAG TLC Scanner 3. Quantitative evaluation was performed with WinCats software using deuterium lamp having slit width of 5 × 0.45 mm and an application rate of 150 nL/s.

Validation of method

Validation was performed in terms of linearity, specificity, precision, limit of detection (LOD), limit of quantification (LOQ), robustness, and system suitability by ICH guidelines (CPMP/ICH/381/95).

Linearity

Standard solution of FA (50 to 250 ng/band) and vanillin (50 to 200 ng/band) with varying volumes were applied on TLC plates. A plot of peak area against concentrations and its respective standard deviation (SD) and coefficient of correlation was calculated for both the compounds.

Precision

Precision specifies random errors. Results were expressed in percent relative standard deviation (%RSD < 2). Standard solution of FA (100, 150, and 200 ng/band) and of vanillin (100, 150, and 200 ng/band) were applied. Intra-day precision was evaluated by applying each concentration five times on the same day. Inter-day precision was evaluated by applying each concentration five times on three different days with an interval of 24 h.

Recovery

The recovery was used to determine the accuracy of the method. Recovery of FA and vanillin with three different concentration namely, 50, 100, and 150 ng (n = 3) was performed. Samples after extraction were spiked with standard concentration and applied. Peak areas of standard added to samples were calculated and average percent recovery was estimated. Further average percent recovery was calculated.

Specificity

Specificity was performed to compare the standard FA and vanillin and extract. It was calculated by comparing the Rf of the peak, peak start, peak apex, and peak end of the standard and extract. The spectral scan of both the standard and extract was compared. Spectrum scan accelerated at 100 nm/s with split dimensions 5 × 0.45 mm, micro. Spectral detection for optimum wavelength was calculated in the range 200 to 700 nm.

Robustness

Modifications in mobile phase concentration, mobile phase volume, mobile phase saturation time, and temperature were examined to check the robustness. Standard solutions of FA (150 ng/band) and vanillin (150 ng/band) were applied thrice and %RSD of each compound was calculated.

Limit of detection and limit of quantification

LOD is the lowest amount of compound that can be detected with signal-to-noise ratio of 3:1 and LOQ is the lowest amount of compound which can be quantified by signal-to-noise ratio 10:1 with adequate precision and

Table 2 Recovery of FA and vanillin

Sample	Amount in sample (ng)	Std added (ng)	Total conc. (ng)	Recovery (ng)	%Recovery	Avg. %Recovery
FA	20.54	50	70.54	69.20 ± 0.30	98.47 ± 0.05	98.77
	20.54	100	120.54	119.23 ± 2.2	99.10 ± 1.89	
	20.54	150	170.54	168.42 ±0.29	98.56 ± 0.17	
Vanillin	37.23	50	87.23	84.08 ± 0.38	96.51 ± 0.34	98.45
	37.23	100	137.23	136.15 ± 0.45	99.19 ± 0.30	
	37.23	150	187.23	186.49 ± 2.30	99.65 ± 1.25	

Mean ± standard deviation (n = 3).

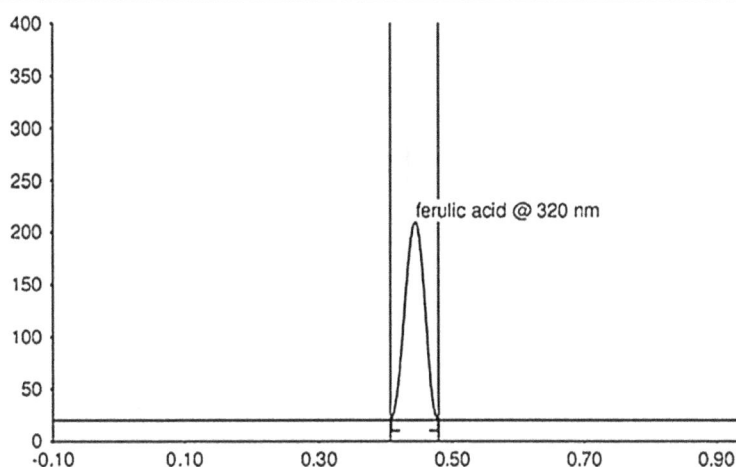

Figure 3 HPTLC chromatogram of standard FA.

specificity. LOD and LOQ of FA and vanillin were calculated.

System suitability

System suitability was executed to check the reproducibility and resolution of the method. Standard solution of both the standards of 150 ng concentration ($n = 5$) was analyzed on the same chromatographic plates. After development, plates were scanned and the peak area of each concentration and their Rf values were calculated.

Results and discussion

A GC method for detection of phenolic compounds is complicated and unsuitable for rapidly analyzing profuse samples and with derivatization step. HPLC-ECD, a new method was developed for the analysis of phenolic compound. However, use of HPLC with ECD is not feasible as a routine analytical method (Takahashi et al. 2013). Even with the HPLC UV detector system, the analysis is time consuming and the quantity of the solvents is the main concern. In the present study, two compounds FA and its bio-transformed product vanillin were quantified using HPTLC. Various mobile phases were screened for proper separation of both the compounds. Well-defined peaks with Rf values 0.48 for FA and 0.56 for vanillin were obtained using toluene/1, 4-dioxan/acetic acid (9:2.5:0.4; v/v) (Olsson et al. 1974). Experimental conditions should be selected when the compounds to be analyzed moves towards or near to the center of the layer (Rf = 0.5)

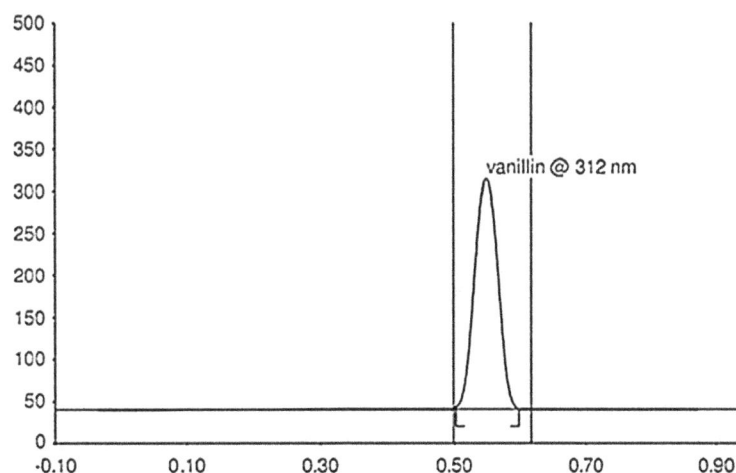

Figure 4 HPTLC chromatogram of standard vanillin.

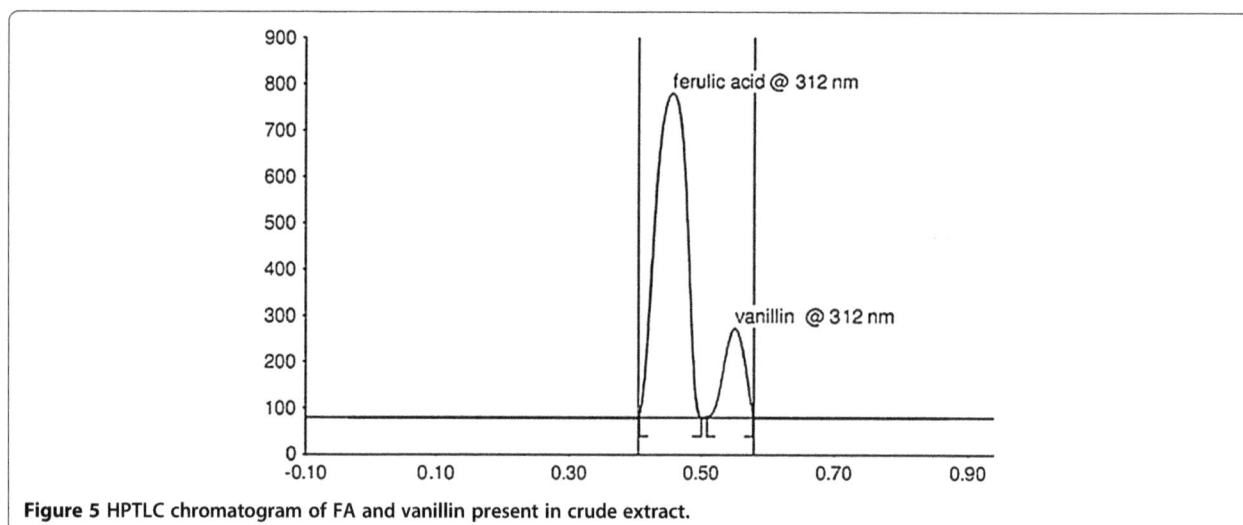

Figure 5 HPTLC chromatogram of FA and vanillin present in crude extract.

(Srivastava 2011). Krishna veni et al. (2013) used methanol/water/glacial acetic acid (20:5:2; v/v) as the mobile phase and resulted with Rf 0.84 for vanillin. For better peak detection and Rf, the polarity can be reduced. Other mobile phases were compared which resulted in tailing of peaks (Sharma et al. 2007) using methanol/water/isopropanol/acetic acid (30:65:2:3; v/v) and inappropriate separation of both the compounds with toluene/ethyl acetate/formaldehyde (6:3:1; v/v) (Srivastava et al. 2008), no identification of vanillin peak using hexane/ethyl acetate (5:2; v/v) (Hennig et al. 2011) and 1-butanol/acetic acid/water (66:17:17; v/v) (Males et al. 2001). Chloroform/methanol/formic acid (85:15:1; v/v) with spraying reagent 2, 4-dinitrophenylhydrazine was used for vanillin detection but resulted in poor peak visualization and separation of vanillin (Mabinya et al. 2006). Sharp peaks were obtained with a presaturation of mobile phase for 20 min. FA and vanillin was quantified using UV detector and scanning at 320 and 312 nm. The peaks corresponding to FA and vanillin in samples had the same retention time when compared to their respective standards.

Linearity

Linearity was achieved with concentrations ranging from 50 to 250 ng/band for FA and 50 to 200 ng/band for vanillin (Figures 1 and 2). The regression equation and correlation coefficient of FA was found to be $y = 37.94 \times X + 621.04$, $R^2 = 0.9975$ with SD = 1.95% and for vanillin $y = 36.016 \times X + 1128.3$, $R^2 = 0.9991$ with SD = 1.60%.

Precision

To get accurate chromatographic results, the precision of the chromatographic method must be analyzed and confirmed whether it is fit for purpose which is adequate

to the analytical requirements and it is evaluated in terms of intra- and inter-day precision. The standard deviation and percent relative standard deviation will evaluate the variation limit of the analysis. The value lower than 2% indicate the method is more precise to variation which assumes that the chromatograph does not malfunction after the system precision testing has been performed (Indrayanto 2011). Peak areas measurement of 100, 150, and 200 ng concentration of FA and vanillin showed %RSD less than 2 as shown in Table 1. Both intra- and inter-day results suggested an excellent method of precision which ensures the objective of the method development phase to be reproducible.

Recovery

Recovery is an important parameter as it offers information about the recovery of the analyte from the sample preparation and the effect of matrix. If the recovery is close to 100% then it implies that the proposed analytical method is free from constant and proportional systematic error (Srivastava 2011). Recovery of FA at three different levels obtained was 98.47%, 99.1%, and 98.75% with 98.77% average recovery and of vanillin was 96.51%, 99.19%, and 99.65% with 98.45% average

Table 3 Specificity of FA and vanillin

Retention factor (Rf)	Peak start	Peak apex	Peak end
FA[a]	0.43	0.48	0.51
Vanillin[a]	0.49	0.56	0.62
FA[b]	0.41	0.47	0.50
Vanillin[b]	0.51	0.56	0.60

[a]Standard ferulic acid and vanillin; [b]crude extracts.

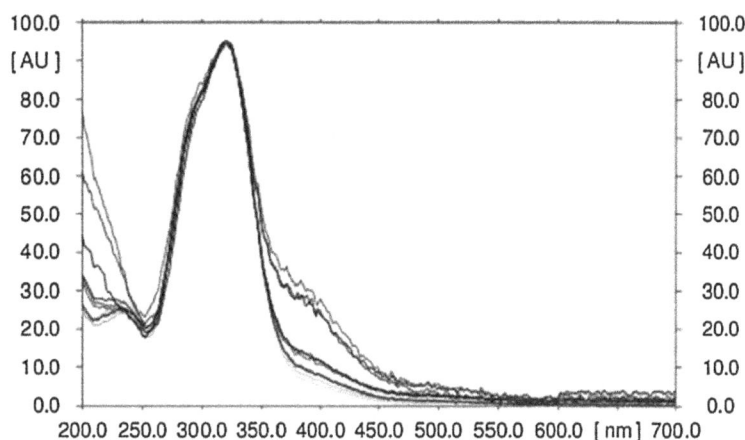

Figure 6 Overlay of UV absorption spectra of standard FA with crude extract.

recovery. The results are shown in Table 2. The percentage recovery was close to 100% which indicated no interference of any other compound and representing the accuracy of the method. This indicates the suitability of the method for the routine analysis.

Specificity

Specificity is a method which provides a response for only a single analyte. This study is performed to check how accurately and specifically the analyte of interest is estimated in the presence of other components with system interference during detection and quantification of analyte (Indrayanto and Yuwono 2010; Kakde et al. 2008). Retention factor values of standard FA and vanillin were compared with sample extract. There was no interference of other peaks as shown in Figures 3, 4, and 5. The standard and sample was compared with

respect to peak start, peak apex, and peak end of the bands which showed the specificity between extracts and standard compound and purity of the peaks (Table 3). Overlay of the standard and sample compound using spectral scan was compared to confirm the specificity (Figures 6 and 7). Spectral scan of both the compounds showed maximum absorption at 320 nm for ferulic acid and 312 nm for vanillin. Thus, results obtained from comparison of peak and spectral scan showed the method is specific for detection of FA and vanillin.

Robustness

Robustness can be described as the ability to reproduce the analytical method under different circumstances and provides an indication of its reliability during normal phase. It was introduced to avoid problems in

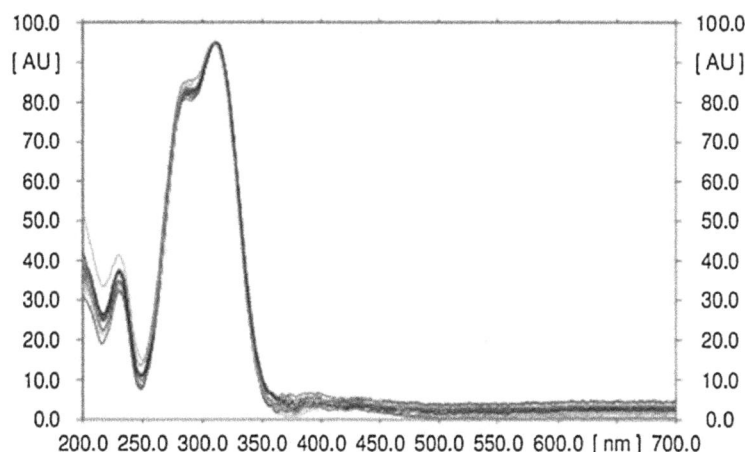

Figure 7 Overlay of UV absorption spectra of standard vanillin with crude extract.

Table 4 Robustness of FA & Vanillin

Parameters	FA		Vanillin	
	SD[a]	%RSD[b]	SD[a]	%RSD[b]
Mobile phase (toluene/1,4-dioxan/acetic acid) (9{±1}:2.5{±1}:0.4{± 0.2}) (v/v)	2.95 ± 0.13	0.039	2.526 ± 0.05	0.039
Mobile phase vols. 10, 12 and 14 ml	3.00 ± 0.09	0.027	3.626 ± 0.12	0.056
Saturation time 10, 15 and 20 min	2.20 ± 0.06	0.027	2.699 ± 0.07	0.058
Temperature 25, 30 and 37°C	2.25 ± 0.12	0.050	3.351 ± 0.10	0.052

[a]SD, standard deviation of peak area ($n = 3$); [b]RSD, percent relative standard deviation ($n = 3$).

inter-laboratory studies and to discover the potentially repairable factors (Van der Hyden et al. 2001). According to the ICH guidelines, the evaluation of robustness should be considered during the development phase and depends on the type of procedure under study. For robustness evaluation by chromatographic method, the acceptance criteria are that, the Rf values of all standards should lie within the acceptance criteria of the precision method by performing variations in considered parameters. Calculations of standard or relative error are common ways to look at the data and departures from deviations in the data will directly affect robustness. Variations made in mobile phase composition, mobile phase volume, saturation time, and temperature showed less %RSD and SD for FA and vanillin by spotting 150 ng/spot ($n = 3$) (Table 4). No significant change in Rf or response to FA and vanillin was observed which indicated robustness of the method. Robustness study has provided valuable information about the quality and reliability of the method and no further development or optimization is necessary.

Limit of detection and limit of quantification

LOD is based on the analyte response sensitivity (response per amount or concentration per time, using either peak height or area), and LOQ is the lowest amount of analyte that can be quantitatively determined in sample with defined precision and accuracy under standard conditions. LOQ is usually a multiple of LOD (Kakde et al. 2008). Standard deviation and slope used in the equations are used to determine LOD and LOQ which is equivalent to instrument sensitivity for the specific analyte, reinforcing that the LOD/LOQ details, are expressed in units of analyte concentration (Apostol et al. 2012). It is important to determine sensitivity using analyte amounts near to their detection limits. LOD and LOQ with signal-to-noise ratio of FA were found to be 13.63 and 45.42 ng/band, respectively. LOD and LOQ of vanillin were found to be 10.59 and 35.30 ng/band, respectively. Sensitivity of the method is evaluated with regard to LOD and LOQ (Kakde et al. 2008). These results indicate the sensitivity of the method which can be used for quantification of the compound.

System suitability

System suitability test (SST) is an integral part of many analytical procedures. The test is based on the conception that, the equipment, electronics, analytical operations, and samples to be analyzed represent an integral system that can be evaluated. System suitability test parameters to be established for a particular procedure depend upon the type of procedure being validated. It is the ability of the analytical method to detect analyte quantitatively in the presence of other components which are expected to be present in the sample and they should be chromatographed along with the analyte to check the system suitability and retention factor of the required analyte (Dolan 2004). On the basis of repeatability relative standard deviations of peak response, SST was analyzed. Retention factor of FA and vanillin were 0.48 and 0.56, respectively. Standard deviation of FA was 2.95 ± 0.13 with 0.039% RSD and standard deviation of vanillin was 3.62 ± 0.12 with 0.056% RSD. The low %RSD indicates the reproducibility and the system suitability of the method.

Conclusion

The simultaneous detection of FA and vanillin by the HPTLC method can be performed as there is noteworthy difference in their retention factor values. The proposed method was developed and validated by ICH guidelines which is simple, rapid, accurate, precise, sensitive, and eco-friendly. The mobile phase selected was toluene/1, 4-dioxan/acetic acid 9:2.5:0.4 (v/v) which resulted in proper peak separation as compared to different mobile phase which were not able to separate the compounds properly. Other chromatographic methods like HPLC, GC, and spectrophotometric mentioned may not be applied for routine check because of the various shortcomings as compared to HPTLC. The total optimized method is therefore useful in both qualitative and quantitative analysis for routine assays in pharmaceutical and food industry within acceptable limits.

Competing interests
The authors declare that they have no competing interests.

Authors' contributions

SH and SD has performed all the experimental and analytical work and drafted the manuscript. The guidelines for all the mentioned part was provided by UA. All authors read and approved the final manuscript.

References

Apostol I, Krull I, Kelner D (2012) Analytical Method Validation for Biopharmaceuticals. Analytical Chemistry. doi:10.5772/52561

Bakshi M, Singh SJ (2002) Development of validated stability-indicating assay methods-critical review. J Pharm Biomed Anal 28:1011–1040

Butehorn U, Pyell U (1996) Micellar electrokinetic chromatography as a screening method for the analysis of vanilla flavorings and vanilla extracts. J Chromatogr A 736:321–332

Chiou A, Karathanos VT, Mylona A, Salta FN, Preventi F, Andrikopoulos NK (2007) Currants (Vitisvinifera L.) content of simple phenolic and antioxidant activity. Food Chem 102:516–522

Constantine DS (2007) Extraction, separation, and detection methods for phenolic acids and flavonoids. J Sep Sci 30:3268–3295

Dolan JW (2004) System suitability. LC troubleshooting, BASi Northwest Laboratory, McMinnville, Oregon, (USA) 17(6):328–332

European Pharmacopoeia (EDQM) (2008) 6th edn. Strasbourg, Council of Europe

Graf E (1992) Antioxidant potential of ferulic acid. Free Radical Biol Med 13:435–448

Gross B, Asther M, Corrieu G, Brunerie P (1993) Production of vanillin by bioconversion of benzenoid precursors by Pycnoporus. U.S. Patent 5262315 B

Hennig L, Garcia GM, Giannis A, Bussmann RW (2011) New constituents of Baccharis genistelloides (Lam.). Pers. Arkivoc 6:74–81

Ho K, Yazana LS, Ismail N, Ismail M (2009) Apoptosis and cell cycle arrest of human colorectal cancer cell line HT-29 induced by vanillin. Cancer Epidem 33:155–160

Huck CW, Stecher G, Scherz H, Bonn G (2005) Analysis of drugs, natural and bioactive compounds containing phenolic groups by capillary electrophoresis coupled to mass spectrometry. Electrophoresis 26:1319–1333

Indrayanto G (2011) Analytical Aspects of High Performance Thin Layer Chromatography. MM. Srivastava edn, High-Performance Thin-Layer Chromatography (HPTLC), Springer-Verlag Berlin Heidelberg

Indrayanto G, Yuwono MS (2010) TLC: Validation of Analyses. In. Cazes J Encyclopedia of Chromatography, 3rd edn, Taylor & Francis Group, London

Kakde RB, Kotak VH, Kale DL (2008) Estimation of bisoprolol fumarate in pharmaceutical preparations by HPTLC. Asian J Res Chem 1(2):70–73

Krishna Veni N, Meyyanathan SN, Reddy AA, Sompura SA, Elango K (2013) Analysis of Vanillin In Food Products By High Performance Thin Layer Chromatography. J Adv Sci Res 4(1):48–51

Lomascolo A, Stentelaire C, Asther M, Lesage-Meessen L (1999) Basidiomycetes as new biotechnological tools to generate natural aromatic flavours for the food industry. Trends Biotechnol 17:282–289

Mabinya LV, Mafunga T, Brand JM (2006) Determination of ferulic acid and related compounds by thin layer chromatography. Afr J Biotechnol 5:1271–1273

Mabry TJ, Markham KR, Thomas MB (1970) The Systematic Identification of Flavonoids, 1st edition. Springer, New York, NY, USA

Macheix JJ, Fleuriet A, Billot J (1990) Fruit Phenolics. CRC Press, Bota Raton, FL

Males Z, Medic-Saric M (2001) Optimization of TLC analysis of flavonoids and Phenolic acids of Helleborus atrorubens Waldst. et Kit. J Pharm Biomed Anal 24(3):353–9

Olsson L, Samuelson O (1974) Chromatography of aromatic acids and aldehydes and phenols on cross-linked polyvinylpyrrolidone. J Chromatogr 93:189–199

Priefert H, Rabenhorst J, Steinbuchel A (2001) Biotechnological production of vanillin. Appl Microbiol Biotechnol 56:296–314

Prinjaporn TN, Namthip N, Poomrat R, Weena S, Orawon C (2013) Simple and Rapid Determination of Ferulic Acid Levels in Food and Cosmetic Samples Using Paper-Based Platforms. Sensors 13:13039–13053

Raisi A, Aroujaliana A, Kaghazchia T (2008) Multicomponent pervaporation process for volatile aroma compounds recovery from pomegranate juice. J Membr Sci 322:339–348

Rakchoy S, Suppakul P, Jinkarn T (2009) Antimicrobial effects of vanillin coated solution for coatingpaperboard intended for packaging bakery products. As J Food Ag-Ind 2:138–147

Rao SR, Ravishankar GA (1999) Biotransformation of isoeugenol to vanilla flavour metabolites and capsaicin in suspended and immobilized cell cultures of Capsicum frutescens: study of the influence of β-cyclodextrin and fungal elicitor. Process Biochem 35:341–348

Renger B (1993) Quantitative planar chromatography as a tool in pharmaceutical analysis. J AOAC Int 76:7–13

Renger B (1998) Contemporary thin layer chromatography in pharmaceutical analysis. J AOAC Int 81:333–339

Sharma UK, Sharma N, Gupta AP, Kumar V, Sinha AK (2007) RP-HPTLC densitometric determination and validation of vanillin and related Phenolic compounds in accelerated solvent extract of Vanilla planifolia. J Sep Sci 30:3174–3180

Sostaric T, Boyce MC, Spickett EE (2000) Analysis of volatile components in vanilla extract and flavorings by solid-phase microextraction and gas chromatography. J Agric Food Chem 48:5802–5807

Srivastava MM (2011) An Overview of HPTLC. In: A Modern Analytical Technique with Excellent Potential for Automation, Optimization, Hyphenation, and Multidimensional Applications. High-Performance Thin-Layer Chromatograpy (HPTLC), Springer-Verlag Berlin Heidelberg

Srivastava SK, Singh AP, Rawat AKS (2008) Pharmacognostical and phytochemical evaluation of Lycopodium clavatum stem. J Sci Ind Res 67:228–232

Takahashi M, Sakamaki S, Fujita A (2013) Simultaneous analysis of Guaiacol and vanillin in a vanilla extract by using High Performance Liquid Chromatography with Electrochemical detection. Biosci. Biotechnol. Biochem 77(3):595–600

Tilay A, Bule M, Kishenkumar J, Annapure U (2008) Preparation of ferulic acid from agricultural wastes: its improved extraction and purification. J Agric Food Chem 56:7644–8

Tilay A, Bule M, Annapure U (2010) Production of Biovanillin by One-Step Biotransformation Using Fungus Pycnoporous cinnabarinus. J Agric Food Chem 58:4401–4405

Van der Hyden Y, Nijhuis A, Smayers-Verbeke J, Vandeginste BMG, Massart DL (2001) Guidance for robustness/ruggedness test in method validation. J Pharm Biomed Anal 24:723–753

Wu SL, Chen JC, Li CC, Lo HY, Ho TY, Hsiang CY (2009) Vanillin Improves and Prevents Trinitrobenzene Sulfonic Acid-Induced Colitis in Mice. J Pharmacol Exp Ther 330:370–376

Xu F, Sun RC, Sun JX, Liu CF, Heb BH, Fan JS (2005) Determination of cell wall ferulic and p-coumaric acids in sugarcane bagasse. Anal Chim Acta 552:207–217

Zheng L, Zheng P, Sun Z, Bai Y, Wang J, Guo X (2007) Production of vanillin from waste residue of rice bran oil by Aspergillus niger and Pycnoporus cinnabarinus. Bioresour Technol 98:1115–1119

7

Synthesis of alumina, titania, and alumina-titania hydrophobic membranes via sol–gel polymeric route

Amany Abd AL-Azem Gaber[1][*], Doreya Mohamed Ibrahim[1], Fawzia Fahm Abd-Almohsen[2] and Elham Mohamed El-Zanati[3]

Abstract

Nanometer TiO_2-Al_2O_3 composite membranes were synthesized through the sol–gel polymeric reaction of $TiCl_4$ and $AlCl_3$ in the presence of acrylic-acrylamide copolymer as a template. The dried samples were characterized by DTA, TGA, FTIR, XRD, and TEM to determine the thermal behavior, chemical composition, crystal structure, shape, and size of the particles. Octyltrichlorosilane was chosen as a silane coupling agent to increase the hydrophobic nature of the prepared membranes. The morphological structure, hydrophobic nature, water permeability, and desalination efficiency of the prepared membranes were studied by SEM, contact angle, permeability, and NaCl rejection coefficient ($R\%$) measurements. The crystal structure of titania and alumina particles in the composite was affected by the $AlCl_3$ and $TiCl_4$ feed ratio. As the titania concentration increased, the average particle size of the composite particles became larger and the uniformity of the membrane layer decreased. The alumina (75%)-titania (25%) composite (AT25) showed a uniform crack-free membrane layer with a pore diameter of 12.9 nm and a porosity of 21.46%, with great hydrophobic nature, and with contact angle reaching 116°. This membrane can withstand calcination temperature up to 700°C, as the alumina and titania were present in their active forms: gamma-alumina and anatase, respectively. The membrane produced from this composite showed a high surface area of 333 m^2/g with a respective particle size of 4.6 nm. Moreover, it showed a high ability to reject NaCl from water with a rejection coefficient of 73% and a high permeation flux of 4.8 l/h m^2 at 75°C.

Background

Ceramic membranes are gaining more and more importance in separation technology, especially in combination with catalytic processes. They have several positive merits especially their chemical resistance, thermal resistance, and high permeability (Schaep et al. 1999; van Gestel et al. 2002, 2003). The main aim of the research work in this field was the production of new nano-porous metal oxide membranes. Thus, great advances were made regarding the development of non-silicate ceramic membranes. Systems like ZrO_2 and TiO_2 were taken into consideration, in particular with respect to their chemical resistance (Schaep et al. 1999; van Gestel et al. 2002, 2003; Shojai and Mantyla 2001). Also, γ-Al_2O_3 and TiO_2 were of

main interest (Xu and Anderson 1993; Larbot et al. 1994; Wildman et al. 1994; Puhlfürß et al. 2000). These membranes have high selectivity against small macromolecules. The reduction in pore size from ultrafiltration to nano-filtration range was enabled by changing the method of synthesis and the precursors used from the colloidal to the polymeric sol–gel technique.

Alumina membranes based on the application of a template polymer were produced over decades (Benfer et al. 2001; Richter et al. 1997; Benfer et al. 2004) with varying pore sizes and permeation rates. However, there was a current limitation for the practical application of these alumina membranes due to the failure in the production of a complete crack-free layer by the sol–gel technique. The partial kinetic γ- to α-alumina phase transformation occurs upon calcination of the alumina membrane layer at temperatures above 600°C. Phase transformation takes place by coalescence of small (γ-alumina) particles into

* Correspondence: amany1gaber@yahoo.com
[1]Ceramic Department, National Research Centre, Cairo, Egypt
Full list of author information is available at the end of the article

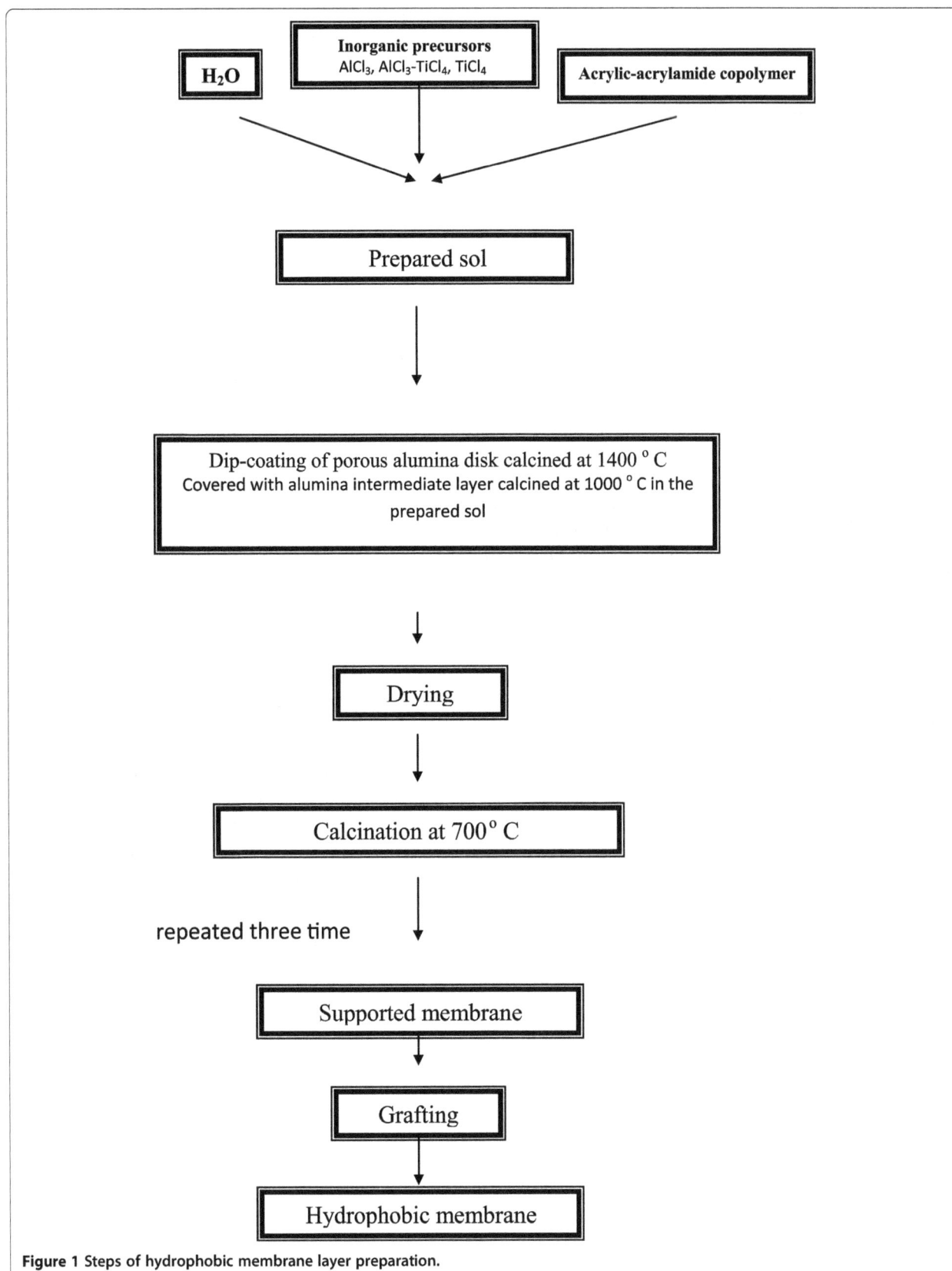

Figure 1 Steps of hydrophobic membrane layer preparation.

larger (α-alumina) grains, accompanied by considerable grain and pore growth. This was practically overcome by calcination at a minimum temperature of 600°C to obtain well-defined, mechanically stable layers of alumina membranes (Gaber 2007). The effect of phase transformation and accompanying grain growth can be avoided as suggested by Kumar, by retarding its occurrence to a temperature above the normal calcination temperature. It has been suggested that the presence of a second phase decreases the sub-coordination number of the prepared particles in the nano-composite matrix (Sekulic et al. 2004; Kumar 1993; Zhang and Banfield 1999). The presence of titania as a second phase to form an alumina-titania composite membrane retards the γ-alumina transformation and keeps it in its amorphous phase, avoiding its transformation into α-alumina phase; at the same time, the presence of alumina keeps the titania in its stable form as anatase phase.

The present work aims at preparing alumina-titania composite membranes that can withstand temperature up to 700°C. The prepared membrane surfaces were modified by octyltrichlorosilane to render them hydrophobic for desalination purposes. The properties and microstructure of the prepared membranes before and after modification were characterized.

Methods

Materials
Pure chemical reagents were selected to prepare the required membranes. The following precursors were used: aluminum chloride ($AlCl_3$) was supplied by Aldrich (St. Louis, MO, USA), titanium chloride ($TiCl_4$) by Fluka Chemika (Buchs, Swizerland), aluminum hydroxide ($Al(OH)_3$) by Arabian Medical & Scientific Lab. Sup. Co. (Dubai, United Arab Emirates), ammonium persulfate and acrylic and acrylamide monomers by Merk-Schuchardt (Darmstadt, Germany), polyvinyl alcohol by German, and octyltrichlorosilane by Aldrich.

Method of preparation of the membranes
The method of membrane preparation is demonstrated by the flow chart in Figure 1.

Preparation of the acrylic-acrylamide copolymer
Acrylic-acrylamide was polymerized on laboratory scale via a free radical method to obtain the copolymer Gaber AA (2007). Preparation of alumina membranes by sol–gel polymeric route 658 M.Sc Thesis, Cairo University. The following shows the reaction of formation:

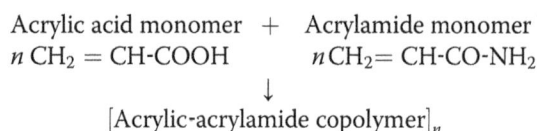

$$\text{Acrylic acid monomer} + \text{Acrylamide monomer}$$
$$n\,CH_2 = CH\text{-}COOH \qquad n\,CH_2 = CH\text{-}CO\text{-}NH_2$$
$$\downarrow$$
$$[\text{Acrylic-acrylamide copolymer}]_n$$

Table 1 Composition of the prepared membranes

Membrane symbol	Type of inorganic salts	Concentration of inorganic salts (mol%)
A	$AlCl_3$	100% $AlCl_3$
T	$TiCl_4$	100% $TiCl_4$
AT25	$AlCl_3$-$TiCl_4$	75% $AlCl_3$
		25% $TiCl_4$
AT50	$AlCl_3$-$TiCl_4$	50% $AlCl_3$
		50% $TiCl_4$
AT75	$AlCl_3$-$TiCl_4$	25% $AlCl_3$
		75% $TiCl_4$

Preparation of the alumina support
Supports in the form of disks with the following dimensions: diameter 25 mm and thickness 2 mm, were processed from α-alumina powder (commercial alumina) with a mean particle size ≤10 μm and 2 wt% polyvinyl alcohol as organic binder under a uniaxial press and a pressure of 200 MPa. The specimens were dried and then first fired in a muffle furnace in air at a rate of 2°C/min up to 500°C and maintained for 2 h at this temperature to eliminate the organic binder. Heating was then continued at a rate of 4°C/min up to 1,400°C for 4 h and then cooled to room temperature.

Preparation of the alumina suspension
Fine α-alumina powder was first prepared by calcining chemically pure $Al(OH)_3$ at 1,200°C for 3 h. The obtained powder was used to prepare a homogeneous and stable suspension by the addition of 0.5 ml of ammonia solution, 10 g of acrylic-acrylamide copolymer, and 6.6 g of 3.5 wt% polyvinyl alcohol solution; 1.08 g of this dispersing agent was added to 1 g of the calcined α-alumina powder and well stirred for 1 h, followed by dispersing in an ultrasonic bath for another 1 h.

The prepared suspension was poured on the surface of the alumina support, homogenized to form a uniform layer of about 3 μm thick, dried for 24 h at 80°C, and then fired at 1,000°C for 3 h at a heating rate of 1.5°C/min.

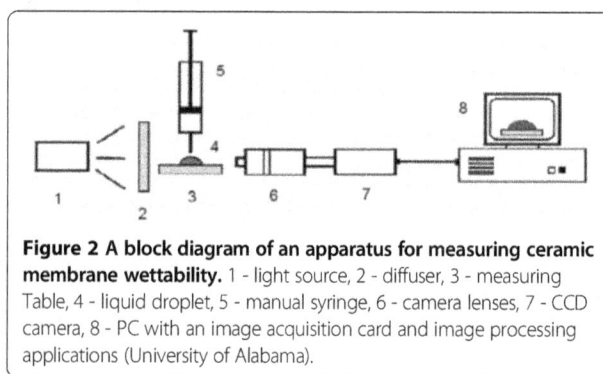

Figure 2 A block diagram of an apparatus for measuring ceramic membrane wettability. 1 - light source, 2 - diffuser, 3 - measuring Table, 4 - liquid droplet, 5 - manual syringe, 6 - camera lenses, 7 - CCD camera, 8 - PC with an image acquisition card and image processing applications (University of Alabama).

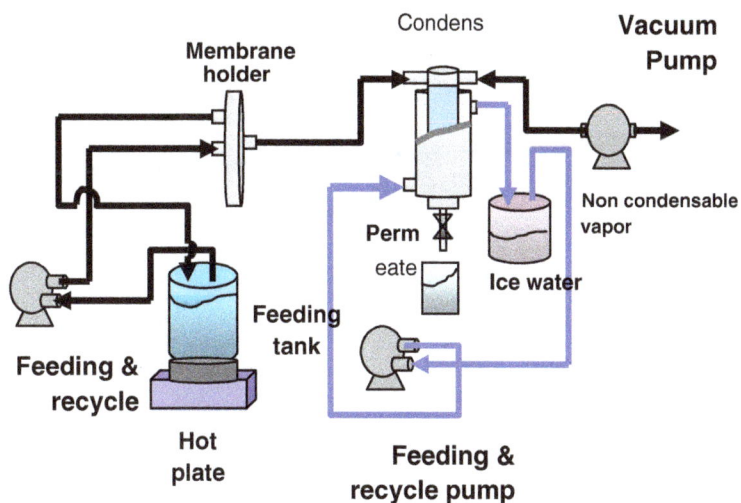

Figure 3 Vacuum membrane distillation system (flow diagram).

Preparation of the membrane layer

The salt solution of AlCl$_3$ and TiCl$_4$ (alumina 100% and titania 100%) as well as AlCl$_3$-TiCl$_4$ mixed oxides (75%:25%, 50%:50%, and 25%:75%) were prepared by dissolving the calculated ratio equivalent to 12 mol. The prepared solid solutions were added dropwise to an equivalent weight of 1 mol of the acrylic-acrylamide monomer that was kept constant in all batches as demonstrated in Table 1. The reaction proceeds at room temperature in an acidic media at pH 3 with continuous

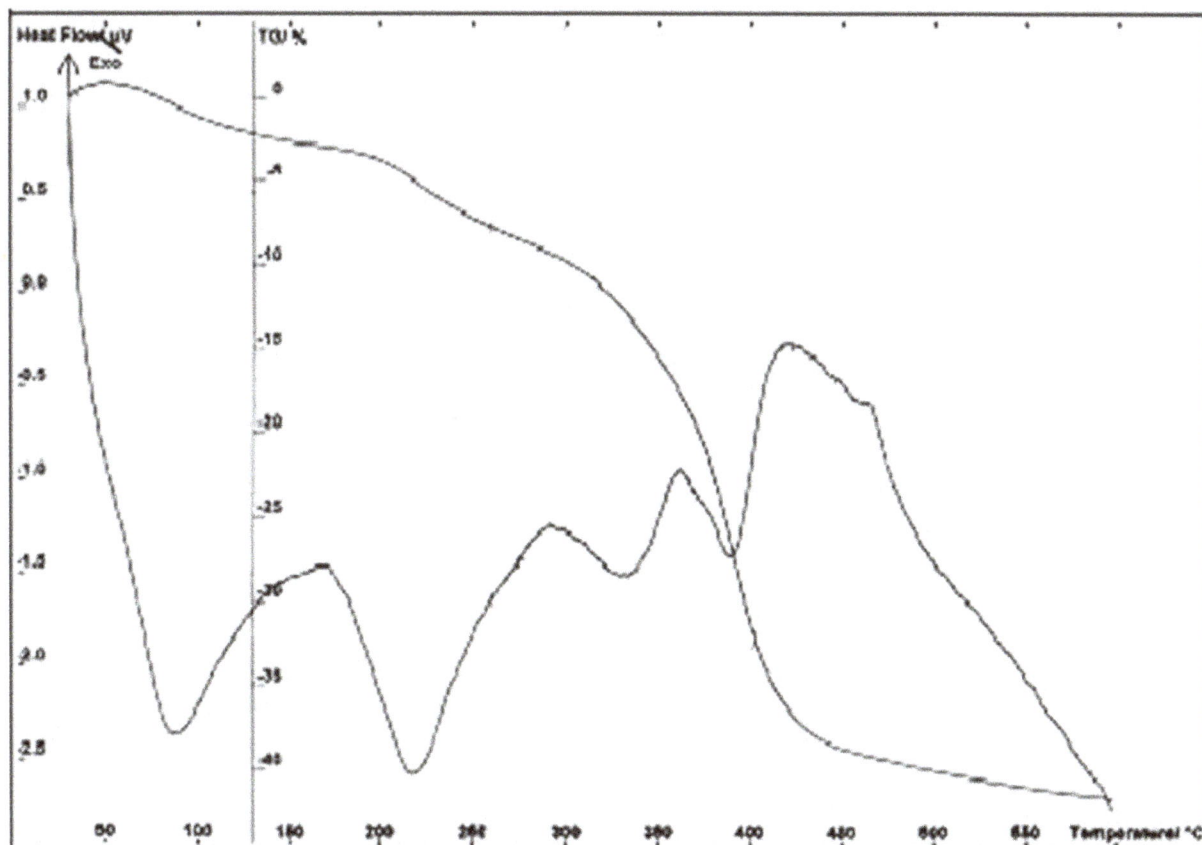

Figure 4 Thermal analysis of the acrylic-acrylamide copolymer.

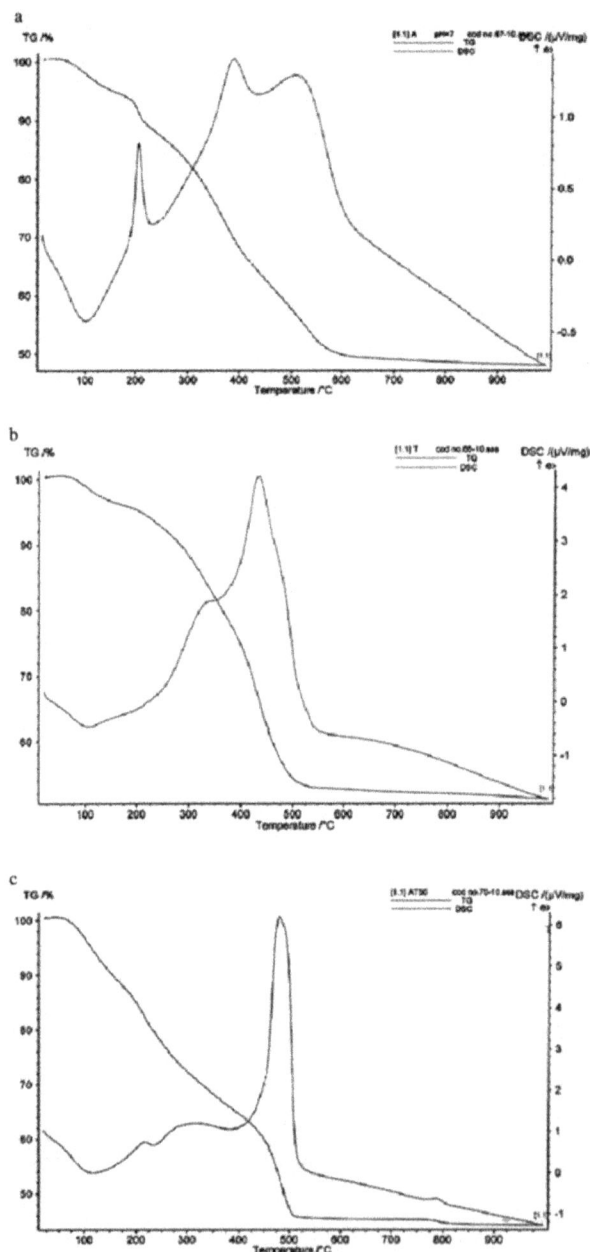

Figure 5 DSC and TGA curves of acrylic-acrylamide copolymers incorporated with (a) Al^{3+} (A), (b) Ti^{4+} (T), and (c) Al^{3+}-Ti^{4+} (AT50).

Table 2 Temperatures of the DSC peaks of the free polymer and those incorporated with Al^{3+} and Ti^{4+}

Material	Endothermic peak temperature (°C)				Exothermic peak temperature (°C)			
	First	Second	Third	Fourth	First	Second	Third	Fourth
Free polymer	85	217	334	389	420	-	-	-
+Al^{3+}	102	-	-	-	207	388	508	-
+Al^{3+} and Ti^{4+}	118	232	-	-	479	787	-	-
+Ti^{4+}	106	-	-	-	433	-	-	-

Table 3 Temperatures of the main weight loss steps in the TGA curves of the polymers

Material	Main steps							
	Step I		Step II		Step III		Step IV	
	Temperature (°C)	Weight loss (%)	Temperature (°C)	Weight loss (%)	Temperature (°C)	Weight loss (%)	Temperature (°C)	Weight loss (%)
Free polymer	50 to 179	8	179 to 218	12	308 to 450	80		
+Al³⁺	75 to 162.5	5.8	163 to 242.5	6.6	243 to 637	38.77	637 to 1,000	16.26
+Al³⁺ and Ti⁴⁺	50 to 175	12	175 to 378	22.3	378 to 550	20.42	775 to 1,000	1.27
+Ti⁴⁺	75 to 175	4.4	175 to 375	14.4	375 to 570	28.7	570 to 1,000	1.57

stirring. A gel layer was deposited on the surface of the support by a dipping procedure. The obtained gel layers were left to dry at room temperature for 24 h followed by drying for 24 h at 80°C. Finally, calcination of the prepared membranes took place at 700°C for 3 h in a temperature-programmable furnace with heating and cooling rates of 1.5°C/min. The deposition of the membrane layer was repeated three times as demonstrated in the flow chart in Figure 1.

Grafting process

Organo-silane products are used in surface modification to provide a convenient and stable means to create a hydrophobic ceramic surface and tailor the effective pore size (Miller and Koros 1990; Caro et al. 1998; Castricum et al. 2005; Javaid et al. 2001; Abidi et al. 2006; Hyun et al. 1996; Leger et al. 1996; Randon and Paterson 1997). Alkyl, chloro-alkyl, or fluoro-alkyl silanes of varying carbon chain lengths can be used to provide chemical affinity, to improve the separation performance, and to provide a

specific degree of pore size reduction (Javaid et al. 2001). The prepared membranes were grafted using two different organo-silane compounds, namely octyltrichlorosilane and γ-aminopropyl-trimethoxysilane, to select the appropriate one for the process. The membrane samples were immersed in the silane solution of different concentrations (2, 5, and 10 vol.% in ethanol) at room temperature (25°C) and then dried at 70°C for 24 h. The procedure was repeated twice for different time intervals: 24 and 72 h, giving a total of 96 h of immersion time. This procedure was used to characterize hydrophobicity and also grafting efficiency. After the immersion, the membranes were rinsed with ethanol two times to remove any unreacted chemicals from the membranes and dried at 70°C for 24 h. Finally, the membranes were stored at room temperature ready for characterization (Krajewski et al. 2006).

Methods for characterization

Thermal analysis, comprising both differential scanning calorimetry (DSC) and thermogravimetric analysis (TGA),

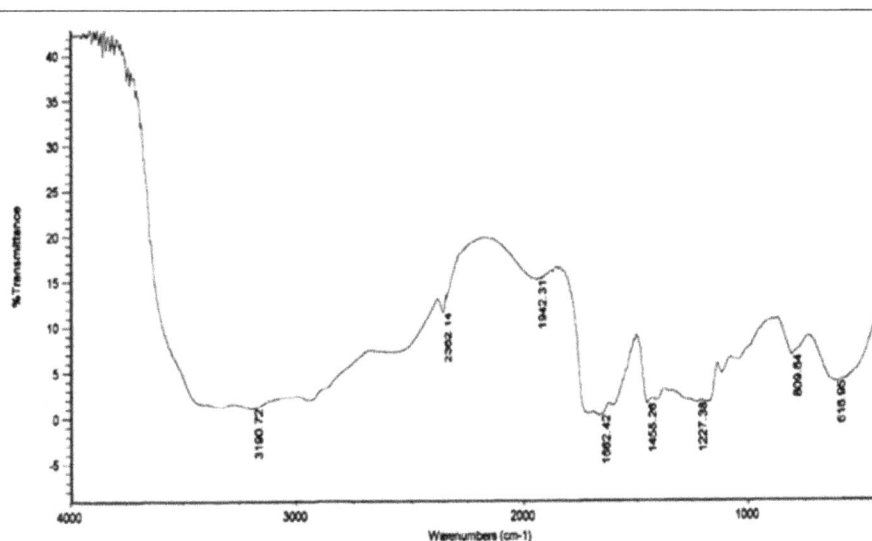

Figure 6 FTIR spectrum of the acrylic-acryl amide copolymer.

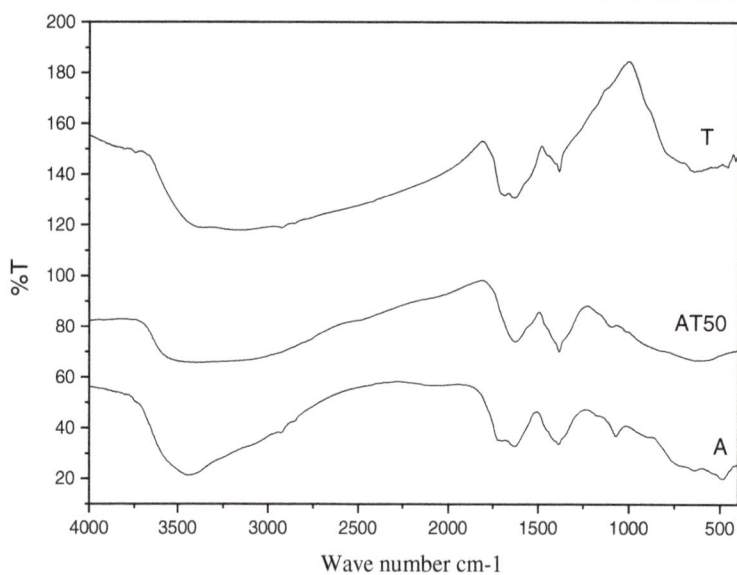

Figure 7 FTIR spectra of different gels of alumina (A), titania (T), and alumina-titania (AT50).

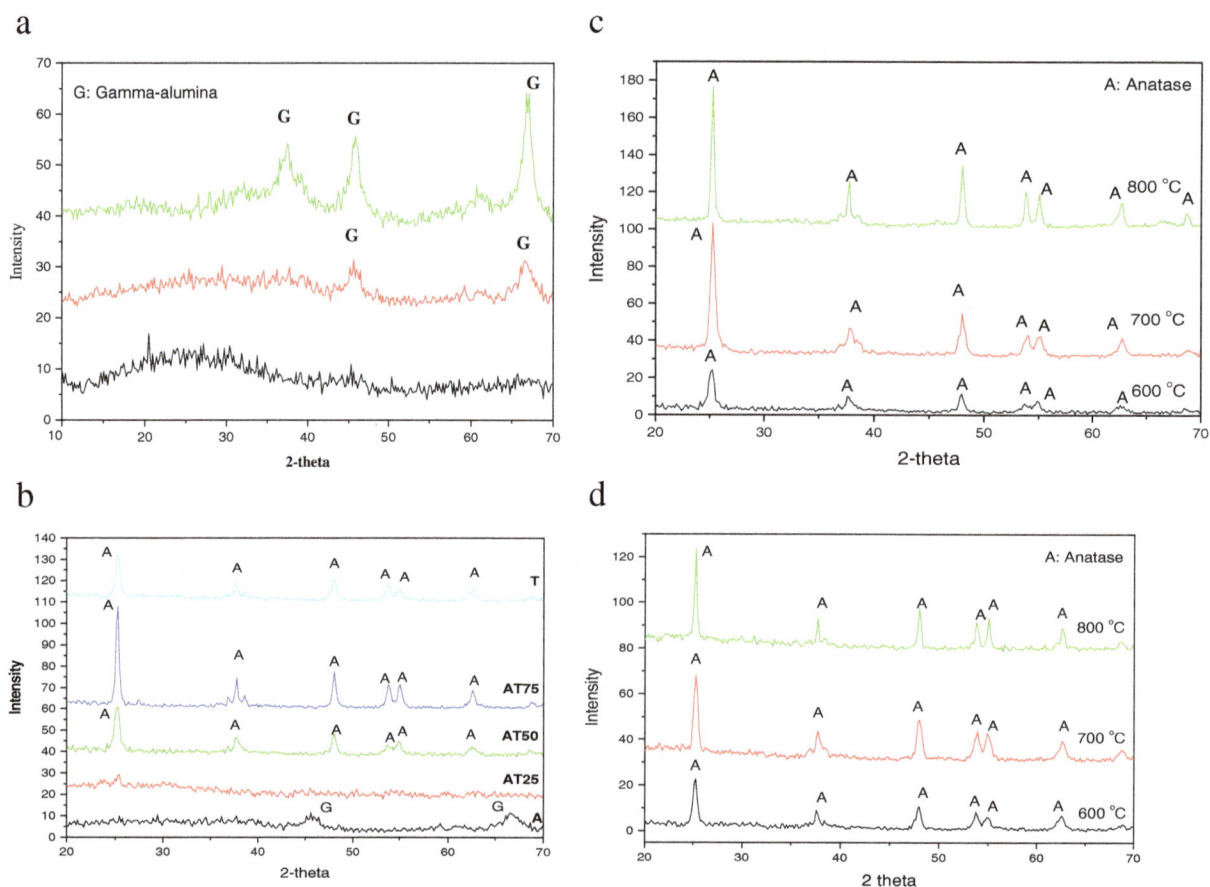

Figure 8 XRD patterns of the samples. (a) Alumina (A) powder calcined at 600°C, 700°C, and 800°C. **(b)** Alumina (A), alumina-titania (AT25, AT50, and AT75), and titania (T) membranes calcined at 700°C, where G is gamma-alumina and A is anatase. **(c)** Alumina-titania (AT50) membrane calcined at 600°C, 700°C, and 800°C. **(d)** Titania (T) membrane calcined at 600°C, 700°C, and 800°C.

was carried out on the acrylic-acrylamide copolymer and the dried membranes using a Setaram Labsys TM TG-DSC16 system (Newark, CA, USA).

Fourier transform infrared (FTIR) spectroscopy equipment (MB154S, Bomem, Quebec, Canada) was used to determine the main bonds in the copolymer and the effect of the introduced inorganic cations to the polymer structure on the spectra of the different groups.

X-ray diffraction analysis was carried out to characterize the respective alumina and titania phases developed in the membrane powder calcined at 600°C, 700°C, and 800°C utilizing Bruker D8 (Madison, WI, USA) and Cu Kα radiation. Scanning was carried out at a rate of 1° per minute in the 2θ range between 5° and 70°.

The surface area measurements were performed using Quantachrome Instruments NOVA Automated Gas Sorption version 1.12 (Boynton Beach, FL, USA). N_2 isotherms were performed at 77 K using a Coulter SA3 analyzer (Fullerton, CA, USA). The respective surface area values were calculated using the Brunauer-Emmett-Teller (BET) equation.

A transmission electron microscope (model JEOL JEM-1230, Akishima-shi, Japan) was used to examine the membrane powders with respect to their particle size and shape.

The distribution of pore size, pore area, and pore volume developed in the prepared membranes was determined using a Hg porosimeter (Type No. 9810). The chamber was first evacuated to a pressure less than 10 psia and then subjected to the introduction of a non-wetting liquid (mercury), under a hydraulic pressure of 14 to 415 Pa, corresponding to pore radii from approximately 2 nm to approximately 200 μm.

The morphological characteristics of the membrane surface and the thickness of the prepared layer after and before the grafting process were examined using scanning electron microscopy (SEM) equipment (Philips XL30, Amsterdam, The Netherlands). The method is based on directing a fine-focused electron beam accelerated under a maximum potential difference of 30 kV to scan the surface and microstructure of the specimen displayed on a cathode ray screen. The microstructure is then photographed at a magnification between × 200 and × 50,000.

The surface of the prepared membranes was treated to produce a kind of surface modification to maximize its degree of hydrophobicity by eliminating the existence of small, hydrophilic pores. This approach has been achieved through the treatment with chloro-alkyl silanes that enhanced surface flow and solution diffusion.

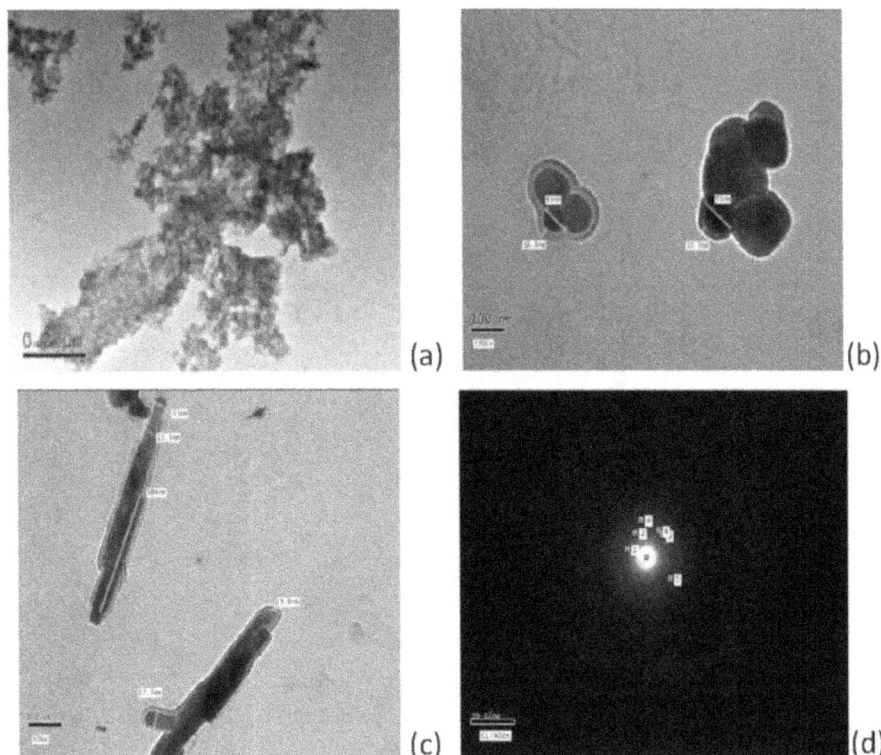

Figure 9 TEM images (a, b, c) and electron diffraction pattern (d) of the alumina (A) membrane powder fired at 700°C.

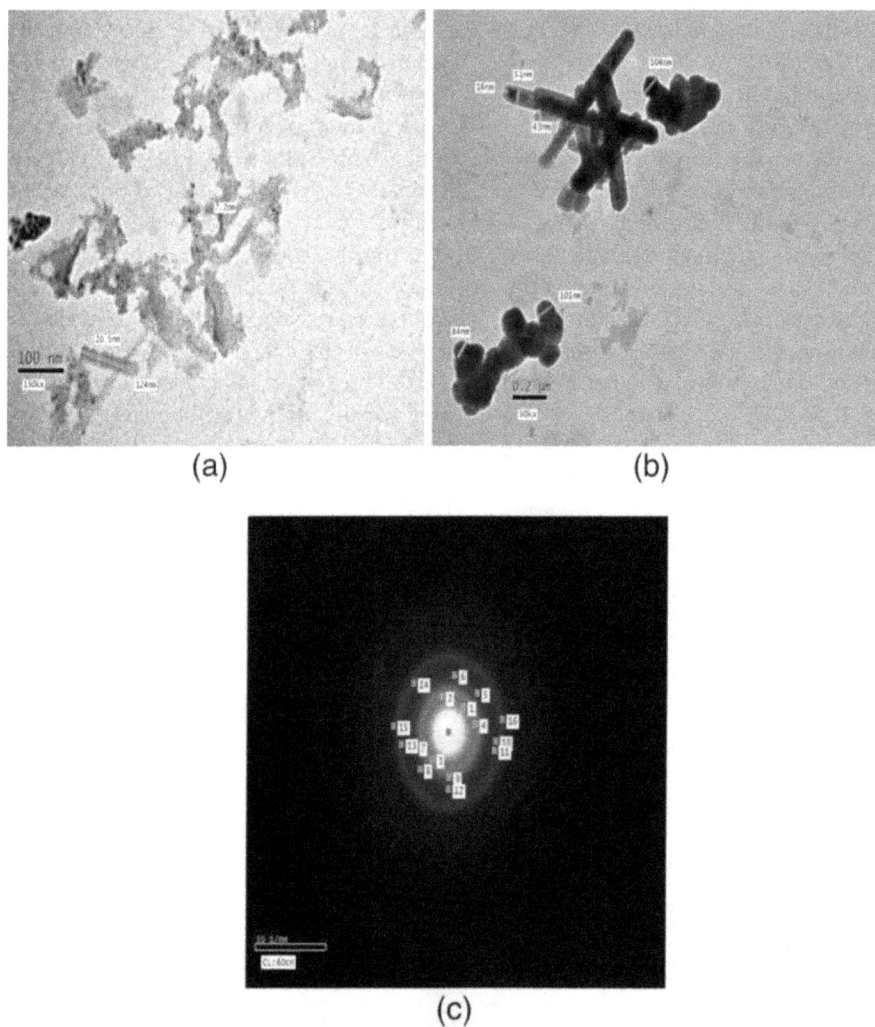

Figure 10 TEM images (a, b) and electron diffraction pattern (c) of the alumina-titania (AT50) membrane powder fired at 700°C.

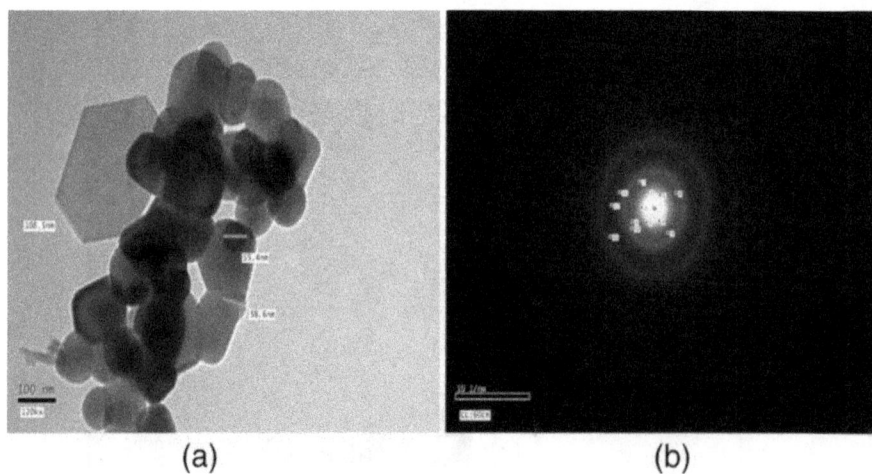

Figure 11 TEM image (a) and electron diffraction pattern (b) of the titania (T) membrane powder fired at 700°C.

The hydrophobic character of the prepared membranes was checked by measuring the contact angles of a sessile waterdrop on the membrane samples using a goniometer apparatus (Figure 2).

Water flux, permeability measurements, and salt rejection efficiency of the prepared membranes were performed using a homemade pilot plant, as shown in Figure 3.

The salt rejection efficiency of the prepared membranes was measured using a Hanna model conductivity electrode (model: HI99301). The retention coefficient (R_{NaCl}) was calculated according to the following equation:

$$R_{NaCl} = \{[CF_{NaCl} - CP_{NaCl}]/CF_{NaCl}\} \times 100\%,$$

where CF and CP denote the concentration of NaCl in both feed and permeate, respectively.

The desalination experiments were performed using the different prepared flat membranes, namely alumina (A), alumina-titania composite (AT25, AT50, AT75), and titania (T). A fixed flow rate (10 ml/s) and vacuum pressure (−0.8 bar) were used in the process. Three aqueous NaCl feed solutions were as follows: 2,000, 3,000, and 5,000 ppm.

The NaCl solutions were prepared and heated at different temperatures (45°C, 55°C, 65°C, and 75°C). The salt concentration of the permeate was measured in order to determine the respective retention coefficient. The temperature of the cooling condenser was maintained at 7°C.

Results and discussion

Thermal analysis

The TGA and DSC of the acrylic-acrylamide copolymer alone and those incorporated with Al^{3+} or Ti^{4+} cations are shown in Figures 4 and 5, respectively. Weight loss and destruction of the acrylic-acrylamide copolymer take place in three steps: loss of water (moisture) followed by a gradual dissociation of the copolymer that ends by the combustion of the copolymer at 450°C.

The DSC of the copolymer reveals four endothermic peaks. The glass transition temperature of the copolymer is at 85°C, followed by its melting point at 217°C. The third and fourth peaks at 334°C and 389°C, respectively, are due to dissociation of the copolymer according to the polymer molecular weight. Decomposition of the copolymer occurs as an exothermic peak at 420°C.

Figure 5a,b,c and Tables 2 and 3 show the TGA and DSC of the acrylic-acrylamide copolymer incorporated with alumina, titania, and alumina-titania composite, respectively. It was found that the thermogram of the acrylic-acrylamide copolymer incorporated with alumina, titania, and alumina-titania composite represents

Table 4 Surface area measurements for the different membrane powders calcined at 700°C

Sample ID	Type of membrane	Temperature (°C)	Surface area (m²/g)	Particle size (nm)
A	Alumina (100 mol%)	700	481.2	3.28
AT25	Alumina (75 mol%)-titania (25 mol%)	700	333	4.63
AT50	Alumina (50 mol%)-titania (50 mol%)	700	201.9	7.69
AT75	Alumina (25 mol%)-titania (75 mol%)	700	175.1	8.81
T	Titania (100 mol%)	700	324.9	4.98

three stages of weight loss, as demonstrated before and illustrated in Table 3.

From Figure 5a, the glass transition temperature increased to 102°C and the softening point increased to 206.5°C. Also, the polymer was completely degraded at 508°C. Figure 5b shows that the glass transition temperature and the softening point of the acrylic-acrylamide copolymer coupled at 106.1°C, and the polymer was completely combusted at 570°C. Figure 5c shows that the glass transition temperature and the softening point of the acrylic-acrylamide copolymer were at 117.9°C and 232.2°C, respectively, while the polymer was combusted at 478.8°C.

It is clear that all reaction temperatures: glass transition, softening point, and combustion, of the copolymer are shifted to higher temperatures. These increases are due to the reaction that occurred between the metal oxide and copolymer.

Fourier transform infrared spectroscopy

The IR spectrum of the acrylic-acrylamide copolymer is displayed in Figure 6. A broad band occurs at 2,500 to 3,500 cm^{-1} which is due to the combination of two broad bands corresponding to the stretching vibration of the amide group and the stretching vibration of the carboxylic group. The main bands corresponding to the presence of the C = O group occur at 2,362 and 1,662 cm^{-1}. The bending vibrations of O-H and N-H

Table 5 Results of the surface area of the alumina membrane powders calcined at 600°C, 700°C, and 800°C

Sample ID	Type of membrane	Temperature (°C)	Surface area (m²/g)	Particle size (nm)
A	Alumina (100%)	600	812	1.89
A	Alumina (100%)	700	481.2	3.28
A	Alumina (100%)	800	282.7	5.99

Table 6 Pore size distribution of the different membranes

Sample symbol	Total intrusion volume (ml/g)	Total pore area (m²/g)	Bulk density (g/ml)	Average pore diameter (μm)	Apparent density (g/ml)	Total porosity (%)
Support	0.2025	4.863	0.0914	2.2924	4.2786	46.42
Hydrophobic support	0.1756	4.087	0.1719	2.3728	4.0677	41.67
Intermediate layer	0.1547	3.116	0.2163	2.4669	3.9889	38.16
A	0.0951	9.080	2.9666	0.0419	4.1316	28.27
AT25	0.0785	24.258	2.7355	0.0129	3.4830	21.46
AT50	0.0971	8.273	2.9119	0.0248	4.0595	28.27
AT75	0.0344	5.546	2.9833	0.0469	3.3249	34.32
T	0.0998	35.464	2.5678	0.0113	3.3425	25.03

groups attached to the polymer are found at 1,027 and 810 cm^{-1}, respectively, while the main bands related to the rocking and bending vibrations of the C-H bond are detected at 617 and 1,455 cm^{-1}.

The IR spectra of the acrylic-acrylamide copolymer gels dried at 80°C, incorporated with one or two cations, e.g., Al^{3+}, Ti^{4+}, and Al^{3+}-Ti^{4+}, are shown in Figure 7.

The high-frequency part of the spectrum is dominated by a broad band occurring between 3,000 and 3,500 cm^{-1} which is a characteristic of the -OH stretching mode of -COOH groups in the 'acrylic-acrylamide copolymer'

template polymer. The corresponding deformation modes appear in the range of 1,384 to 1,388 cm^{-1}.

The IR spectra of the substituted cations with the functional groups of the template polymer are more or less similar with only slight variation. This indicates that the same reactions between the metal oxide and copolymer are taking place.

The bands at the range 624 to 659 cm^{-1} in the substituted copolymer spectra are attributed to the different inorganic cations' R^+-(O-C)- stretching vibrations, where R^+ = Al^{3+} and Ti^4.

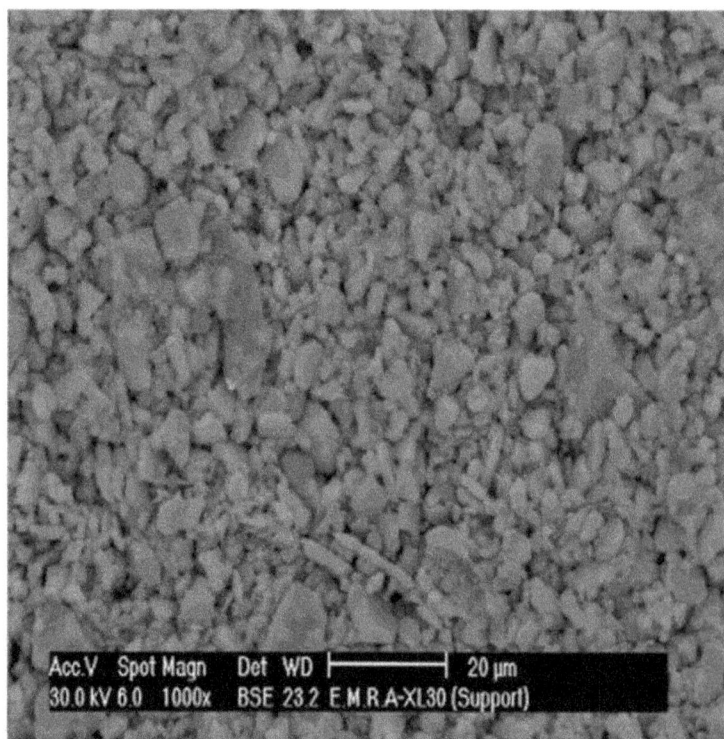

Figure 12 SEM image of the alumina support.

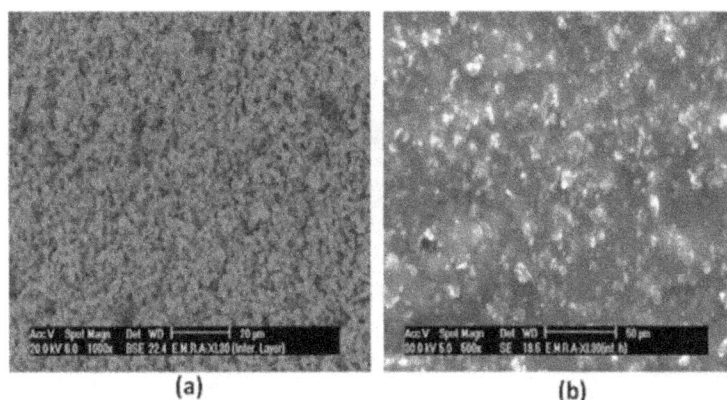

Figure 13 SEM images of both the (a) non-grafted and (b) grafted alumina intermediate layer.

The bands detected at 1,627 to 1,631 cm^{-1} correspond to the stretching mode of the $C = O$ functional group, whereas the NH and OH stretching vibrations occur in the same range 3,300 cm^{-1}. Therefore, these bands failed to be distinguished from one another.

X-ray diffraction analysis

The X-ray diffraction (XRD) patterns of the different samples prepared using different molar ratios of the inorganic precursors ($AlCl_3$ and $TiCl_4$) added to the template polymer (acrylic-acrylamide copolymer) and subjected to a calcination reaction at temperatures between 600°C and 800°C for 3 h are displayed in Figure 8a,b,c,d.

The XRD patterns of the alumina (A) powders heat-treated at different temperatures: 600°C, 700°C, and 800°C, were ill crystalline at 600°C, whereas the γ-alumina phase started to appear at 700°C showing an increase in the peak intensity at 800°C, as shown in Figure 8a.

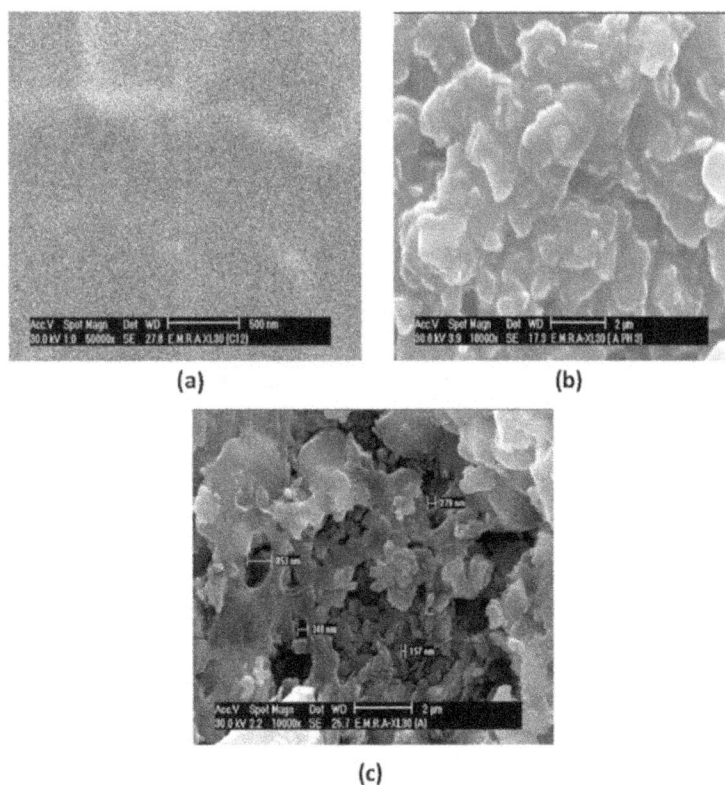

Figure 14 SEM images of the alumina membranes calcined at different temperatures: (a) 600°C, (b) 700°C, and (c) 800°C.

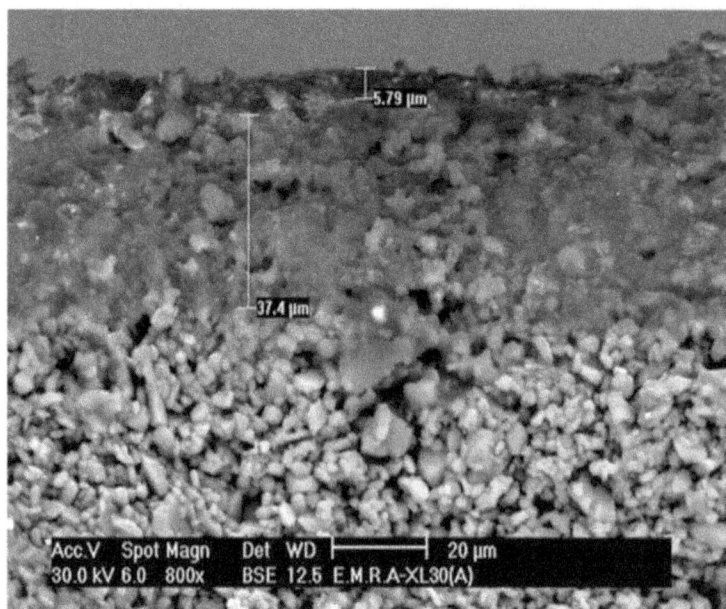

Figure 15 Cross section of the alumina membrane calcined at 700°C.

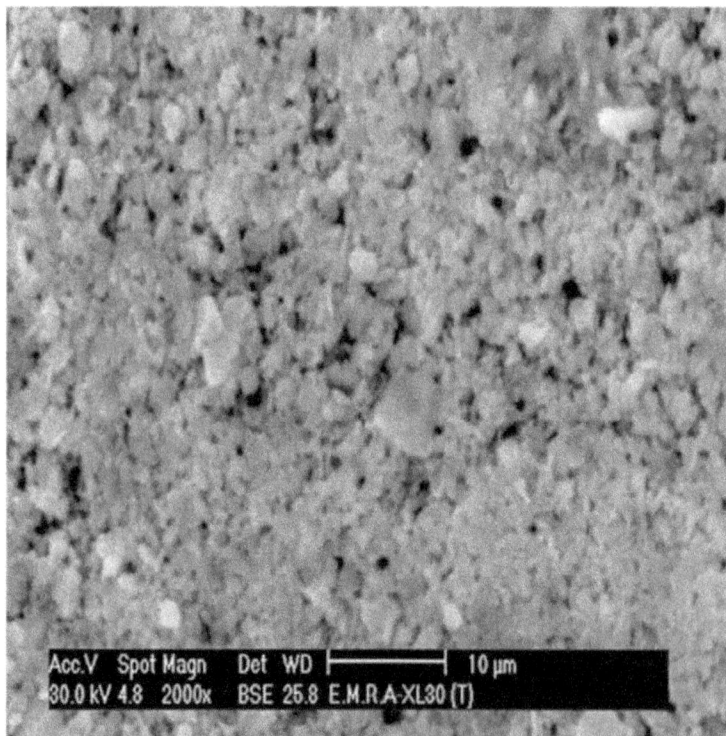

Figure 16 Titania membrane calcined at 700°C.

The XRD patterns of the membrane powders formed by alumina (A), alumina-titania (AT25, AT50, and AT75), and titania (T) were heat-treated at 700°C are shown in Figure 8b. The XRD pattern of alumina indicates a small peak depicted at $2\theta = 67°$ denoting the start of formation of the γ-alumina phase.

The XRD patterns of alumina-titania with different molar ratios of $AlCl_3/TiCl_4$: 75%:25%, 50%:50%, and 25%:75%, exhibit a characteristic peak at $2\theta = 25°$, attributed to the anatase phase beside that of γ-alumina. The intensity of the anatase peak increases with the increase of the proportion of titania concentration; as a result, the crystallization of the γ-alumina phase is retarded.

The XRD patterns of the alumina-titania (AT50) powders heat-treated at different temperatures are shown in Figure 8c. The alumina is ill crystalline at 600°C, with the start of formation of the γ-alumina phase at 700°C and 800°C. On the other hand, the titania crystallized as anatase in all powders heat-treated at 600°C up to 800°C. The peak intensity increases with the increase of the temperature of the treatment.

The XRD patterns of the titania (T) powders in Figure 8d show the anatase phase at 600°C up to 800°C. The intensity of the anatase peaks increases with the increase of the temperature of the treatment.

Transmission electron microscopy

Figures 9, 10, and 11 demonstrate the shapes of particles and overall appearance based on transmission electron microscopy of the prepared alumina, titania, and alumina-

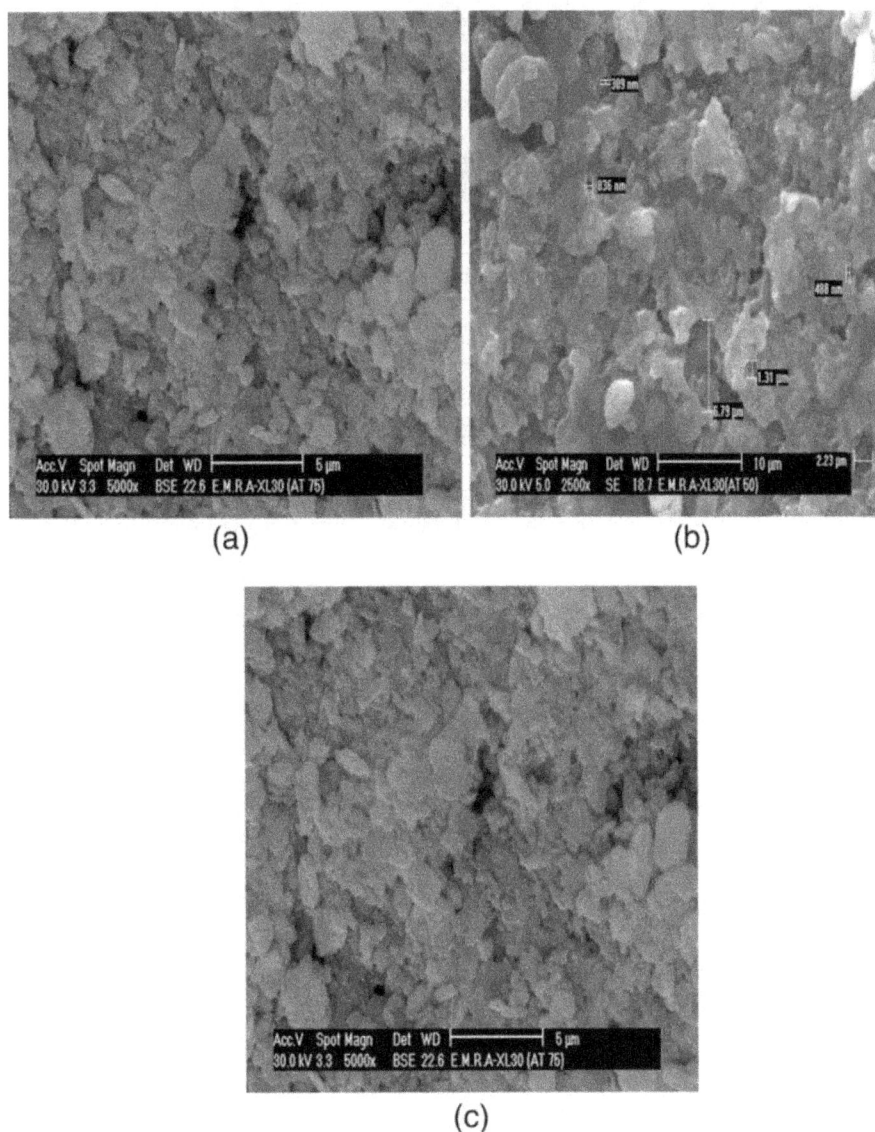

Figure 17 Alumina-titania composite membranes with different concentrations calcined at 700°C. (a) Alumina (75 mol%)-titania (25 mol%) (AT25) membrane. **(b)** Alumina (50 mol%)-titania (50 mol%) (AT50) membrane. **(c)** Alumina (25 mol%)-titania (75 mol%) (AT75) membrane.

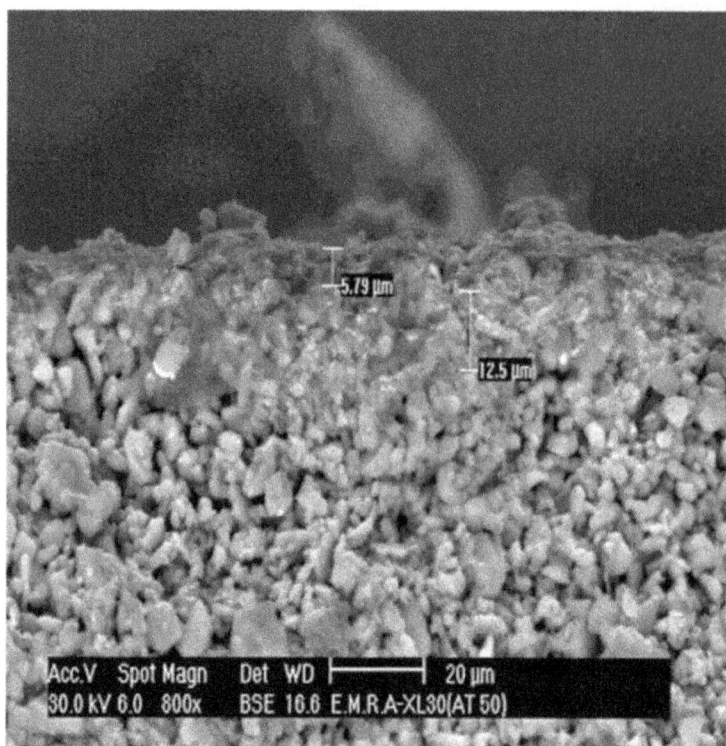

Figure 18 Cross section of the alumina-titania composite (AT50) membrane calcined at 700°C.

titania composite membrane powders heat-treated at 700°C for 3 h.

The TEM images of the alumina powder are shown in Figure 9a,b,c,d. Figure 9a shows a kind of agglomeration of the grains. The structure of the template polymer precursor was preserved by the substitution of the alumina cation as evident from the scattered dendrites. Figure 9b,c shows that the shape of the alumina grains ranged between spherical and rodlike with a size ranging from 65 to 95 nm. The electron diffraction pattern of the powder showed diffuse rings indicating the ill-crystalline nature of the grains with the presence of some spots presenting γ-alumina as demonstrated in Figure 9d.

The TEM images and electron diffraction pattern of the alumina-titania composite (AT) powder are shown in Figure 10a,b,c. The grains are agglomerated and arranged in a manner preserving the previous structure of the polymer, as demonstrated in Figure 10a, with a size ranging between 7 and 125 nm indicating the very fine nature of the powder. Figure 10b shows the shape of the particles that ranged between spherical and rodlike, with a size ranging between 16 and 104 nm. On the other hand, the electron diffraction pattern of the powder shows the presence of diffuse rings attributed to the amorphous nature of the alumina, besides the presence

of spots indicating the anatase phase of titania, as shown in Figure 10c.

The TEM image and electron diffraction pattern of the titania (T) membrane powder in Figure 11a,b show agglomerates of the nano-grains with a size ranging

Table 7 Contact angle measurements of the alumina support modified with two different silane agents: C3 and C8

Number	Sample ID	Concentration of silane/ethanol solution (vol.%)	Side	CA (deg)	Average time (s)
1	C3 (2 vol.%)	2	Front	86.2	
			Back		8
2	C3 (5 vol.%)	5	Front		5
			Back		5
3	C3 (10 vol.%)	10	Front		6
			Back		11
4	C8 (2 vol.%)	2	Front	102.2	
			Back	115.7	
5	C8 (5 vol.%)	5	Front	116.3	
			Back	111.5	
6	C8 (10 vol.%)	10	Front	107.4	
			Back	106.1	

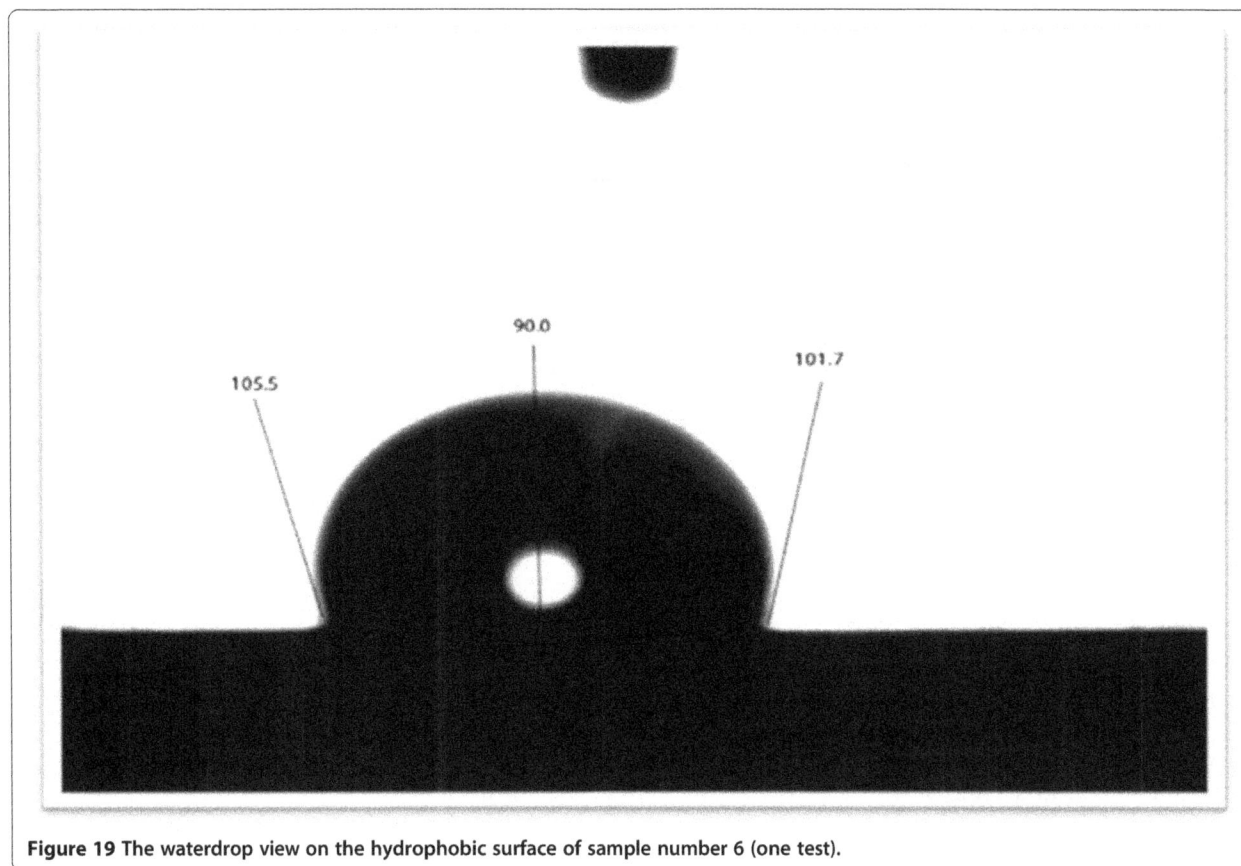

Figure 19 The waterdrop view on the hydrophobic surface of sample number 6 (one test).

between 55 and 108 nm indicating the fine nature of the powder. Particles are either spherical or hexagonal shaped. The electron diffraction pattern of the titania powder shows spots indicating the crystallization of the anatase phase.

Specific surface area

The results of the different membrane powders obtained after firing at 700°C in Table 4 indicate that the values of the specific surface area are affected by the type and molar ratio of the inorganic precursors reacted with the copolymer.

Powders of the alumina membranes heat-treated at 600°C, 700°C, and 800°C gave the following values for the specific surface area: 812, 481, and 282.7 m^2/g, respectively, whereas the calculated particle sizes were 1.89, 3.198, and 5.889 nm, as shown in Table 5.

Powders of the alumina-titania composite heat-treated at 700°C showed a decrease in the values of the specific surface area with the increase in the concentration of titania precursors. Coarsening of the grains took place as evident from the calculated values recorded which increased from 4.6318 to 8.813 nm, as shown in Table 4.

Pore size distribution

The porosity and pore size distribution measurements of the prepared membranes are greatly affected by the alumina-titania ratios while those modified by octyltrichlorosilane show a slight decrease in the respective porosities and pore size measurements, as demonstrated in Table 6. This indicates that the organo-silane agent does not affect the whole structure, but only affect the surface properties.

The change in the average pore diameter of the support on grafting recorded was between 2.29 and 2.37 μm and accompanied by a decrease in the total porosity from 46.42% to 41.67%.

The recorded pore diameters of the alumina (A), alumina-titania (AT25, AT50, and AT75), and titania (T)

Table 8 Wetting angle measurements for the different grafted membranes

Membrane ID	Contact angle (deg)
A	Approximately 119
AT50	Approximately 120
T	Approximately 123

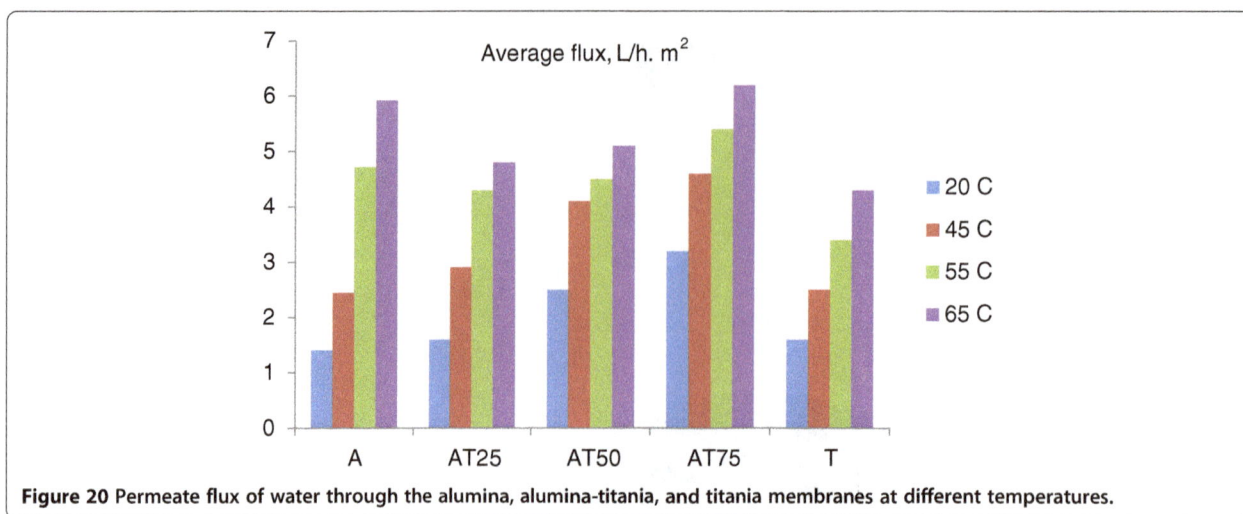

Figure 20 Permeate flux of water through the alumina, alumina-titania, and titania membranes at different temperatures.

membranes are in the following sequence: 41.9, 12.9, 46.9, 24.8, and 11.3 nm, with respective porosity of 21.46%, 28.27%, 34.32%, and 25.03%.

Scanning electron microscopy

Microstructures of the main layers as well as the cross sections of the prepared membranes are shown in Figures 12, 13, 14, 15, 16, 17, and 18.

The SEM image in Figure 12 shows the surface of the alumina support specimen fired at 1,400°C. The alumina grains with a size between 3 and 5 μm show a coarse columnar to platy shape that is randomly oriented giving a porous microstructure with a rough and pitted surface. The interstices between the grains are filled with smaller ones about 1 to 2 μm.

The SEM images in Figure 13 show the outer surface of the grafted and non-grafted intermediate layer. The SEM image in Figure 13a shows the alumina support specimen covered with an α-alumina intermediate layer (non-grafted sample) and fired at 1,000°C. The coarse alumina grains are totally covered by the intermediate layer with a grain size ranging between 0.2 and 0.5 μm with connected pores giving a smooth surface. The SEM image in Figure 13b shows the alumina support specimen covered with α-alumina intermediate layer, fired at 1,000°C, and grafted using octyltrichlorosilane. The covering layer displays the details of the underlying structure. No distinct behavior was spotted on the grafted surface.

The SEM images of the composite and monophase membranes in Figures 14, 15, 16, 17, and 18 show the effect of controlling the temperature profile of heat treatment and the concentration of the second phase on the elimination of microcracks and pinholes in the produced membranes to reduce the stresses originating from the removal of volatiles and the accompanying shrinkage.

The alumina membrane treated at 600°C in Figure 14a shows uniform and discrete layers. Increasing the temperature to 800°C, as shown in Figure 14c, leads to the formation of pinholes and cracks with coarsening of the grains through the agglomeration of the alumina particles to reach a size ranging between 348 and 853 nm. Figure 14b, on the other hand, shows the improvement of the surface of the membrane layer heated at 700°C, where these defects were diminished as possible with the presence of large alumina particles.

The SEM image of the cross section of the alumina (A) membrane in Figure 15 shows two different layers on top of the support: an intermediate layer with a thickness of 37.4 μm followed by the alumina membrane layer with a thickness of 5.7 μm.

The SEM image of the titania membrane heat-treated at 700°C in Figure 16 shows the uniformity of the surface that completely covers the alumina support.

The effect of the addition of titania as a second component to form the composite membrane is shown in Figures 17 and 18.

Table 9 Permeate flux of water through the alumina, alumina-titania, and titania membranes at different temperatures

Temperature (°C)	Average flux (l/h m²)				
	A	AT25	AT50	AT75	T
20	1.4	1.6	2.5	3.2	1.51
45	2.5	2.9	4.1	4.6	2.5
55	4.7	4.3	4.5	5.4	3.4
65	5.9	4.8	5.1	6.2	4.3

The effect of the content of titania in the composite on the uniformity of the membrane layer is shown in Figure 17. A uniform surface of the alumina-titania composite (AT25) membrane heat-treated at 700°C is shown in Figure 17a. AT50 and AT75, on the other hand, show a kind of non-uniformity that might be generated by the stresses arising from the start of conversion of anatase to rutile phase, and this conversion is usually accompanied by grain growth of the latter phase, as shown in Figure 17b,c.

The SEM cross-sectional image of the alumina-titania composite (AT50) membrane as an example of the alumina-titania composite samples is shown in Figure 18. Two different layers appear on top of the support. The support is covered by an intermediate layer with a thickness of 12.5 μm followed by the alumina-titania composite membrane layer with a thickness of 5.7 μm.

The SEM image of the surface of the alumina-titania (AT25) membrane showed a uniform crack-free top layer with the least pore diameter of 0.0129 μm as demonstrated from the pore size distribution results.

Contact angle measurements

In the present work, two different organo-silane compounds, namely γ-aminopropyl-trimethoxysilane (C3) and octyltrichlorosilane (C8), were selected to carry out the surface modification.

The grafted membranes (alumina (A), alumina-titania composite (AT), titania (T)) obtained by immersion in a silane solution of different concentrations (2, 5, and 10 vol.%) in an ethanol solution at room temperature 25°C were tested by measuring the contact angle developed on the surface. Also, these membranes were subjected for water permeation and water desalination. Therefore, the degree of water permeability and the rejection coefficient (R%) of the modified membranes were measured.

The results obtained shown in Table 7 represent an average of three readings for the tested membranes. An example of the drop formation and testing measurements is demonstrated in Figure 19.

The measured contact angles of the non-grafted supports are lower than 90°. Accordingly, they are considered hydrophilic and likely to absorb water. On the other hand, the measured contact angles of three alumina support samples grafted using γ-aminopropyl-trimethoxysilane denoted by C3 (2, 5, and 10 vol.%) are demonstrated in Table 7.

Accordingly, octyltrichlorosilane (C8, 5 vol.%) was selected to graft the prepared ceramic membranes for the desalination measurements including water flux and rejection coefficient (R%) measurements for each membrane.

Table 10 The retention coefficient values of NaCl solutions through alumina, alumina-titania, and titania membranes

NaCl concentration (ppm)	Feed/permeate temperature (°C)	Retention coefficient (%)				
		A	AT25	AT50	AT75	T
2,000	45:7	19.58	26.30	28.51	11.5	10.67
	55:7	21.57	29.56	31.77	17.11	27.54
	65:7	32.52	41.55	38.69	19.17	38.96
	75:7	35.24	46.55	42.77	30.52	42.93
3,000	45:7	26.2	28	30.79	15.31	24.27
	55:7	45.24	36.22	39.10	28.11	43.69
	65:7	47.62	44	46.43	29.32	53.79
	75:7	50.82	47.25	48.88	30.67	58.09
5,000	45:7	34.44	53.02	32.99	16.87	53.58
	55:7	49.77	56.11	46.43	37.65	54.91
	65:7	51.39	63.58	60.49	40.09	56.23
	75:7	54.26	72.59	70.26	47.43	61.57

The wetting angles of the different grafted membranes using 5 vol.% octyltrichlorosilane (C8) indicated that the contact angle values recorded are independent of the membrane type as they show more or less the same contact angle, as shown in Table 8.

Vacuum membrane distillation experiments
Water permeation process

The measured values of water flux through the prepared membranes depend on the temperature difference between the feed and permeate sides, as shown in Figure 20. Thus, the alumina membrane showed a gradual increase in water flux from 1.4 to 3.9 l/h m^2 when the temperature was raised gradually from 20°C to 65°C.

The results in Table 9 compare water fluxes through the different grafted membranes (alumina (A), alumina-titania (AT25, AT50, AT75), titania (T)). It is evident from these results that water flux slightly depends on the pore diameter of the used membrane. The water fluxes of 1.58 and 1.5 l/h m^2 measured at 20°C were recorded through the AT25 and T membranes with an average pore diameter of 12.9 and 11.3 nm, respectively.

These values were smaller than those reported for other alumina (A) and alumina-titania composite types

Table 11 Comparison between values of retention coefficient of NaCl solution (5,000 ppm at 75°C) using the different membranes

	Membrane type				
	A	AT25	AT50	AT75	T
Retention coefficient (%)	54.26	72.59	70.26	47.43	61.57

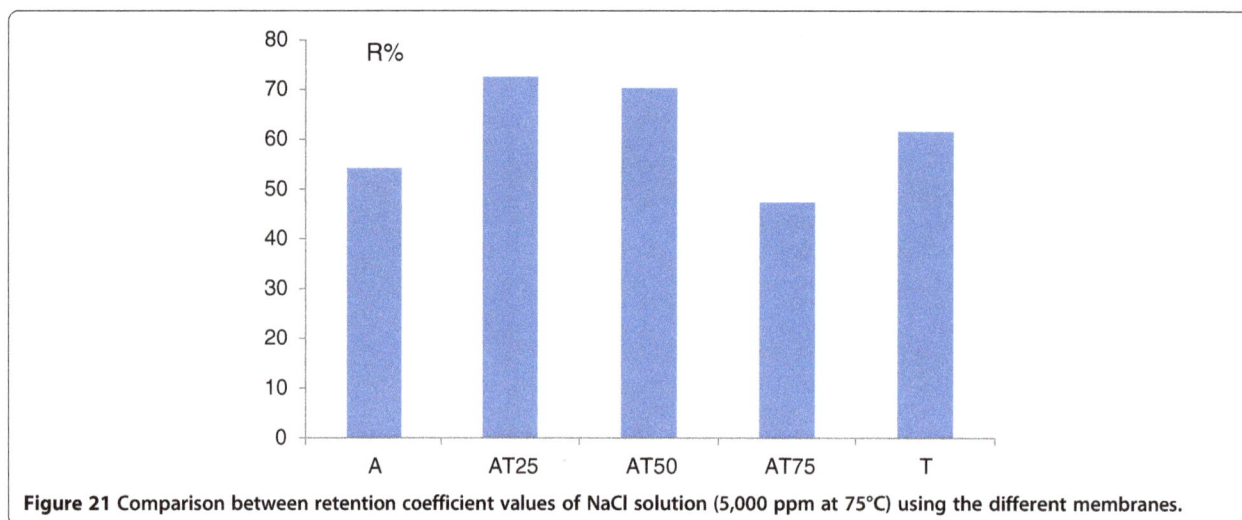

Figure 21 Comparison between retention coefficient values of NaCl solution (5,000 ppm at 75°C) using the different membranes.

(AT50 and AT75) of 4, 2.5, and 4.2 l/h m^2 measured at 20°C with an average pore diameter of 41.9, 24.8, and 46.9 nm, respectively.

Desalination process

The retention coefficient values ($R\%$) of the different grafted membranes are presented in Table 10 which depended strongly on the temperature difference between the feed and the permeate side and on the concentration of the NaCl solution. The alumina membrane shows a retention coefficient of 34, 49.7, 51.39, and 54.26 at a temperature difference of 45:7, 55:7, 65:7, and 75:7, respectively.

The retention coefficient values ($R\%$) showed an increase by increasing the concentration of the NaCl solution. The retention coefficient ($R\%$) of the alumina membrane increased from 35.24% to 54.2% by increasing the NaCl solution concentration from 2,000 to 5,000 ppm.

The alumina-titania composite (AT25 and AT50) and titania (T) membranes showed a higher ability to reject the NaCl salt from water showing a retention coefficient of 72.59%, 70.26%, and 61.57%, respectively, while the alumina-titania composite AT75 showed a lower retention coefficient of 47.43%.

Figure 21 and Table 11 show the salt retention (R_{NaCl}) during the membrane distillation process using the different grafted membranes (A, AT25, AT50, and T) at the temperature difference of 75:7 using NaCl solution of 5,000 ppm as a feed solution. It can be seen that the salt retention coefficient in the MD process with the different prepared grafted membranes is close to 75%. This can be explained by the fact that some of the biggest pores were wetted and limited transport of NaCl solution could occur.

Conclusions

The study of the preparation of membranes via the application of the acrylic-acrylamide copolymer as template was successful in overcoming the presence of cracks through the different additions. It was possible to obtain membrane layers of uniform nano-pore size and porosities between 25% and 37% fired at 700°C. The crystal and morphological structures of the alumina-titania membranes were affected by the AlCl$_3$ and TiCl$_4$ feed ratio. The addition of titania succeeded in hindering the crystallization of the alumina phases and eliminating the possibility of the accompanying cracking. The polymeric route using acrylic-acrylamide copolymer as a template polymer led to preparation of membranes with ill-crystalline nature at 600°C that started to crystallize at 700°C which showed high surface area values as well as nano-pore size and mesoporosities. The results of water permeation showed that there is an upper limit for the addition of titania. The final supported membranes prepared using alumina-titania (AT25 and AT50) precursors showed uniform layers without cracks. The alumina-titania composite (AT) membranes showed a pore size of 13 to 46 nm, porosity of 21% to 34%, and water permeability of 2 to 8 l/h m^2/bar. These membranes can be used for ultrafiltration purposes, such as pretreatment of water desalination and concentration of aqueous solutions (fruit juice, sugar solution). The polymeric sol–gel method used in this study to produce different hydrophobic alumina-titania membranes which utilized chloride salts of aluminum and titanium using acrylic-acrylamide as a template polymer and octyltrichlorosilane as a grafting agent is promising and can be used for different membranes.

Competing interests

The authors declare that they have no competing interests.

Authors' contributions

AMANY Gaber carried out the membrane prepration studies and drafted the manuscript. Doreya Ibrahim: participated in the design of the study and revese the manuscrpt. Fawzia Fahim: prepared the template polymer used in the study. Elham ELZANZTI: measure the permeability performance of the different prepared membranes. All authors read and approved the final manuscript

Author details

[1]Ceramic Department, National Research Centre, Cairo, Egypt. [2]Polymers Department, National Research Centre, Cairo, Egypt. [3]Chemical Engineering Department, National Research Centre, Cairo, Egypt.

References

Abidi N, Sivade A, Bourret D, Larbot A, Boutevin B, Guida-Pietrasanta F, Ratsimihety A (2006) Surface modification of mesoporous membranes by fluoro-silane coupling reagent for CO_2 separation. J Membr Sci 270:101

Benfer S, Popp U, Richter H, Siewert C, Tomandl G (2001) Development and characterization of ceramic nanofiltration membranes. Sep Purif Tech 22 (23):231–237

Benfer S, Árki P, Tomandl G (2004) Ceramic membranes for filtration applications —preparation and characterization. Adv Eng Mater 6(7):495–500

Caro J, Noack M, Kolsch P (1998) Chemically modified ceramic membranes. Micropor Mesopor Mat 22:321

Castricum HL, Sah A, Mittelmeijer-Hazeleger MC, ten Elshof JE (2005) Hydrophobisation of mesoporous γ-Al_2O_3 with organochlorosilanes— efficiency and structure. Microspor Mesopor Mat 83:1

Gaber AA (2007) Preparation of alumina membranes by sol-gel polymeric route. M.Sc Thesis, Cairo University

Hyun SH, Jo SY, Kang BS (1996) Surface modification of γ-alumina membranes by silane coupling for CO_2 separation. J Membr Sci 120:197–206

Javaid A, Hughey MP, Varutbangkul V, Ford DM (2001) Solubility-based gas separation with oligomer-modified inorganic membranes. J Membr Sci 187:141

Krajewski SR, Kujawski W, Bukowska M, Picard C, Larbot A (2006) Application of fluoroalkylsilanes (FAS) grafted ceramic membranes in membrane distillation process of NaCl solutions. J Membr Sci 281:253–259

Kumar K-NP (1993) Nanostructured ceramic membranes; layer and texture formation. Ph.D. Thesis, University of Twente, Enschede, The Netherlands, p 113

Larbot A, Alami-Younssi S, Persin M (1994) Preparation of γ-alumina nanofiltration membrane. J Membr Sci 97:167

Leger C, Lira HDL, Paterson R (1996) Preparation and properties of surface modified ceramic membranes. Part III. Gas permeation of 5 nm alumina membranes modified by trichloro-octadecylsilane. J Membr Sci 120:187

Miller JR, Koros WJ (1990) The formation of chemically modified g-alumina microporous membranes. Sep Sci Technol 25:1257

Puhlfürß P, Voigt A, Weber R, Morbe M (2000) Microporous TiO_2 membranes with a cut off <500 Da. J Membr Sci 174:123

Randon J, Paterson R (1997) Preliminary studies on the potential for gas separation by mesoporous ceramic membranes modified by tri-chlorooctadecylsilane. J Membr Sci 120:187

Richter H, Piorra A, Tomandl G (1997) Developing of ceramic membranes for nanofiltration. Key Eng Mater 132–136:1715–1718

Schaep J, Vandecasteele C, Peeters B, Luyten J, Dotremont C, Roels D (1999) Characteristics and retention properties of a mesoporous γ-Al_2O_3 membrane for nanofiltration. J Membr Sci 163:229

Sekulic J, Magraso A, ten Elshof JE, Blank DHA (2004) Influence of ZrO_2 addition on microstructure and liquid permeability of mesoporous TiO_2 membranes. Micropor Mesopor Mat 72:49–57

Shojai F, Mantyla TA (2001) Chemical stability of yttria doped zirconia membranes in acid and basic aqueous solutions: chemical properties, effect of annealing and ageing time. Ceram Int 27:299–307

van Gestel T, Vandecasteele C, Buekenhoudt A, Dotremont C, Luyten J, Leysen R, van der Bruggen B, Maes G (2002) Alumina and titania multilayer membranes for nanofiltration: preparation, characterization and chemical stability. J Membr Sci 207:73

van Gestel T, Vandecasteele C, Buekenhoudt A, Dotremont C, Luyten J, van der Bruggen B, Maes G (2003) Corrosion properties of alumina and titania NF membranes. J Membr Sci 214:21

Wildman DL, Peterson RA, Anderson MA, Hill CG (1994) Investigation of titania membranes for nanofiltration. In: Proceedings of the ICIM94. Worcester Polytechnic Institute, Worcester, p 111

Xu Q, Anderson MA (1993) Sol-gel route to synthesis of microporous ceramic membranes: thermal stability of TiO_2–ZrO_2 mixed oxides. J Am Ceram Soc 76:2093–2097

Zhang H, Banfield JF (1999) Synthesis and applications of TiO_2 nanoparticles. Am Mineral 84:528.7.A

8

Kinetic and Thermodynamic Spectrophotometric Technique to Estimate Gabapentin in Pharmaceutical Formulations using Ninhydrin

Farhan Ahmed Siddiqui[1*], Nawab Sher[2], Nighat Shafi[1], Hina Shamshad[3] and Arif Zubair[4]

Abstract

Background: Simple and sensitive spectrophotometric method is described based on the reaction of drug (gabapentin) with ninhydrin in pure form and in pharmaceutical preparations.

Methods: Complex formed during this reaction is measured at 575 nm as a function of time. Kinetic study involve initial-rate, rate-constant and fixed-time (80 minutes) procedures to determine the concentration of the drug.

Results: Drug was studied in the concentration range of 10-30 μgmL^{-1} showing correlation coefficient 0.9997, 0.9970 and 0.9990 for initial rate, rate constant and fixed time respectively. Limit of detection (LOD) and limit of quantification (LOQ) was found to be 0.13 and 0.04 nana grams respectively. The variables affecting the reactions were optimized and the developed method was validated according to ICH guidelines.

Conclusion: The proposed method has been efficiently applied to the estimation of gabapentin in pharmaceutical formulation with first-class recovery (98.3-101.4%). Thermodynamic parameters were studied i.e., association constants and standard free energy changes were determined by Benesi–Hildebrand equation while, Gibbs free energy change for the complex was also estimated.

Keywords: Spectrophotometric determination; gabapentin; ninhydrin and charge transfer complex

Background

The new anti-convulsant drug gabapentin (1-(aminomethyl)cyclo-hexaneacetic acid) is a GABA analogue. It was originally developed for the treatment of epilepsy, and currently, gabapentin is widely used to relieve pain, especially neuropathic pain, it is indicated in the treatment of epilepsy and neuropathic pain, also in the treatment of bipolar disorder and may be effective in reducing pain and spasticity in multiple sclerosis. Gabapentin is a γ-aminobutyric acid (GABA) analogue that does not bind to GABA receptors or alter GABA metabolism in the brain (Goldlust et al. 1995). Its action is attributed to the irreversible inhibition of the enzyme GABA-transaminase, thus preventing the physiological degradation of GABA in the brain (Ouellet et al. 2001). Analytical methods reported for its determination consist of high-performance liquid chromatography (HPLC) (Jiang & Li 1999; Tang et al. 1999; Chollet et al. 2000; Ifa et al. 2001; Ratnaraj & Patsalos 1998; Wad & Kramer 1998), spectrofluorimetry (Belal et al. 2002; Hassan et al. 2001), gas chromatography–mass spectrometry (GC–MS) (Kushnir et al. 1999; Van Lentea & Gatautis 1998), capillary electrophoresis (Rada et al. 1998) and spectrophotometry applying Hantzsch reaction (al-Zehouri et al. 2001). So far, no traces of any attempts have been found for determination of gabapentin by colorimetric method and the literature is still starving for such analytical procedures. There are number of methods for determination of gabapentin in literature (Manera et al. 2009; Lin et al. 2004; Jia et al. 2012; Ribeiro et al. 2007; Abdulrahman & Basavaiah 2011; Abdulrahman & Basavaiah 2012; Jalali et al. 2007; Hegde et al. 2009; Patel et al. 2011; Siddiqui et al. 2010).

Reactions with ninhydrin (NIN) has been widely used to analyze and characterize amino acids, thiophen and proteins as well as numerous other NIN positive

---

* Correspondence: farhanchemist@gmail.com
[1]Faculty of Pharmacy, Federal Urdu University Arts, Science and Technology, Karachi 75300, Pakistan
Full list of author information is available at the end of the article

compounds in biomedical, clinical, food, forensic, histo-chemical, microbiological, nutritional and plant studies (Friedman 2004). It has been extensively used in the determination of the compounds of pharmaceutical importance applied to their kinetic studies (Rahman & Azmi 2001a; Campins-Falco et al. 1996; Arayne et al. 2008). Present study describes a direct, sensitive and precise spectrophotometric method simpler than the existing UV and HPLC methods that is free from such experimental variables as extraction step for the determination of gabapentin in reference material and pharmaceutical formulations by means of developing charge transfer complex with NIN.

No interference was observed in the assay of gabapentin from common excipients in levels found in pharmaceutical formulations. The method rely on the use of simple and inexpensive technique but give out sensitivity analogous to that procured by sophisticated and expensive techniques such as HPLC, and are validated as per ICH recommendations (ICH Topic Q2(R1) 2005). The kinetic approach for determining gabapentin in commercial dosage form, using NIN as a reagent, confer simplicity and rapidity as the procedure simply require heating and cooling of the reaction mixture. During this study the reaction conditions and application of the methods for determination of gabapentin in pharmaceutical formulations have been established, in addition, the association constant, stoichiometric ratio of reactants and the standard free energy changes ($\Delta G°$) were determined.

Our present study suggests kinetic and thermodynamic spectrophotometric procedure for the determination of gabapentin in pharmaceutical formulations. The methods are based on the reaction of primary amino group of gabapentin with NIN.

Experimental
Apparatus
Shimadzu 1601 double beam UV–visible spectrophotometer possessing a fixed slit width (2 nm) with quartz cells of 10 mm path length connected to a PIV computer loaded with Shimadzu UVPC version 3.9 software were used to record the absorption spectra.

Materials and reagents
All reagents were of analytical grade. Gabapentin pure drug was obtained from Godecke AG, Darmstadt, Germany under license of Park-Davis (Pvt.) Ltd. Karachi, Pakistan. Gabin® capsules 200 mg (PharmEvo Pharmaceutical Company (Pvt.) Ltd., Karachi, Pakistan), Gaba® capsules 100 mg (Nabi Qasim Pharmaceuticals (Pvt) Ltd., Karachi, Pakistan), Gabaplus® capsules 100 mg (Platinum Pharma (Pvt.) Ltd., Karachi, Pakistan) and Neupentin® capsules 400 mg (Highnoon Pharma (Pvt.)

Ltd., Karachi, Pakistan) were purchased from the market. Ninhydrin was purchased from Merck Schuchardt OHG, Darmstadt, Germany. HPLC grade methanol was from fisher scientific UK.

General procedure
Preparation of standard stock solutions
Solution of 0.1 mgmL^{-1} gabapentin was prepared in water by dissolving 10 mg of gabapentin in 100 mL of purified water and stored in a cool (<25°C) and dark place. Ninhydrin reagent was 2 mgmL^{-1} in methanol and was prepared fresh daily.

Method
Aliquots of 1 mL of stock solution corresponding to 100 μgmL^{-1} of gabapentin were transferred into heating tubes. 2 mL of 1% NIN solution was added and heated on boiling water bath for 2 hours, after cooling the mixture was transferred into 25 mL volumetric flask and diluted to volume with distilled water. Increase in absorbance at 575 nm was recorded as a function of time against the reagent blank at room temperature (spectra 1). The initial rate of reaction at different concentrations was calculated from the initial slope of absorbance time curve. The calibration curves were constructed by plotting logarithm of initial-rate of reaction versus logarithm of molar concentration, rate-constant versus final concentration and absorbance measured at a fixed-time versus final concentration of gabapentin.

Procedures for pharmaceuticals formulation
Twenty capsules of each formulation were weighed and powdered. The powder equivalent to 10 mg of gabapentin was dissolved in 100 mL of water to give 0.1 mg mL^{-1} of gabapentin. The procedure was continued as described under general procedures.

Stoichiometric study
Job's method of continuous variation (Rose 1964) was employed. Master equimolar solution of gabapentin was prepared in water whereas NIN was prepared in methanol and made up to volume with the same solvent. A series of 10 mL portions of master solution of gabapentin with NIN was made up comprising different complementary proportions (0:10, 1:9, 2:8......9:1) in 10-mL calibrated flasks. The absorbance of the resulting solutions were measured at the wavelength of maximum absorption after the appropriate time against reagent blanks treated similarly.

Interference from excipients
Samples were prepared by mixing 50 mg of gabapentin with various amounts of common excipients such as

glucose, lactose, talc powder, magnesium stearate, pyr-rolidone, HPMC (hydroxypropylmethylcellulose) and starch. The procedure was continued as described under general procedures.

Results and discussion

Gabapentin exhibits a very low UV absorption, with $A_{1cm}^{1\%}$ at 276 nm = 6.5 (Abdellatef & Khalil 2003) and as a result poor sensitivity will be achieved by conventional UV spectrophotometric methods. There was a critical need to develop a spectrophotometric method that could quantitate gabapentin in pharmaceutical formulations.

Reaction with Ninhydrin (NIN)

Ninhydrin reagent is used for the determination of an aliphatic primary amine or an amino acid group (Friedman 2004; Rahman & Azmi 2001a; Campins-Falco et al. 1996; Arayne et al. 2008; Rahman & Azmi 2001b; Nobrega Jde et al. 1994; Molnar-Perl & Pinter-Szakacs 1989). The presence of an aromatic ring exhibits the response; the exhibition increases if the amino group is nearer to the ring. The end product of NIN reaction with amino acid (Ruhemanns purple) give best color in methanol, however water can be used as good option in case when extraction of the active molecule is compromised. The reaction mixture is heated for a short while and is measured at maximum wavelength 568 nm which is dependent on solvent system and reaction condition (Görög 1995).

Gabapentin interacts with NIN in pure methanol via oxidative deamination of the primary amino group followed by the condensation of the reduced NIN to form the purple colored reaction complex with λ_{max} at 575 nm (Figures 1 and 2).

Gabapentin was found to be competent of reacting with NIN only at higher temperatures. Maximum color was obtained by heating on a water bath at $70 \pm 5°C$ for 80 minutes. Prolonged heating decreased the chromogenic intensity, so the reaction time should be controlled. Different solvents such as water, ethanol, methanol, isopropanol, and acetonitrile have been tried, but the best results were obtained with methanol.

Optimization of reaction

The reaction between gabapentin and ninhydrin in methanol resulted in the formation of blue colored complex. At 70°C, the intensity of color increased with time and became stable after 80 minutes.

Kinetic studies

Initial rate method In order to study the kinetic parameters of the proposed reactions, the initial rate of the reaction was determined by using time curve (from the measurement of the slope of the initial tangent to the absorbance). Concentration of NIN was kept constant and the reaction was studied at different concentrations of gabapentin to establish the order of reaction with respect to gabapentin. For each run, a plot of log $A_¥/A_¥-A_t$ versus time was a straight line indicating a first order reaction. The first order rate constant was also estimated from the slopes of the above plot.

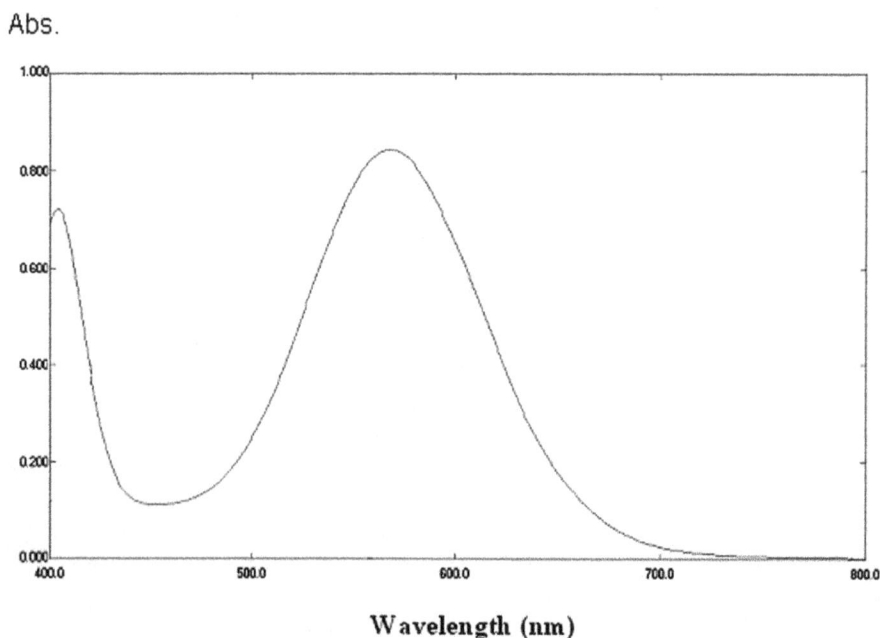

Figure 1 Absorption spectra of the reaction products of gabapentin with NIN.

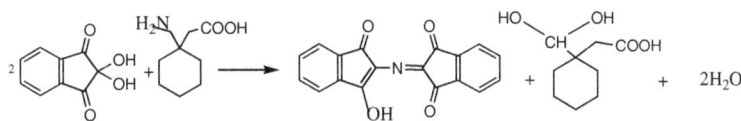

Figure 2 Suggested reaction pathway between gabapentin and NIN.

Similarly to establish order of reaction with respect to NIN, all subsequent investigations were conducted with fixed concentration of gabapentin and varied concentrations of NIN. The first order kinetics was also confirmed by plot of log $A_¥/A_¥-A_t$ versus time. The initial rate of reaction under pseudo-first order conditions would obey the following equation:

$$Rate = dA/dt = k'C^n$$

Where, "k'" is the pseudo-first order rate constant, "C" is the concentration of gabapentin, "n" is the order of reaction. The above equation may be written in the logarithmic form as,

$$Log\ rate = log\ k' + n\ log\ C$$

Linear regression analysis was used to calculate slope, intercept and correlation coefficient (Table 1). The regression of log rate versus log C gave a linear regression equation,

$$Log\ rate = log\ k' + 0.01018\ log\ C$$

The value of "n" in the regression equation also indicated the first order reaction with respect to gabapentin concentration. The calibration curve constructed in the range of 10-30 μgmL^{-1} (absorbance of different concentrations of gabapentin versus time) showed a linear relationship.

Rate-constant method The rate constant values analogous to different concentrations of gabapentin were calculated by plotting the slopes of log $A_¥/A_¥-A_t$ versus time under pseudo-first order conditions (Table 2). The calibration graph was constructed by plotting rate constant against the concentration of gabapentin, and a linear response in the concentration range of 10-30 μgmL^{-1} were observed. Consequent data is presented in Table 2.

Fixed time method A single concentration of gabapentin was monitored at 575 nm against reagent blank at a pre selected fixed time. A plot of absorbance versus initial concentration of gabapentin was calibrated at fixed time (20, 40, 60 and 80 minutes). Regression equations were developed keeping working standards in view and important analytical parameters have been calculated (Table 3) which were found to be in acceptable limits for correlation coefficient, intercept and slope at all fixed time. It is hence suggested that any fixed time can be used for assay of gabapentin.

The high values of correlation coefficients resulting from regression equations demonstrate reliable linearity of the methods. The values of slopes of the regression equations of the proposed methods indicate good sensitivity. The small values of the standard deviation address the precision of the calibration data points around the line of regressions for all the proposed procedures. Independent repeatability studies were performed of the proposed methods with five replicates for each method (Table 4). The obtained data shows that the methods can be applied to dosage formulations with accuracy and precision (Table 5).

Stoichiometry of the reaction
On observing the molar ratio of the gabapentin with NIN using Job's method of continuous variation (Rose 1964), it was found to be 1:2 for NIN.

Thermodynamic studies
Association constants and standard free energy changes
The association constants were determined for the interaction of gabapentin with NIN using Benesi–Hildebrand equation (Benesi & Hidelbrand 1949) was 1.418×10^3.

$$\frac{Ca}{A} = \frac{1}{\varepsilon} + \frac{1}{Kc \cdot \varepsilon} \cdot \frac{1}{Cb}.$$

Table 1 Statistical and regression data of proposed method

	Initial Rate	Rate Constant	Fixed Time
Intercept	0.0021	−0.22284	−0.0028
Slop	0.01018	0.014626	0.0129
r^2	0.9994	0.9990	0.9999
Correlation coefficient (**r**)	0.9997	0.9970	0.9990

Table 2 Method of rate constant

Concentration μgmL^{-1}	Calculated Value of Rate Const (slope) Min^{-1}
10	0.0147
14	0.0146
18	0.0146
20	0.0146
30	0.01463

Table 3 Regression characteristics of gabapentin concentration at different time interval

(Fixed Time)	20	40	60	80
Intercept	−0.002	−0.0022	−0.0034	−0.0036
Slope	0.0112	0.0124	.0114	0.0115
Correlation coefficient (**r**)	0.9990	0.9992	0.9998	0.9999

where *Ca* and *Cb* are the concentrations of the acceptor and donor respectively, *A* is the absorbance of the complex, ε is the molar absorptivity of the complex and K_c is the association constant of the complex.

Straight line was obtained by plotting *Ca* versus *A* and Gibbs Free energy change for the complex was calculated to be (-4.947) by using equation as given below (Martin et al. 1969).

$$\Delta G^\circ = -2.303 \, R \, T \, log \, K_C$$

Where ΔG° is the free energy change of the complex (kJ mol^{-1}), R the gas constant (1.987 cal mol^{-1} deg^{-1}), T the temperature in Kelvin (273 +°C) and K_c is the association constant of drug-acceptor complexes (1 mol^{-1}).

Linearity, accuracy and precision

Linearity, accuracy and precision were assessed for the method in the range of 10 to 30 μgmL^{-1}. Regression statistics were calculated for the colorimetric procedures and linear regression plots showed the directly proportional relationship of absorbance over Beer's law range given in Tables 1 and 4. The table also shows the results of the statistical analysis of the experimental data, such as the slopes, the intercepts, the Square of correlation coefficients obtained by the linear least-squares treatment of the results.

Five different concentrations of gabapentin were prepared, each solution was analyzed in five replicate to evaluate the accuracy and precision of the methods.. The mean Standard Deviation and% relative standard

deviation (%RSD) as depicted in Table 4 were found to be in the acceptable range of (0.0793 – 0.8376) and (0.494 – 0.8317) respectively.

It was observed that at specific wavelength the absorption intensity was dependent upon the concentration of gabapentin. It was observed that Beer's law was followed in all cases with very small range of intercept values (-0.0028 to 0.0021) and slopes ranged from (0.01018 to 0.0146) for the concentration ranges as described in Table 1. The correlation coefficient values were found to be in the range of 0.9970 – 0.9997 using the least-square method.

Specificity

The interference of excipients, additives and other substances present in formulation and the affect of degradation products of gabapentane on the proposed method were experimentally observed. Ionization potential of the donor and the electron affinity of the acceptor are the two main parameters which influenced the energy of complex. The basic nature of gabapentin due to charge transfer is responsible for its specificity to the reaction. Hence a degradation product of gabapentin does not have specificity for the reaction as they lack the basicity. The percentage recoveries as shown in Table 6 confirmed that there was no interference from any excipient present in the formulation for the proposed method.

Limit of detection (LOD) and limit of quantification (LOQ)

The theoretically determined values of LOD and LOQ for gabapentin with NIN were cross checked by actual analysis of these concentrations using proposed methods. LOD of gabapentin with NIN 0.04 μg mL^{-1} while LOQ were 0.13 μg mL^{-1}.

Analysis of pharmaceutical dosage forms

The determination of gabapentin in formulation was carried out using the proposed charge transfer spectrophometric method along with the reference

Table 4 Accuracy and precision of proposed method

Amount	Initial Rate		Rate Constant		Fix Time	
	Found	% Recover	Found	% Recover	Found	% Recover
10	10.05	100.5	9.96	9.96	10.1	101
14	14.14	101	13.95	9.96	14.15	101
18	18.22	101.22	18.17	10.09	17.98	99.8
20	19.86	99.3	20.22	10.11	20.2	101
30	30.41	101.36	29.85	9.98	30.17	100
Mean		100.6778		10.01575		100.70
STD		0.837361		0.079303		0.4987
RSD		0.831723		0.791779		0.494

STD = Standard deviation, RSD = Relative standard deviation

Table 5 Determination of gabapentin in pharmaceuticals formulations by proposed

	Ini. Rate		Rate Constant		Fix Time		Reference method	
	Gabaplus 100 mg cap (Platanium)							
Taken	Found	%Rec	Found	%Rec	Found	%Rec	Found	%Rec
100	100.78	100.78	99.38	99.38	101.30	101.3	99.2	99.2
100	99.540	99.54	100.84	100.84	98.88	98.88	101.4	101.4
100	101.230	101.23	98.41	98.41	99.40	99.4	100.66	100.66
100	98.670	98.67	101.28	101.28	100.66	100.66	98.3	98.3
100	100.230	100.23	99.63	99.63	99.30	99.3	100.7	100.7
Mean	100.090	100.09	99.91	99.908	99.91	99.908	100.05	100.052
STD	1.014	1.01417	1.16	1.15662	1.02	1.023191	1.27	1.26512
RSD	1.013	1.013263	1.16	1.157685	1.024133	1.024133	1.264459	1.26446
T-Test	0.72		0.83		0.94			
F-Test	1.26		1.39		1.05			
	Gabin 200 mg cap (PharmEvo)							
Taken	Found	%Rec	Found	%Rec	Found	%Rec	Found	%Rec
200	201.300	100.65	202.20	101.1	199.30	99.65	202.2	101.1
200	200.680	100.34	199.30	99.65	201.50	100.75	197.9	98.95
200	198.950	99.475	198.80	99.4	200.80	100.4	198.6	99.3
200	199.200	99.6	201.30	100.65	201.40	100.7	200.6	100.3
200	198.300	99.15	200.80	100.4	199.40	99.7	200.6	100.3
Mean	199.686	99.843	200.48	100.24	200.48	100.24	199.98	99.99
STD	1.254	0.627092	1.41	0.704805	1.07	0.533151	1.73	0.86342
RSD	0.628	0.628079	0.70	0.703117	0.531875	0.531875	0.86351	0.86351
T-Test	0.68		0.94		0.73			
F-Test	1.25		1.48		1.17			
	Neupentin 400 mg cap (Highnoon)							
Taken	Found	%Rec	Found	%Rec	Found	%Rec	Found	%Rec
400	400.800	100.2	398.40	99.6	398.50	99.625	402.87	100.718
400	402.100	100.525	397.50	99.375	401.20	100.3	400.96	100.24
400	398.600	99.65	401.50	100.375	400.90	100.225	397.5	99.375
400	399.400	99.85	402.80	100.7	401.20	100.3	398.2	99.55
400	398.200	99.55	398.80	99.7	400.90	100.225	404.3	101.075
Mean	399.820	99.955	399.80	99.95	400.54	100.135	400.77	100.192
STD	1.616	0.404042	2.24	0.56097	1.15	0.287554	2.92	0.73106
RSD	0.404	0.404224	0.56	0.561251	0.287167	0.287167	0.729663	0.72967
T-Test	0.74		0.68		0.84			
F-Test	1.39		1.47		1.14			
	Gaba 100 mg cap (NabiQasim)							
Taken	Found	%Rec	Found	%Rec	Found	%Rec	Found	%Rec
100	101.200	101.2	98.58	101.2	101.33	101.33	101.2	101.2
100	99.800	99.8	99.64	99.8	99.66	99.66	98.96	98.96
100	100.600	100.6	110.80	100.6	98.44	98.44	99.47	99.47
100	100.700	100.7	100.33	100.7	101.30	101.3	100.22	100.22
100	99.500	99.5	101.20	99.5	100.66	100.33	99.32	99.32

Table 5 Determination of gabapentin in pharmaceuticals formulations by proposed *(Continued)*

Mean	100.360	100.36	100.11	100.36	100.28	100.278	99.83	99.834
STD	0.695	0.694982	1.03	0.694982	1.23	1.230577	0.89	0.8919
RSD	0.692	0.692489	1.03	0.692489	1.227166	1.227166	0.892481	0.89248
T-Test	0.65		0.88		0.94			
F-Test	1.37		1.62		1.08			

method (Abdellatef & Khalil 2003) using the same samples. Similar accuracy and precision were observed for the calculated and theoretical values (95% confidence) of the proposed and official methods as no remarkable difference was observed for the t and F tests. From Table 5 it is apparent that the present method can be followed for the analysis of these drugs in their single dosage forms. The recoveries in the range from 98.3 to 101.4% clearly showed no interference of any excipients of formulation.

Spectroscopic studies
Infrared spectra
The IR spectra of gabapentin+Nin Complex showed neither the expected doublet of primary NH_2 in the region $3200 - 3400$ cm^{-1} nor the usual carbonyl stretch of COOH near 1710 cm^{-1}. Instead multiple peaks were observed in the region $2500 - 3000$ cm^{-1} that can be attributed to ammonium ion (NH_3^+), the asymmetric and symmetric peaks of carboxylate ion were observed at 1600 and 1400 cm^{-1} coincide with the one observed in amino acids (Wright & Vanderkooi 1997) and NH_3^+ bending at 1550 cm^{-1} conclude that the gabapentin exists in zwitterionic form. Our studies match up to the already reported infrared absorptions of gabapentin (Chimatadar et al. 2007).

NIN produced two broad bands at 3300 and 3250 cm^{-1} and a C-O stretching at 1061 cm^{-1} signify the presence of two OH groups. The carbonyl gave two peaks in the region 1660 to 1760 cm^{-1}. Aromatic resonance appeared at 750 cm^{-1} (Arayne et al. 2008; Charles & Pouchert 1989; Charles & Pouchert 1981).

Primary amines to give Ruhemann's Purple complex with NIN (Arayne et al. 2008). The formation of the complex was evidenced by comparing the spectra of complex with parent reactant. Many of the functionalities of NIN and gabapentin were found absent which confirms the formation of complex. The doublet of

Table 6 Recovery of Gabapentin in presence of different excipient

	Pyrro	Lactose	Talc	Mag Stea	Starch	HPMC
Initial Rate	99.46	99.39	100.26	99.87	101.2	98.96
Rate Constant	98.92	100.66	100.33	99.55	101.47	99.1
Fixed Time	100.43	99.24	101.27	98.92	99.37	100.84

carbonyl in NIN changed significantly into one single sharp peak at 1680 cm^{-1} and the broad band of O-H shifted to 3400 cm^{-1}.

Nuclear magnetic resonance spectra
The ^{1}H NMR spectra of gabapentin showed two $-CH_2$ peaks at Δ 2.443 and Δ 2.873 ppm and the cyclohexyl protons appeared in the region of Δ 1.365–1.585 ppm. The likely peak of NH_2 near Δ 2 ppm and that of carboxylic OH near Δ 11 ppm were not observed but one peak of NH_3^+ at 4.849 Δ ppm was observed, may be as suggested earlier, due to zwitterion formation. Same is also reported in literature (Chimatadar et al. 2007). NIN exhibited two singlets at Δ 7.240 and Δ 7.446 ppm for the four protons of the aromatic group and a singlet at Δ 1.52 ppm for two protons of the OH group. This coincides with the reported studies (Arayne et al. 2008; Charles & Pouchert 1981). By studying the ^{1}H-NMR spectrum of the gaba-NIN complex it was found that the NH_2 protons completely diminished and the broad multiplet appearing between Δ 7.42 and Δ 8.163 ppm showing eight aromatic CH protons. A singlet at Δ 4.803 ppm represents the enolic OH proton. The above results were found in accord with UV and IR spectra, confirming the proposed structure.

Conclusion
The data given above divulge that the proposed methods are easy, accurate and sensitive with good precision and accuracy. With these methods, one can do the analysis with pace at low cost without losing accuracy. The proposed methods can be used as alternative methods to the reported ones for the routine determination of gabapentin in pharmaceutical formulations. This encourages their successful use in routine analysis of these drugs in quality control laboratories.

Competing interests
The authors declare that they have no competing interests.

Authors' contributions
FAS designed, coordinated and carried out experiments the study. NS, NS and HS carried out experiments, FAS, NS, NS, HS and AZ drafted the manuscript. All authors read and approved the final manuscript.

Acknowledgements
Valuable comments of two anonymous reviewers are acknowledged.

Author details

[1]Faculty of Pharmacy, Federal Urdu University Arts, Science and Technology, Karachi 75300, Pakistan. [2]Department of Chemistry, University of Karachi, Karachi 75270, Pakistan. [3]Research Institute of Pharmaceutical Sciences, Faculty of Pharmacy, University of Karachi, Karachi 75270, Pakistan. [4]Department of Environmental Sciences, Federal Urdu University Arts, Science and Technology, Karachi 75300, Pakistan.

References

Abdellatef HE, Khalil HM (2003) Colorimetric determination of gabapentin in pharmaceutical formulation. J Pharmaceut Biomed Anal 31:209–214

Abdulrahman SAM, Basavaiah K (2011) Sensitive and selective spectrophotometric determination of gabapentin in capsules using two nitrophenols as chromogenic agents. Int J Anal Chem 2011:1–9. Article ID 619310. doi:10.1155/2011/619310

Abdulrahman SAM, Basavaiah K (2012) Highly sensitive spectrophotometric method for the determination of gabapentin in capsules using sodium hypochloride. Turk J Pharm Sci 9:113–126

al-Zehouri J, al-Madi S, Belal F (2001) Arzneimittel-forsch 51:97

Arayne MS, Sultana N, Siddiqui FA, Mirza AZ, Zuberi MH (2008) Spectrophotometric techniques to determine tranexamic acid: Kinetic studies using ninhydrin and direct measuring using ferric chloride. J Mol Struc 889:475–480

Belal F, Abdine H, Al-Majed A, Khalil NY (2002) Spectrofluorimetric determination of vigabatrin and gabapentin in urine and dosage forms through derivatization with fluorescamine. J Pharm Biomed Anal 27:253–260

Benesi HA, Hidelbrand J (1949) A Spectrophotometric investigation of the Interaction of Iodine with Aromatic Hydrocarbons. J Am Chem Soc 71:2703

Campins-Falco P, Sevillano-Cabza A, Gallo-Martinez L, Bosch-Reig F (1996) A comparison of various calibration techniques applied to the ninhydrin-cefoxitin determination. Anal Chim Acta 324:199

Chimatadar SA, Basavaraj T, Thabaj KA, Nandibewoor ST (2007) J Mol Catal A Chem 267(1-2):65–71

Chollet DF, Goumaz L, Juliano C, Anderegg G (2000) Fast isocratic high-performance liquid chromatographic assay method for the simultaneous determination of gabapentin and vigabatrin in human serum. J Chromatogr B 746:311–314

Friedman M (2004) Applications of the ninhydrin reaction for analysis of amino acids, peptides, and proteins to agricultural and biomedical sciences. Agric Food Chem 52:385–406

Goldlust A, Su TZ, Welty DF, Taylor CP, Oxender DL (1995) Effects of anticonvulsant drug gabapentin on the enzymes in metabolic pathways of glutamate and GABA. Epilepsy Res 22:1–11

Görög S (1995) Ultraviolet–Visible Spectrophotometry in Pharmaceutical Analysis. CRC Press, New York, p 318

Hassan EM, Belal F, Al-Deeb OA, Khalil NY (2001) Spectrofluorimetric determination of vigabatrin and gabapentin in dosage forms and spiked plasma samples through derivatization with 4-chloro-7-nitrobenzo-2-oxa-1,3-diazole. J AOAC Int 84:1017–1024

Hegde RN, Kumara Swamy BE, Shetti NP, Nandibewoor ST (2009) Electro-oxidation and determination of gabapentin at gold electrode. J Electroanal Chem 635:51–57

ICH Topic Q2(R1) (2005) Validation of analytical procedures: text and methodology. Current step 4 version parent guideline dated 27 October 1994 (Complementary Guideline on Methodology dated 6 November 1996 incorporated in November 2005)

Ifa DR, Falci M, Moraes ME, Bezerra FA, Moraes MO, de Nucci G, (2001) Gabapentin quantification in human plasma by high-performance liquid chromatography coupled to electrospray tandem mass spectrometry. Application to bioequivalence study. J Mass Spectro 36:188–194

Jalali F, Arkan E, Bahrami G (2007) Preparation of a gabapentin potentiometric sensor and its application to pharmaceutical analysis. Sens Actuat B: Chem 127:304–309

Jia S, Lee HS, Choi MJ, Hyun Sung S, Sang BH, et al. (2012) Non-derivatization method for the determination of gabapentin in pharmaceutical formulations, Rat serum and Rat urine using high performance liquid chromatography coupled with charged aerosol detection. Curr Anal Chem 8:159–167

Jiang Q, Li S (1999) Rapid high-performance liquid chromatographic determination of serum gabapentin. J Chromatogr B 727:119–123

Kushnir MM, Crossett J, Brown PI, Urry FM (1999) Analysis of gabapentin in serum and plasma by solid-phase extraction and gas chromatography-mass spectrometry for therapeutic drug monitoring. J Anal Toxicol 23:1–6

Lin FM, Kou HS, Wu SM, Chen SH, Wu HL (2004) Capillary electrophoresis analysis of gabapentin and vigabatrin in pharmaceutical preparations as ofloxacin derivatives. Anal Chim Acta 523:9–14

Manera M, Miro M, Ribeiro MF, Estela JM, Cerda V, et al. (2009) Rapid chemiluminometric determination of gabapentin in pharmaceutical formulations exploiting pulsed-flow analysis. Luminescence 24:10–14

Martin AN, Swarbrick J, Cammarata A (1969) Physical Pharmacy, 3rd edition. Lee & Febiger, Philadelphia, PA, p 344

Molnar-Perl I, Pinter-Szakacs M (1989) Spectrophotometric determination of tryptophan in intact proteins by the acid ninhydrin method. Anal Biochem 177:16–19

Nobrega Jde A, Fatibello-Filho O, Vieira Ida C (1994) Flow injection spectrophotometric determination of aspartame in dietary products. Analyst 119:2101–2104

Ouellet D, Bockbrader HN, Wesche DL, Shapiro DY, Garofalo E (2001) Population pharmacokinetics of gabapentin in infants and children. Epilepsy Res 47:229–241

Patel B, Patel J, Singh H, Patel B (2011) Extractive spectrophotometric methods for the determination of gabapentin in pharmaceutical dosage forms. Int J Pharma Sci Drug Res 3:197–201

Pouchert JC (1981) The Aldrich library of infrared spectra, Volume 2, 2nd edition. Aldrich Chemical Company, University of California

Pouchert JC (1983) The Aldrich library of NMR Spectra, 2 Volume Set, 2nd edition. Bookseller: Mountainview Books, Hopeland, PA, USA

Rada P, Tucci S, Perez J, Teneud L, Chuecos S, Hernandez L (1998) In vivo monitoring of gabapentin in rats: a microdialysis study coupled to capillary electrophoresis and laser-induced fluorescence detection. Electrophoresis 19:2976–2980

Rahman N, Azmi SNH (2001a) Spectrophotometric method for the determination of amlodipine besylate with ninhydrin in drug formulations. IL Farmaco 56:731–735

Rahman N, Azmi SN (2001b) Farmacokinetics 56:731–735

Ratnaraj N, Patsalos PN (1998) A high-performance liquid chromatography micromethod for the simultaneous determination of vigabatrin and gabapentin in serum. Ther Drug Monit 20:430–434

Ribeiro MF, Santos JL, Lima JL (2007) Piezoelectric pumping in flow analysis: application to the spectrophotometric determination of gabapentin. Anal Chim Acta 600:14–20

Rose J (1964) Adv Physico-Chem Exp. Pittman, London, p 54

Siddiqui FA, Arayne MS, Sultana N, Qureshi F, Mirza AZ, et al. (2010) Spectrophotometric determination of gabapentin in pharmaceutical formulations using ninhydrin and pi-acceptors. Eur J Med Chem 45:2761–2767

Tang PH, Miles MV, Glauser TA, DeGrauw T (1999) Automated microanalysis of gabapentin in human serum by high-performance liquid chromatography with fluorometric detection. J Chromatogr B 727:125–129

Van Lentea F, Gatautis V (1998) Cost-efficient use of gas chromatography–mass spectrometry: a "piggyback" method for analysis of gabapentin. Clin Chem 44:2044–2045

Wad N, Kramer G (1998) Sensitive high-performance liquid chromatographic method with fluorometric detection for the simultaneous determination of gabapentin and vigabatrin in serum and uein. J Chromatogr B 705:154–158

Wright WW, Vanderkooi JM (1997) Use of IR absorption of the carboxyl group of amino acids and their metabolites to determine pKs, to study proteins, and to monitor enzymatic activity. Biospectroscopy 3:457–467

9

Correction of spike contribution for strontium isotopic measurement by thermal ionization mass spectrometry: a test for spike-standard mixed solutions

Chang-sik Cheong[1*], Youn-Joong Jeong[1] and Sung-Tack Kwon[2]

Abstract

Background: The Rb-Sr isotope system has long been used for radiometric dating and petrogenetic investigation. The concentrations of Rb and Sr could be precisely measured by isotope dilution thermal ionization mass spectrometry combined with chemical purification of these elements. For the simultaneous measurement of Sr isotopic composition and isotope dilution, the contribution from the added spike should be carefully corrected.

Findings: Reliable $^{87}Sr/^{86}Sr$ ratios of the spike-standard mixed solutions were obtained using the new mass bias factor calculated on the basis of measured Sr isotopic ratios. This correction yielded reasonable $^{87}Sr/^{86}Sr$ ratios for overspiked standard solutions whose spike fractions reaching 25 wt.%.

Conclusions: The correction procedure described in this study shows that the simultaneous measurement of Sr isotopic composition and isotope dilution is available for the case that the spike proportion in the sample-spike mixture is significantly high ($^{84}Sr/^{86}Sr > 3.7$). The principle of this correction protocol can also be applied to other isotope systems such as Sm-Nd and Lu-Hf pairs.

Keywords: Rb-Sr; Thermal ionization mass spectrometry; Isotope dilution; Spike contribution

Findings

Introduction

Rubidium-87 decays to stable ^{87}Sr by emission of β^- particle with a decay constant of $1.420 (\pm0.010) \times 10^{-11}$ years^{-1} (Steiger and Jäger 1977) which corresponds to a half-life of 48.8×10^9 years. It is notable that this International Union of Geological Sciences-accepted decay constant is being considered to be high by 1% to 2% as summarized in Begemann et al. (2001). Rubidium and strontium belong to the groups IA and IIA, respectively. They are easily fractionated from each other through geological processes such as partial melting and igneous and metamorphic mineral growth. Therefore, the ^{87}Rb-^{87}Sr isotope system has long been used for radiometric dating and petrogenetic investigation (Faure and Mensing 2005).

The traditional thermal ionization mass spectrometry (TIMS) is still regarded as the benchmark technique to measure Rb-Sr isotope ratios. By TIMS, the inter-elemental ratio cannot be directly measured but is obtained through isotope dilution (Moore et al. 1973), a method of analyzing chemical substances by the addition of isotopically enriched spike to the sample. Considering the inhomogeneous distribution of Rb and Sr in most geological samples, simultaneous measurement of Sr isotopic composition and isotope dilution is essential. In this case, inevitable contribution from the spike should be carefully corrected.

This study evaluates the effectiveness of correction protocol to measure $^{87}Sr/^{86}Sr$ ratio in a series of mixture of ^{84}Sr-enriched spike and standard solution. It has been tested whether a reasonable $^{87}Sr/^{86}Sr$ ratio could be obtained for overspiked standard solutions of which spike fractions reach 45 wt.%.

* Correspondence: ccs@kbsi.re.kr
[1]Division of Earth and Environmental Sciences, Korea Basic Science Institute, Ochang, Chungbuk 363-883, Republic of Korea
Full list of author information is available at the end of the article

Availability and requirements

Preparation of spike and standard solution

The ^{84}Sr-enriched isotope spike and standard solutions were prepared at the Korea Basic Science Institute (KBSI) in Ochang. In the following, all errors are quoted on the basis of 2 σ standard error, unless stated otherwise.

The spike, $SrCO_3$ form, was provided by the Oak Ridge National Laboratory (batch number = 236,201, order number = 65-0056). It was dissolved in hot 10% HNO_3 and diluted to about 15 µg/g solution with 5% HNO_3. The AnApure^{TM} ICP standard of 1,002 (±10) mg/L Sr (lot no. AEP-130-726) was diluted to 21.480 µg/g solution in 2% HNO_3 (the specific gravity of 2% HNO_3 = 1.028 g/mL) and then was admixed with the spike solution. Ten mixed solutions were prepared with mixing proportions (spike/standard) ranging from about 1:1.2 to 1:70 in weight.

Instrumental analysis

The Rb-Sr isotopic analysis was conducted by using a Phoenix (Isotopx) TIMS, Cheshire, CW, UK, installed at the KBSI. This instrument is equipped with eight movable Faraday collectors and one fixed axial channel where the ion beam intensities can be measured with either a Faraday collector or an ion counting Daly detector.

In this study, all required isotopes were simultaneously detected on Faraday collectors. The sensitivity on ^{88}Sr was typically around 3 V (10^{11} Ω resistors). The strontium isotope measurements of the standard and spike-standard mixed solutions were performed with a multi-dynamic mode (Lenz and Wendt 1976) in which the Faraday collectors were set to simultaneously detect ^{84}Sr (axial), ^{86}Sr (H2), ^{87}Sr (H3), and ^{88}Sr (H4) for the first static run, and ^{84}Sr (L2), ^{86}Sr (H1), ^{87}Sr (H2), and ^{88}Sr (H3) for the second run. One measurement consists of 5 blocks of 12 cycles with an integration time of 10 s. The mass bias was exponentially normalized to ^{86}Sr/^{88}Sr = 0.1194. The mean multi-dynamic ^{87}Sr/^{86}Sr acquired for NBS987 was 0.710252 ± 0.000007 ($n = 7$) during the course of this study.

The isotopic composition of ^{84}Sr-enriched spike was measured with a multi-static mode (100 cycles, 5 blocks, integration time = 10 s) in which the Faraday collectors were set to detect ^{84}Sr (axial), ^{86}Sr (H2), ^{87}Sr (H3), and ^{88}Sr (H4). In this measurement, the instrumental mass fractionation was not normalized.

Results and discussion

Five measurements for the ^{84}Sr spike yielded an average ^{84}Sr/^{88}Sr of 561.4 ± 0.9, ^{86}Sr/^{88}Sr of 0.7661 ± 0.0010, and ^{87}Sr/^{88}Sr of 0.1819 ± 0.0030, respectively. Therefore, the ^{84}Sr enrichment and atomic weight of the spike are calculated to be 83.9242 and 99.65 at.%, respectively. Although the instrumental mass fractionation was not

corrected during the TIMS measurement, this enrichment value is well matched with the suggested value (99.64 ± 0.01%, Tracy 1999). The exponentially normalized multi-dynamic measurement of the Sr standard yielded an average ^{87}Sr/^{86}Sr ratio of 0.707630 ± 0.000009 ($n = 5$).

The Sr isotope ratios measured for the spike-standard mixed solutions have been normalized to ^{86}Sr/^{88}Sr = 0.1194. This mass bias correction is not valid because the ^{86}Sr/^{88}Sr of the added spike was significantly shifted from the natural value through the enrichment processes from 0.1194 to 0.7661. The first step for the correction of spike contribution is to determine a new mass bias factor (α_{new}) from the measured Sr isotope ratios. In the following, 's' denotes the normal Sr standard, 't' denotes the Sr spike, and 'm' and 'c' represent the measured and corrected values, respectively. The $(86t/86s)$ can be calculated using $(84/86)m$, $(84/86)s$, and $(84/86)t$:

$$\left(\frac{84}{86}\right)_m = \frac{84_s + 84_t}{86_s + 86_t} = \frac{\frac{84_s}{86_s} + \frac{84_t}{86_s}}{1 + \frac{86_t}{86_s}}$$
$$= \frac{\left(\frac{84}{86}\right)_s + \frac{86_t}{86_s} \times \left(\frac{84}{86}\right)_t}{1 + \frac{86_t}{86_s}}$$

$$\left(\frac{86_t}{86_s}\right) = \frac{\left(\frac{84}{86}\right)_m - \left(\frac{84}{86}\right)_s}{\left(\frac{84}{86}\right)_t - \left(\frac{84}{86}\right)_m},$$

$$\left(\frac{88_t}{88_s}\right) = \frac{\frac{88_t}{86_t} \times 86_t}{\frac{88_s}{86_s} \times 86_s}$$

Because the measured 84/86 ratio used in the above calculation has an uncertainty due to incorrect normalization to 86/88 = 0.1194, the $86t/86s$ should be recalculated after determination of the new mass bias factor (see below).

The $(86/88)s$ can be reduced by using $(86/88)m$, $(88t/88s)$, and $(86/88)t$:

$$\left(\frac{86}{88}\right)_m = \frac{\left(\frac{86}{88}\right)_s + \frac{88_t}{88_s} \times \left(\frac{86}{88}\right)_t}{1 + \frac{88_t}{88_s}},$$

$$\left(\frac{86}{88}\right)_s = \left(\frac{86}{88}\right)_m \times \left(1 + \frac{88_t}{88_s}\right) - \left(\frac{86}{88}\right)_t \times \frac{88_t}{88_s}$$

The mass fractionation can now be accurately corrected using the calculated $(86/88)s$. The exponential law (Russel et al. 1978) yields a mass bias factor before (α_{old}) and after (α_{new}) the spike correction as the following:

$$\alpha_{old} = \frac{\ln\left(\frac{0.1194}{\left(\frac{86}{88}\right)_m}\right)}{\ln\left(\frac{M_{86}}{M_{88}}\right)}, \alpha_{new} = \frac{\ln\left(\frac{0.1194}{\left(\frac{86}{88}\right)_s}\right)}{\ln\left(\frac{M_{86}}{M_{88}}\right)},$$

where 'M' denotes the mass of the isotope.

Table 1 Correction results for the spike-standard mixed solutions

	86/88$_m$	% SE	84/86$_m$	% SE	84/86$_c$	87/86$_m$	% SE	87/86$_s$	2 σ SE	Spike wt.%
Mix 1	0.12090	0.0068	8.4583	0.0050	8.5427	0.705574	0.0011	0.707582	0.000016	45.1
Mix 2	0.12034	0.0089	3.6918	0.0094	3.7076	0.706777	0.0009	0.707634	0.000013	25.9
Mix 3	0.12030	0.0048	2.4858	0.0051	2.4929	0.707068	0.0010	0.707640	0.000014	18.9
Mix 4	0.12032	0.0049	1.9667	0.0050	1.9711	0.707165	0.0009	0.707615	0.000013	15.5
Mix 5	0.11982	0.0179	1.5658	0.0187	1.5686	0.707292	0.0010	0.707644	0.000014	12.6
Mix 6	0.12016	0.0016	1.2043	0.0022	1.2059	0.707349	0.0010	0.707618	0.000014	9.9
Mix 7	0.11983	0.0034	0.7787	0.0030	0.7794	0.707469	0.0008	0.707638	0.000011	6.5
Mix 8	0.11976	0.0143	0.4234	0.0147	0.4236	0.707568	0.0010	0.707653	0.000014	3.4
Mix 9	0.12023	0.0185	0.2831	0.0103	0.2832	0.707593	0.0010	0.707646	0.000014	2.1
Mix 10	0.11983	0.0145	0.2071	0.0173	0.2072	0.707575	0.0010	0.707610	0.000014	1.4
Average[a]								0.707633		
SD[a]								0.000015		
2σ SE[a]								0.000010		

[a]The result of mix 1 is excluded.

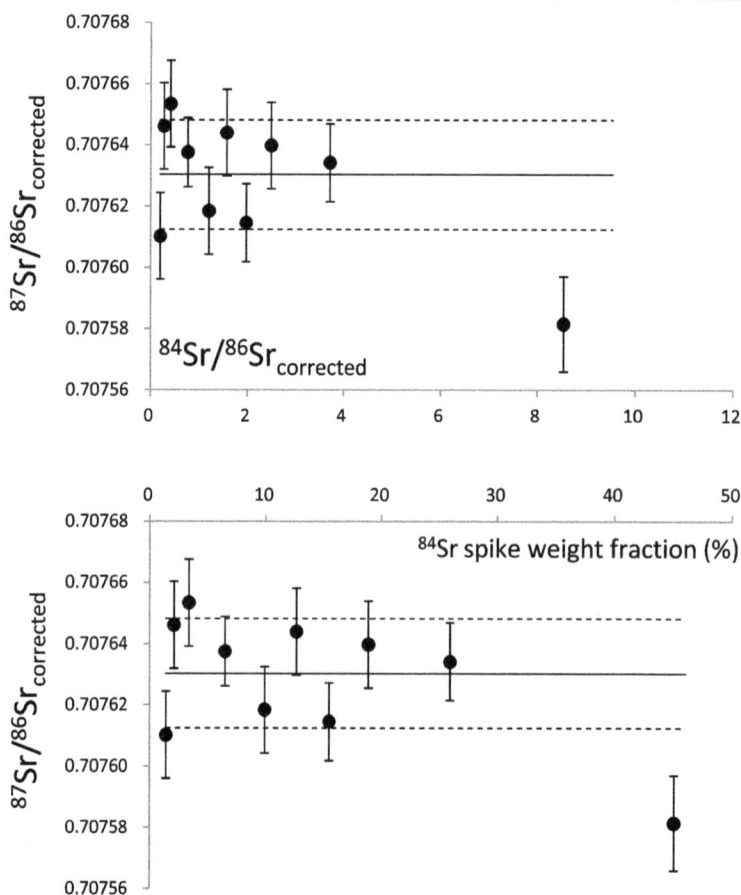

Figure 1 Plots of corrected ^{87}Sr/^{86}Sr as a function of ^{84}Sr/^{86}Sr and weight fractions of the spike. Solid and dashed lines represent an average ^{87}Sr/^{86}Sr and 2 σ standard deviation of the unspiked standard data, respectively. Error bars are based on within-run 2 σ standard error.

The newly corrected (84/86) ratio used for isotope dilution is yielded as the following:

$$\left(\frac{84}{86}\right)_{\text{instrumentally measured}} = \left(\frac{84}{86}\right)_{c(\text{old})} \times \left(\frac{M_{86}}{M_{84}}\right)^{\propto_{\text{old}}}$$

$$\left(\frac{84}{86}\right)_{c(\text{new})} = \left(\frac{84}{86}\right)_{\text{instrumentally measured}} \times \left(\frac{M_{84}}{M_{86}}\right)^{\propto_{\text{new}}}$$

The newly corrected (84/86) ratios of the ten mixed solutions yielded a mean Sr concentration of 15.271 ± 0.031 µg/g for the [84]Sr-enriched spike prepared in this study.

Also, the (87/86)c can be newly calculated using measured Sr isotope ratios as the following.

$$\left(\frac{87}{86}\right)_{c\ (\text{new})} = \left(\frac{87}{86}\right)_{\text{instrumentally measured}} \times \left(\frac{M_{87}}{M_{86}}\right)^{\propto_{\text{new}}}$$

Actually, $\left(\frac{87}{86}\right)_{\text{instrumentally measured}}$

$$= \left(\frac{87}{86}\right)_{c\ (\text{old})} \times \left(\frac{M_{86}}{M_{87}}\right)^{\propto_{\text{old}}}$$

Finally, the (87/86)c(new) is used for the calculation of the (87/86)s:

$$\left(\frac{87}{86}\right)_s = \left(\frac{87}{86}\right)_{c\ (\text{new})} \times \left(1 + \frac{86_t}{86_s}\right) - \left(\frac{87}{86}\right)_t \times \frac{86_t}{86_s}\ \text{because}\ \left(\frac{87}{86}\right)_m$$

$$= \frac{87_s + 87_t}{86_s + 86_t} = \frac{\frac{87_s}{86_s} + \frac{87_t}{86_s}}{1 + \frac{86_t}{86_s}} = \frac{\left(\frac{87}{86}\right)_s + \frac{86_t}{86_s} \times \left(\frac{87}{86}\right)_t}{1 + \frac{86_t}{86_s}}\ \text{(it is noted}$$

that 86t/86s can be recalculated on the basis of newly corrected 84/86).

Table 1 summarizes the spike correction results for the ten spike-standard mixed solutions. The corrected [87]Sr/[86]Sr ratios of the mixed solutions are displayed in Figure 1 with the measured values of the unspiked standard. As shown in Figure 1, the protocol described in this study successfully corrected the spike contribution in the case that the spike fraction in the mixture reaches 25 wt.% ([84]Sr/[86]Sr$_{\text{mixture}}$ > 3.7). It is not clear why the corrected [87]Sr/[86]Sr ratio for mix 1 solution (spike fraction = 45.1 wt.%) deviates from the unspiked standard value. The corrected [87]Sr/[86]Sr ratios of nine mixed solutions (mix 2 to mix 10) yield an indistinguishable average of 0.707633 ± 0.000010 from the unspiked value (0.707630 ± 0.000009). There is no trend between the corrected [87]Sr/[86]Sr and the spike fraction (or [84]Sr/[86]Sr$_{\text{mixture}}$) in the range from 1.4 to 25.9 wt.%. It is noted that the principle of this correction protocol can also be applied to other isotope systems such as Sm-Nd and Lu-Hf pairs, as briefly interpreted in the study of Cheong and Kwon (2010).

Competing interests

The authors declare that they have no competing interests.

Acknowledgements

This study was supported by the KBSI grant (G34200).

Author details

[1]Division of Earth and Environmental Sciences, Korea Basic Science Institute, Ochang, Chungbuk 363-883, Republic of Korea. [2]Department of Earth System Sciences, Yonsei University, Seoul 120-749, Republic of Korea.

References

Begemann F, Ludwig KR, Lugmair GW, Min K, Nyquist LE, Patchett PJ, Renne PR, Shin CY, Villa IM, Walker RJ (2001) Call for an improved set of decay constants for geochronological use. Geochim Cosmochim Acta 65:111–121

Cheong CS, Kwon ST (2010) Calibration of Sm-Nd mixed spike by Teflon powder method. J Anal Sci Tech 1:30–36

Faure G, Mensing TM (2005) Isotopes: Principles and applications, 3rd edn. John Wiley & Sons, Hoboken

Lenz H, Wendt I (1976) Use of a double collector for high-precision isotope ratio measurements in geochronology. Adv Mass Spectrom 7A:565–568

Moore LJ, Moody JR, Barnes IL, Gramlich JW, Murphy TJ, Paulsen PJ, Shields WR (1973) Trace determination of rubidium and strontium in silicate glass standard reference materials. Anal Chem 45:2384–2387

Russel WA, Papanastassiou DA, Tombrello TA (1978) Ca isotope fractionation on the earth and other solar system materials. Geochim Cosmochim Acta 42:1075–1090

Steiger RH, Jäger E (1977) Subcommission on geochronology: convention on the use of decay constants in geo- and cosmochronology. Earth Planet Sci Lett 36:359–362

Tracy JG (1999) High-purity enrichment of [84]Sr. Nucl Instrum Methods Phys Res Sect A 438:1–6

10

Spectroscopic characterization of *in vitro* interactions of cetirizine and NSAIDS

Hina Shamshad[1*], M Saeed Arayne[1] and Najma Sultana[2]

Abstract

Background: Cetirizine (anti-allergy agent) and non-steroidal anti-inflammatory drugs (NSAIDs; anti-inflammatory agents) are co-administered drugs. Cetirizine, a P-glycopretein substrate may be affected by the use of NSAIDs. In the present work, quantification of cetirizine in the presence of commonly co-administered NSAIDs such as diclofenac sodium, ibuprofen, flurbiprofen, tiaprofenac acid, meloxicam and mefenamic acid were studied using the RP-HPLC technique.

Methods: A high-throughput HPLC method for the analysis of cetirizine was developed, validated in the presence of NSAIDs and was further used to study the interactions of cetirizine in the presence of NSAIDs at four different pH levels. Purospher Star, C18 column (5 μm, 25 cm × 0.46 cm) with a mobile phase of methanol/water (90:10 v/v, pH adjusted to 3.5) at a flow rate of 1.0 mL/min and a wavelength of 240 nm was used.

Results: The synthesis of cetirizine in the presence of NSAIDs was carried out, and complexes were characterized using infrared (IR) and nuclear magnetic resonance (NMR) techniques. The method was found to be applicable in serum and was found useful for therapeutic purposes. The differences in availabilities of cetirizine with NSAIDs at three pH levels clearly indicated the interactions of afore mentioned drugs.

Conclusions: The findings suggested further studies on the co-administration of these two drugs simultaneously in order to know the pharmacokinetic and pharmacodynamic profiles of the drugs. It is highly recommended to have a suitable time lapse between the oral uses of these drugs.

Keywords: Cetirizine; Drug interaction; HPLC method; NSAIDs

Background

Second- and third-generation antihistamines are P-glycoprotein substrates. Drugs that affect the P-glycoprotein may lead to drug-drug interactions (Scott and Kelly 2003; Jarkko et al. 2006; Renwick 1999). Cetirizine being a P-glycoprotein substrate may interact with commonly co-administered drugs such as NSAIDs that may affect the P-glycoprotein expression (Lee et al. 2007), as celecoxib and diclofenac, were found to inhibit the function of P-glycoprotein (Wageh et al. 2004). It has been established that synergistic effect was exhibited by the combined use of cetirizine with nimesulide (Rewari and Gupta 1999). Moreover, cetirizine was found to possess analgesic activity in mice (Priya et al. 2013). Cetirizine and mefenamic acid combination was also developed for the treatment of respiratory disorder (Philip and Philip 2010). Nimesulide and cetirizine combination was also prepared which was found to possess anti-leukotriene, antihistamine, anti-allergy, and anti-inflammatory actions (Singh and Jain 2003). Drug interactions of cetirizine have also been reported in literature (Ihsan et al. 2005; Arayne et al. 2010a; Sultana et al. 2010).

Simultaneous HPLC method for the determination of paracetamol, phenylpropanolamine hydrochloride, and cetirizine was reported; however, the mobile phase consisted methanol and disodium hydrogen phosphate dihydrate buffer which could be corrosive to the column (Suryan et al. 2011). Another simultaneous method of paracetamol, acetyl salicylic acid, mefenamic acid, and cetirizine was achieved using disodium hydrogen phosphate buffer and acetonitrile combination which could once again be corrosive and expensive altogether (Freddy and Dharmendra 2010). Separation method of ibuprofen, phenylephrine HCl, and cetirizine from soft gels was

---
* Correspondence: chemdoc9@gmail.com
[1]Research Institute of Pharmaceutical Sciences, Department of Pharmaceutical Chemistry, Faculty of Pharmacy, University of Karachi, Karachi 75270, Pakistan
Full list of author information is available at the end of the article

reported using the mobile phase of acetonitrile and hexanosulphonate (Cosmes and Rodriguez 2012). Simultaneous determination of cetirizine and aceclofenac was achieved by using mobile phase of acetonitrile and heptane sulphonic acid (Padmavathi and Niranjan 2011). Nimesulide, cetirizine, and pseudoephedrine hydrochloride separation was done by using acetonitrile/phosphate buffer/triethyl amine as the mobile phase (Jain et al. 2012). Our group also reported methods of simultaneous determination of cetirizine with anti-diabetic drug (Arayne et al. 2010b) and with H_2 receptor antagonists (Sultana et al. 2010).

It is clearly evident from the above literature that most of the simultaneous methods used acetonitrile as solvent which is quite expensive. In others, buffers were also used which is column corrosive. In order to quantify the drugs and understand the degree of interactions, a fast, least expensive, efficient HPLC method was required, which could be used for therapeutic purposes and could also be employed for routine analysis work.

So, in the present work, cetirizine method was developed and validated in the presence of NSAIDs such as diclofenac sodium, ibuprofen, flurbiprofen, meloxicam, and mefenamic acid using the RP-HPLC method. The method was further used to study the interactions of the cetirizine in the presence of NSAIDs at three pH levels, i.e., 4, 7.4, and 9. Cetirizine complexes were also synthesized with interacting drugs. The synthesized complexes were characterized by their physical parameters as well as by the techniques of infrared (IR) and nuclear magnetic resonance (NMR).

Methods

Materials

Raw materials used were of pharmaceutical purity and formulations as cetirizine (Zyrtec), mefenamic acid (Ponstan), diclofenac sodium (Voren), flurbiprofen (Froben), meloxicam (Melfex), tiaprofenic acid (Surgam), and ibuprofen (Brofen) were purchased from local markets. Analytical grade reagents were used during the whole experimental procedures. Methanol of HPLC grade (TEDIA®, USA) and other reagents included were hydrochloric acid, sodium hydroxide, sodium chloride, potassium dihydrogen orthophosphate, disodium hydrogen orthophosphate, ammonium chloride, 10% NH_3 solution, phosphoric acid 85% (Merck, Darmstadt, Germany) were utilized.

Equipment

Shimadzu HPLC system (Kyoto, Japan) equipped with LC-10 AT VP pump, with a 20-μl loop, Purospher® Star, RP-18 endcapped (5 μm) column and SPD-10 A VP UV-vis detector was utilized. IR studies were carried out using a Shimadzu Model Fourier transform infrared (FTIR) Prestige-21 spectrophotometer. Spectral treatment was performed using Shimadzu IR solution 1.2 software. The ^{1}H-NMR spectra were recorded on a Bruker AMX 500 MHz

spectrometer (Madison, WI, USA) using TMS as an internal standard.

Method development

Optimized conditions for separation

The chromatographic analysis was performed at laboratory temperature (25°C) with isocratic elution. The optimized conditions for the separation of the eluents were achieved by using the mobile phase of methanol/water 90:10 monitored by UV detection 240 nm at a flow rate of 1 ml min^{-1} with pH 3.5 adjusted by orthophosphoric acid. The samples from these solutions were injected in to the system six times.

Reference standard solutions

Stock reference standard solutions of all drugs were prepared by dissolving appropriate amounts of each drug in a mobile phase to yield concentrations of 100 μg ml^{-1}. For calibration curve studies, serial dilutions in the concentration range of 50 to 3.12 μg ml^{-1} were injected in triplicate.

Pharmaceutical dosage form samples

Commercially available pharmaceutical formulations of the respective brands were evaluated by groups of 20 tablets for each drug and dissolved in mobile phase according to the labeled claim. The samples from this solution were injected into the system in triplicate.

Standard drug plasma solutions

The supernatant obtained by centrifuging blood samples was deprotonated by acetonitrile, spiked daily with working solutions, and chromatographed.

Method development protocol

Certain parameters such as mobile phase composition and pH, flow rate, diluents of solutions, and wavelength of analytes were altered in order to achieve symmetrical and well-resolved peaks at a reasonable retention time.

Method validation

All validation steps were carried out according to the ICH guidelines such as system suitability, selectivity, specificity, linearity (concentration-detector response relationship), accuracy, precision, and sensitivity, i.e., detection and quantification limit.

System suitability

System suitability was assessed by examining the six replicates of the drugs at a specific concentration for repeatability, peaks symmetry (symmetry factor), theoretical plates, resolution, and capacity factors.

Specificity

The drugs were spiked with pharmaceutical formulations containing different excipients.

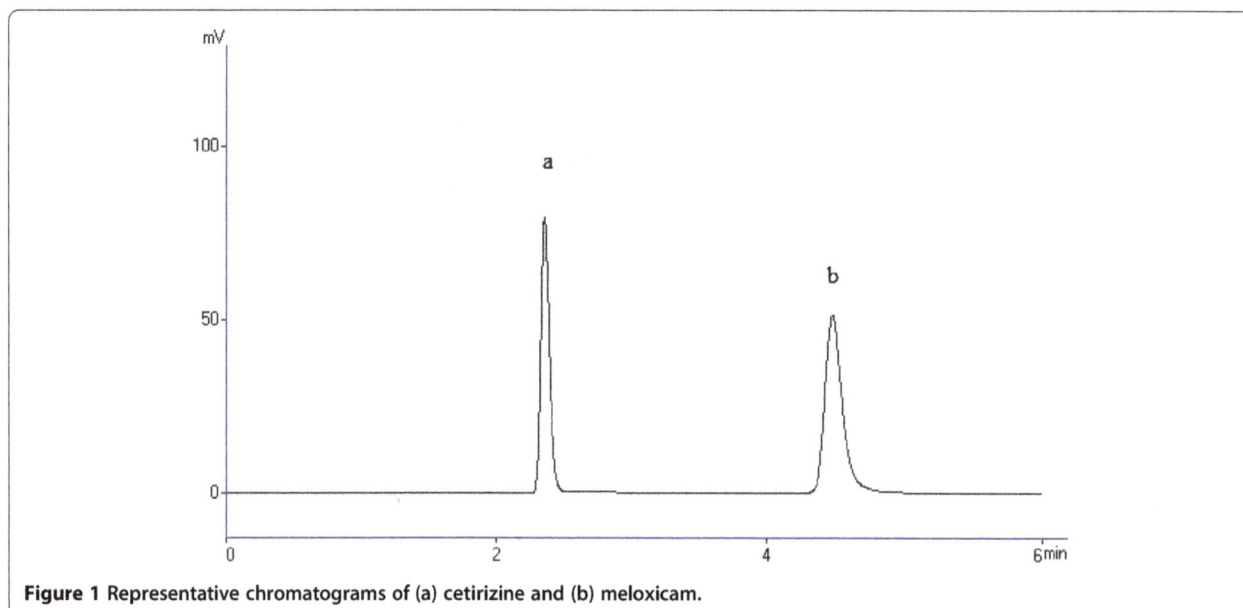

Figure 1 Representative chromatograms of (a) cetirizine and (b) meloxicam.

Linearity

The linearity of the method was evaluated at different concentrations. Linear correlation coefficient, intercept, and slope values were calculated for statistical analysis.

Accuracy

The accuracy of the method was established at three concentration levels (80%, 100%, and 120%) in triplets, and percent recovery (%recovery) was calculated in each case.

Precision

Six replicates of a concentration range were injected to system on two different non-consecutive days and percent relative standard deviation (%RSD) was calculated.

Limit of detection and quantification

The LOD and LOQ of the method were calculated.

Drug–drug interaction studies

The 50-µg ml^{-1} solutions of all the drugs alone and those in combination with cetirizine were made and kept on water bath for 120 min at 37°C. Five milliliters of an aliquot was withdrawn after every 15-min interval, after making dilutions was filtered and injected in to the HPLC system in triplicate. The concentration of each drug was determined and %recovery was calculated.

Synthesis of cetirizine and interacting drugs

Different complexes of cetirizine with NSAIDs (diclofenac sodium, flurbiprofen, ibuprofen, meloxicam, mefenamic acid, tirprofenac acid) were synthesized. Equimolar solution

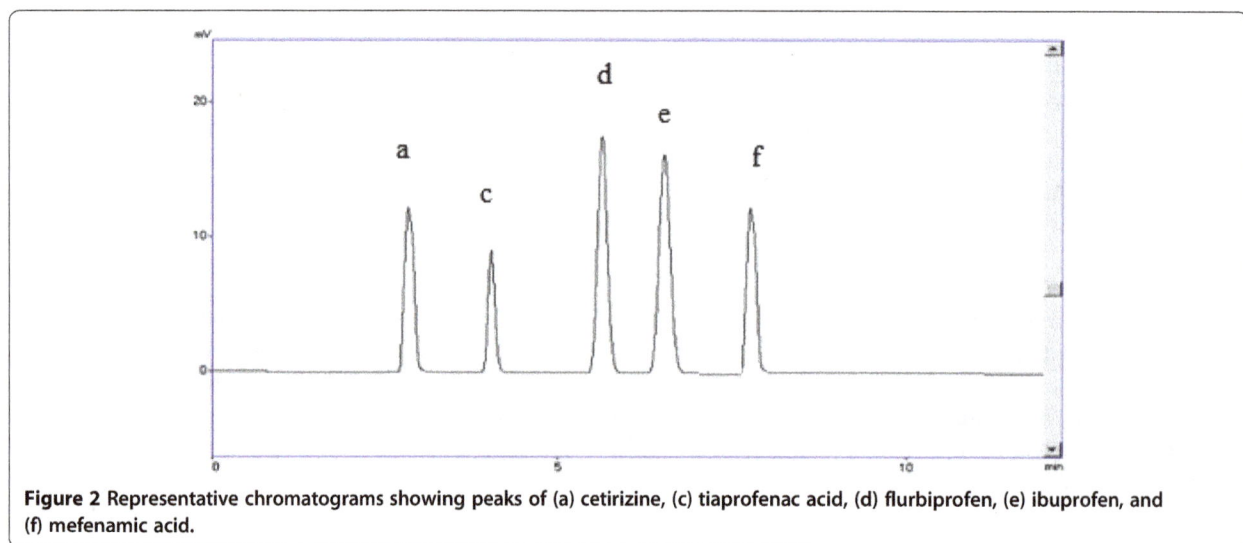

Figure 2 Representative chromatograms showing peaks of (a) cetirizine, (c) tiaprofenac acid, (d) flurbiprofen, (e) ibuprofen, and (f) mefenamic acid.

Table 1 Regression statistics and sensitivity of the proposed method

Drugs	r^2	LOQ ($\mu g\ ml^{-1}$)	LOD ($\mu g\ ml^{-1}$)
Tiaprofenac acid	0.998	0.47	0.14
Diclofenac sodium	0.999	0.56	0.24
Flurbiprofen	0.999	0.7	0.76
Ibuprofen	0.998	1.78	0.53
Mefenamic acid	0.997	0.81	0.24
Meloxicam	0.997	0.16	0.05

of each NSAIDs solutions were mixed with cetirizine solution and were refluxed for 3 h. They were then filtered and left for drying at room temperature. Melting point and physical characteristics of these complexes were observed.

Spectroscopic studies of complexes
Infrared studies
Cetirizine and its complexes were characterized by FTIR spectrophotometry using the potassium bromide disc method in the region of 400 to 4,000 cm^{-1}. The infrared spectra were recorded as attenuated total reflection (ATR) or smart performer accessory was used for the sample (minimum amount).

^{1}H NMR studies
Proton NMR studies were carried out on a Bruker instrument in deuterated water, methanol, and chloroform using TMS as an internal standard.

Results and discussion
Method development and validation
User friendly method in active, pharmaceutical preparations and in serum by UV detection (240 nm) was developed for cetirizine and tiaprofenac acid, flurbiprofen, ibuprofen and mefenamic acid eluting out simultaneously at 2.5, 3.8, 4.8, 5.30, and 7.1 min, respectively (Figures 1 and 2). Meloxicam and diclofenac sodium eluting out at 4.4 and 5.30 min were determined separately in the presence of cetirizine. The mobile phase consisted of methanol water at a ratio of 90:10 (pH 3.5) and a flow rate of 1 ml min^{-1}. NSAIDs and

Table 2 Accuracy and precision of method

Drugs	Conc. ($\mu g\ ml^{-1}$)	%RSD	%recovery
Cetirizine	80	0.02	101.72
	100	0.52	100.64
	120	0.87	99.62
Tiaprofenac acid	80	0.99	100.44
	100	0.67	101.11
	120	0.47	100.84
Diclofenac sodium	80	0.14	99.83
	100	0.34	102.36
	120	0.56	99.98
Flurbiprofen	80	0.6	97.42
	100	0.87	96.35
	120	0.45	98.11
Ibuprofen	80	0.36	103.55
	100	0.74	104.87
	120	0.88	104.12
Mefenamic acid	80	0.12	102.66
	100	0.14	100.22
	120	0.72	103.99
Meloxicam	80	0.41	100.21
	100	0.21	98.77
	120	0.87	98.14

cetirizine separated efficiently with well-resolved and symmetrical peaks of all the drugs. Linearity was demonstrated by running pharmaceutical standards at seven concentrations over the range of 50 to 3.12 $\mu g\ ml^{-1}$ for two consecutive days. The correlation coefficient in each case was monitored and shown in Table 1.

The mean linear regression equations of tiaprofenac acid, diclofenac sodium, flurbiprofen, ibuprofen, mefenamic acid, and meloxicam were found to be $y = 28,166x + 54,952$, $y = 19,567x + 8,726.8$, $y = 12,759x + 10,846$, $y = 6,296.4x - 6,507.9$, $y = 11,989x + 59,294$, and $y = 19,498x - 8,130$,

Table 3 Intermediate precision of the method

Conc. ($\mu g\ ml^{-1}$)	Cetirizine %RSD		Tiaprofenac acid %RSD		Diclofenac sodium %RSD		Flurbiprofen %RSD		Ibuprofen %RSD		Mefenamic acid %RSD		Meloxicam %RSD	
	Intra	Inter	Intra	Inter	Intra	Inter	Intra	Inter	Intra	Inter	Intra	Inter	Intra	Inter
3.12	0.03	2.25	0.53	1.18	0.8	0.97	0.73	1.72	0.16	1.1	0.45	1.12	0.68	1.1
6.25	0.65	0.24	0.85	0.16	0.78	0.36	0.8	1.55	0.31	1.6	0.87	1.2	0.99	1.12
12.5	0.07	0.82	0.33	0.64	0.62	0.47	0.71	0.34	0.56	0.49	0.12	0.99	0.47	1.14
20	0.21	0.335	0.99	1.12	0.47	0.88	0.38	0.66	0.93	1.87	0.06	0.87	0.64	1.21
25	0.599	0.87	0.74	0.85	0.23	0.29	0.36	0.22	0.12	0.55	0.77	0.64	0.74	1.34
30	0.366	0.85	0.79	0.82	0.69	0.72	0.031	0.85	0.4	0.87	0.87	0.97	0.54	1.65

Table 4 %recoveries of proposed method

Conc. (µg ml⁻¹)	Cetirizine		Tiaprofenac acid		Diclofenac sodium		Flurbiprofen		Ibuprofen		Mefenamic acid		Meloxicam	
	Rec	Fou	Rec	Fou	Rec	Fou	Rec	Fou	Rec	Fou	Rec	Fou	Rec	Fou
3.12	102.3	3.19	100.7	3.14	99.82	3.11	101.8	3.18	105.3	3.28	102	3.19	107.9	3.37
6.25	100.6	6.28	102.3	6.4	98.22	6.14	98.25	6.14	98.32	6.15	108	6.72	102.4	6.4
12.5	100.8	12.61	103.5	12.93	99.63	12.45	96.36	12.05	96.14	12.02	105	13.15	101.5	12.68
20	99.88	19.98	101.6	20.33	102	20.4	98.48	19.7	101.4	20.27	103	20.69	100.3	20.06
25	97.54	24.39	102.7	25.67	103.8	25.95	97.57	24.39	102.7	25.67	103	25.67	99.78	24.95
30	96.21	28.86	99.55	29.87	95.66	28.7	103.7	31.1	103	30.9	101	30.37	97.65	29.3

Rec, %recovery; Fou, found (µg ml⁻¹).

respectively. The coefficients of variation (C.V.%) was less than 3%, and sensitivity of the method was also evaluated. Precision and repeatability of the method was determined covering the entire linearity range on two different days as shown in Table 2. Precision of the method was expressed in %RSD and accuracy of the method as shown in Table 3 was achieved at three concentration ranges.

Robustness was observed by varying the wavelength in the range of 230 to 240 nm; peak areas and retention time changes were also observed. Results clearly indicated that peak areas were influenced less, up to 2% for all the drugs assayed (Table 4). Moreover, the excellent chromatograms with good peak symmetry, unchanged retention times of the drugs in different pH solutions also proved the robustness of the method.

To evaluate the selectivity of developed method for the analysis of formulated products, cetirizine, tiaprofenac acid, flurbiprofen, ibuprofen, mefenamic acid, and meloxicam tablets were analyzed, and chromatograms were compared with the standard solution of these drugs where no interference of excipients was observed.

The method was found to be applicable for therapeutic purposes as the calculated %recovery (Table 5), for all the drugs were found to be in the range of 92.45% to 107.45% by spiking serum samples at five different concentrations.

In vitro interaction studies

The application of the method involved the determination of cetirizine in the presence of NSAIDs at different pH levels. The results showed the increase and decrease in peak area values of NSAIDs when compared with those of alone standards at the same pH levels. The results clearly indicated the changes in availability values of cetirizine and NSAIDs in the presence of each other. From these, it could be stated that %availabilities of NSAIDs were affected in presence cetirizine and vice versa. For further verification of the results, complexes of cetirizine were synthesized with NSAIDs and characterized (Table 6).

Characterization of complexes

Infrared studies The assignments of IR bands were made by comparing the spectra of the pure drugs and interacting species with the complexes. The major absorption bands for the infrared frequencies and the corresponding assignments are discussed.

In comparison with the reported spectra of cetirizine and diclofenac sodium (Ihsan et al. 2005; Moffat (2004); Sultana et al. 2011; Fini et al. 2001), the infrared spectrum of the complex showed that NH dimer from 2,700 to 2,400 cm⁻¹ disappeared and the quaternary nitrogen atom stretching shifted from 3,070 to 3,040 cm⁻¹. Similarly, the aromatic CH and aliphatic CH₂ absorption band ranges shifted from 3,110 to 3,000 and 2,985.6 to 2,914.2 to 3,165 to 3,024 and 2,925.31 to 2,847.61 cm⁻¹, respectively. A modified band appeared at 1,638.14 cm⁻¹ which indicated neutralization of the carboxylic group into a carbonyl group. The δ-bending carbonyl mode shifted from 1,421.57 to 1,200.91 cm⁻¹ to 1,409.31 to 1,237.68 cm⁻¹. From the above results, it has been concluded that, weak charge transfer interaction exists between the doubly charged piperazine moiety in cetirizine and diclofenac.

By comparing the cetirizine-flurbiprofen complex from standard (Ihsan et al. 2005; Moffat 2004; Sultana et al. 2011; Paradkar et al. 2003), the quaternary nitrogen atom stretching shifted from 3,070 to 3,043 cm⁻¹. The

Table 5 Analysis of drugs in serum (%recovery)

	Conc. (µg ml⁻¹)					
	3.12	6.25	12.5	20	25	30
Cetirizine	100.35	102.66	101.54	96.12	96.12	100.54
Tiaprofenac acid	101.36	100.74	100.77	102.45	92.45	98.72
Diclofenac sodium	100.22	101.99	107.45	102.66	100.29	98.76
Flurbiprofen	103.57	98.65	98.64	103.77	107.45	94.45
Ibuprofen	107.45	97.45	99.12	101.44	101	97.11
Mefenamic acid	105.21	96.21	96.11	108	100.12	99.87
Meloxicam	107.28	100.38	99.21	97.65	96.14	95.46

Table 6 Possible structures and characterizations of complexes

Complex	Chemical structure	Appearance	Solubility	Melting point (°C)
Dic-cet		White crystalline	Soluble in methanol, chloroform, and acetonitrile	108
Mef-cet		Off-white amorphous	Soluble in methanol, chloroform, and acetonitrile	Decompose at 210
Mel-Cet		Off-white amorphous	Soluble in methanol, chloroform, and acetonitrile	230
Ibu-cet		Off-white amorphous	Soluble in methanol, chloroform, and acetonitrile	225
Flu-cet		White amorphous	Soluble in methanol, chloroform, and acetonitrile	110

Dic-cet, diclofenac and cetirizine complex; Mef-cet, mefenamic acid and cetirizine complex; Mel-Cet, meloxicam and cetirizine complex; Ibu-cet, ibuprofen and cetirizine complex; Flu-cet, flurbiprofen and cetirizine complex.

NH dimer of amino acid from 2,700 to 2,400 cm^{-1} appeared as a weak signal with respect to cetirizine. Characteristic broad peaks in the range of 2,500 to 3,500 and 2,920 cm^{-1} due to hydrogen bonding and hydroxyl stretching disappeared whereas carbonyl peak shifted from 1,698 to 1,654 cm^{-1} with diminished intensity.

The complex formed between cetirizine and meloxicam showed quaternary nitrogen atom stretching at 3,070 cm^{-1} and NH dimer of amino acid in the region of 2,700 to 2,400 cm^{-1} completely disappeared with respect to cetirizine. Characteristic peaks of meloxicam at 1,620 and 3,292 cm^{-1} for C=O and secondary –NH or –OH stretching disappeared (Sharma et. al. 2005) while other sets of signals were the same.

In the complex of mefenamic acid, NH dimer of amino acid and the quaternary nitrogen atom stretching from 2,700 to 2,400 cm^{-1} and 3,070 to 3,040 cm^{-1} disappeared. Shifting of some measured peaks was observed with respect to mefenamic acid (Derle et al. 2008); peaks of neutralized entity of the carboxylic acid shifted from 1,610 to 1,554.5 and 1,409.9 to 1,292.2 to 1,654 to 1,587 and 1,442 to 1,270 cm^{-1}.

In comparison with IR spectrum of cetirizine (Moffat 2004; Sultana et al. 2011), ibuprofen (Gavrilin and Pogrebnyak 2001) proved that the quaternary nitrogen atom stretching and NH dimer of amino acid from 2,700 to 2,400 and 3,070 to 3,040 cm^{-1} completely disappeared. Strong absorption bands due to the carboxyl group shifted from 1,708 to 1,768.90 cm^{-1}.

^{1}H NMR studies The ^{1}H NMR spectra of cetirizine confirmed the above results. The de-shielding effect was evident in complexes on the aromatic NH proton as the resonance downfield shifted to δ 7.6 ppm. Thus, this proton appeared in the broad multiplet between δ 6.27 and 7.56 ppm showing 16 aromatic CH protons and the 2 NH$^+$ protons. A singlet was observed at δ 3.3 ppm for methyl diphenyl CH proton. Triplet at δ 3.71 ppm was obvious due to four protons on the acyclic CH$_2$ groups adjacent to NH$^+$ in the piperazine ring and at δ 3.36 ppm was observed for the groups adjacent to the nitrogen hydrochloride entity. Another singlet at δ 3.61 ppm with two protons was shown for the CH$_2$ in CH$_2$CH$_2$O entity. The CH$_2$ in the CH$_2$COOH group appeared as a singlet δ 3.71 ppm. A very weak singlet was present at δ 10.8 ppm for the one proton of the carboxylic acid group. In spectra of the mefenamic acid complex, downfield shift was observed for aromatic protons. Triplets at δ 3.16 and 3.51 ppm observed for protons on the acyclic CH$_2$ groups adjacent to NH$^+$ in the piperazine ring. Singlet at δ 10.8 ppm was present for one proton of the carboxylic acid group. Similar result was observed for cetirizine-flurbiprofen complex, i.e., singlet of carboxylic group proton remained at δ 10.8 ppm and downfield shift observed for aromatic

protons. The protons of piperazine were observed at δ 3.31 to 3.50 ppm. The other properties are shown in Table 6.

Conclusion

The present work described the applicability of simultaneous and validated method for the determination and *in vitro* interactions of cetirizine in the presence of NSAIDs as diclofenac sodium, flurbiprofen, ibuprofen, meloxicam, mefenamic acid, and tirprofenac acid. Furthermore, the method was also found to be applicable in serum and was found useful for therapeutic purposes. The differences in availabilities of cetirizine with NSAIDs at three pH levels clearly indicated the interactions of aforementioned drugs. It was further supported by synthesis of complexes and their characterization. The findings suggested further studies on the co-administration of these two drugs simultaneously in order to know the pharmacokinetic and pharmacodynamic profiles of the drugs whether they create synergistic or negative interactions. Till further research is pursued in this direction, it is highly recommended to have a suitable time lapse between the oral uses of these drugs.

Competing interests
The authors declare that they have no competing interests.

Authors' contributions
HS designed, coordinated, and carried out experiments in the study. HS and NS drafted the manuscript. MSA supervised the project. All authors read and approved the final manuscript.

Acknowledgement
The authors are thankful to Dr. Agha Zeeshan Mirza of the Department of Chemistry, University of Karachi for his help with the manuscript.

Author details
[1]Research Institute of Pharmaceutical Sciences, Department of Pharmaceutical Chemistry, Faculty of Pharmacy, University of Karachi, Karachi 75270, Pakistan. [2]Department of Chemistry, University of Karachi, Karachi 75270, Pakistan.

References
Arayne MS, Sultana N, Mirza AZ, Siddiqui FA (2010a) Simultaneous determination of gliquidone, fexofenadine, buclizine and levocetirizine in dosage formulation and human serum by RP-HPLC. J Chromatographic Sci 48:382–385
Arayne MS, Sultana N, Shamshad H, Mirza AZ (2010b) Drug interaction studies of gliquidone with fexofenadine, cetirizine and levocetirizine. Med Chem Res 19:1064–1073
Moffat AC (2004) Clark's isolation and identification of drugs in pharmaceuticals, body fluids, and post-mortem material, 3rd edition. The Pharmaceutical Press, London
Cosmes I, Rodriguez EB (2012) Simultaneous assay and identification of ibuprofen, phenylephrine HCl and cetirizine HCl in Softgels® by liquid chromatography. Research & Development, Banner Pharmacaps, High Point, NC. AAPS 2012-08 02511
Derle DV, Bele M, Kasliwal N (2008) In vitro and in vivo evaluation of mefenamic acid and its complexes with β-cyclodexin and HP- β-cyclodexin. Asian J Pharm 2:30–35

Fini A, Garuti M, Fazio G, Alvarez FJ, Holgado MA (2001) Diclofenac salts. I. fractal and thermal analysis of sodium and potassium diclofenac salts. J Pharm Sci 90:2049–2057

Freddy HH, Dharmendra LV (2010) Simultaneous determination of paracetamol, acetyl salicylic acid, mefenamic acid and cetirizine dihydrochloride in the pharmaceutical dosage form. E-J Chem 7:S495–S503

Gavrilin MV, Pogrebnyak AV (2001) Synthesis, characterization, and evaluation of the local irritant action of an ibuprofen- β-cyclodextrin inclusion complex. Pharm Chem J 35:395–396

Ihsan MK, Barsoum NB, Maha AY (2005) Drug-drug interaction between diclofenac, cetirizine and ranitidine. J Pharm Biomed Anal 37:655–661

Jain DK, Dubey N, Malav P (2012) Simultaneous estimation of nimesulide, cetirizine hydrochloride and pseudoephedrine hydrochloride. Asian J Chem 24:4641–4643

Jarkko R, Joan EH, Lindsey OW, Anand B, John PK, Jeevan RK, Cosette JSS, Joseph WP (2006) In vitro P-glycoprotein inhibition assays for assessment of clinical drug interaction potential of new drug candidates: a recommendation for probe substrates. Drug Metab Dispos 34:786–792

Lee JY, Tanabe S, Shimohira H, Kobayashi Y, Oomachi T, Azuma S, Ogihara K, Inokuma H (2007) Expression of cyclooxygenase-2, P-glycoprotein and multi-drug resistance-associated protein in canine transitional cell carcinoma. Res Vet Sci 83:210–216

Padmavathi N, Niranjan MS (2011) Development and validation of HPLC method for simultaneous estimation of cetirizine dihydrochloride with aceclofenac. IJPRD 4:268–273

Paradkar A, Maheshwari M, Tyagi A, Chauhan B, Kadam SS (2003) Preparation and characterization of flurbiprofen beads by melt solidification technique. AAPS Pharm Sci Tech 4:514–522

Philip YM, Philip M (2010) Combination of cetirizine and mefenamic acid for the treatment of exacerbations of asthma, WO/2010/116127.

Priya M, Sathya NV, Satyajit M, Jamuna RR (2013) Screening of cetirizine for analgesic activity in mice. Int J Basic Clin Pharmacol 2:187–192

Renwick AG (1999) The metabolism of antihistamines and drug interactions: the role of cytochrome P450 enzymes. Clin Exp Allergy 3:116–124

Rewari S, Gupta U (1999) Modification of antihistamine activity of cetirizine by nimesulide. JAPI 47:389–392

Scott CA, Kelly LC (2003) Antihistamines. Med-Psych Drug-Drug Interactions 44:430–434

Sharma S, Sher P, Badve S, Pawar AP (2005) Adsorption of meloxicam on porous calcium silicate: characterization and tablet formulation. AAPS PharmSciTech 6:E618–E625

Singh A, Jain R (2003) European patent specification. EP 1005 865 B1.

Sultana N, Arayne MS, Shamshad H, Mirza AZ, Naz MA, Fatima B, Asif M, Mesaik MA (2011) Synthesis, characterization and biological activities of cetirizine analogues. Spect-Biomed Appl 26:317–328

Sultana N, Arayne MS, Shamshad H (2010) In vitro studies of the interaction between cetirizine and H_2 receptor antagonists using spectrophotometry and reversed-phase high-performance liquid chromatography. Med Chem Res 19:462–474

Suryan AL, Bhusari VK, Rasal KS, Dhaneshwar SR (2011) Simultaneous quantitation and validation of paracetamol, phenylpropanolamine hydrochloride and cetirizine hydrochloride by RP-HPLC in bulk drug and formulation. Int J Pharm Sci Drug Res 3:303–308

Wageh MA, El-S A, El-S M, Ahmed EG (2004) The potential role of cyclooxygenase-2 inhibitors in the treatment of experimentally-induced mammary tumour: does celecoxib enhance the anti-tumour activity of doxorubicin? Pharmacol Res 50:487–498

11

New solid phase extractor based on ionic liquid functionalized silica gel surface for selective separation and determination of lanthanum

Hadi M Marwani[1,2*] and Amjad E Alsafrani[1]

Abstract

Background: Direct determination of metal ions, in particular at ultra-trace concentration, cannot be easily achieved in complex systems by analytical techniques because of the lack of sensitivity and selectivity of these methods. Therefore, an efficient separation step is often required prior to the determination of metal ions for sensitive, accurate, and interference-free determination of metal ions. In accordance, a new solid phase extractor based on silica gel functionalized with ionic liquid (SG-N-PhenacylPyrNTf$_2$) was developed for a selective separation of La(III) prior to its determination by inductively coupled plasma-optical emission spectrometry.

Methods: Immobilization of the ionic liquid on activated silica gel surface was confirmed by both Fourier transform infrared spectroscopy and scanning electron microscope. The concentration of ionic liquid on the surface of activated silica gel was determined based on thermal desorption method. The uptake behavior of the new SG-N-PhenacylPyrNTf$_2$ adsorbent toward metal ions was studied under static conditions by batch mode. The supernatant concentrations of metal ions were directly determined after filtration by inductively coupled plasma-optical emission spectrometry.

Results: Fourier transform infrared spectroscopy and scanning electron microscopy results strongly confirmed the formation of SG-N-PhenacylPyrNTf$_2$ phase. Adsorption isotherm study revealed the preference of SG-N-PhenacylPyrNTf$_2$ over activated silica gel for a selective separation of La(III) prior to its determination by inductively coupled plasma-optical emission spectrometry. Adsorption isotherm data were well fit the Langmuir adsorption model with a maximum adsorption capacity of 165.39 mg g^{-1} for La(III), which was consistent with that (167.08 mg g^{-1}) experimentally obtained from adsorption isotherm study. Kinetic study demonstrated that the adsorption of La(III) on the SG-N-PhenacylPyrNTf$_2$ phase followed the pseudo second-order kinetic model.

Conclusions: Ultimately, the developed method can be applied and effectively utilized for the determination of La(III) in natural water samples with acceptable and reliable results.

Keywords: N-PhenacylPyrNTf$_2$; Silica gel surface; La(III); Adsorption; ICP-OES; Batch mode

Background

Rare earth metals (REMs) have been used in different fields, such as chemical engineering, metallurgy, nuclear energy, optical, magnetic, luminescence, and laser materials, high-temperature superconductors, secondary batteries, and catalysis (Maestro and Huguenin 1995; Gaikwad and Damodaran 1993). Lanthanum is one of the REMs and has received special interest due to its technological importance

and increasing demands for advanced new materials. Present day applications of lanthanum, as a pure element or in association with other compounds, are in super alloys, catalysts, special ceramics, and organic synthesis (Palmieri et al. 2002). However, most of the environmental problems are usually caused by human activities and natural resources. In recent years, this phenomenon is remarkably extended with the population density and growth of technology. There are several contaminants in nature, such as contamination with heavy metals, radionuclides, and lanthanides (Maanan 2008; Awwad et al. 2010). All of these are toxic and harmful to the public health, even at low

* Correspondence: hmarwani@kau.edu.sa
[1]Department of Chemistry, Faculty of Science, King Abdulaziz University, P.O. Box 80203, Jeddah 21589, Saudi Arabia
[2]Center of Excellence for Advanced Materials Research (CEAMR), King Abdulaziz University, P.O. Box 80203, Jeddah 21589, Saudi Arabia

concentration level (Cui et al. 2007). Thus, the most convenient way to overcome these problems is to apply selective extraction techniques, particularly when they exist at ultra-trace concentration level in complex matrix (Zang et al. 2010).

Various extraction techniques were implemented for the quantitative determination of trace metal ions, including liquid-liquid extraction (Khajeh 2011; Farajzadeh et al. 2009), coprecipitation (Komjarova and Blust 2006; Soylak and Erdogan 2006; Saracoglu et al. 2006), ion exchange (Tao and Fang 1998), cloud point extraction (Manzoori et al. 2007; Safavi et al. 2004), and solid-phase extraction (Zhang et al. 2012; Marahel et al. 2011; Duran et al. 2007). Recently, solid-phase extraction (SPE) has been widely used as a separation tool for the speciation of metal ions in environmental samples and has received much attention because of its advantages, such as absence of emulsion, high enrichment factor, disposal cost due to low consumption of reagent, and more importantly environment-friendly (Aydin and Soylak 2007; Simpson 2000). Nevertheless, the main limitation of SPE is the lack of selectivity (Jal et al. 2004), which leads to high interference of the other existing species with the target metal ion. The choice of a proper adsorbent plays an important role in SPE because it can control the analytical parameters, such as selectivity, affinity, and capacity (Cai et al. 2003; Dean 1998). Hence, different surface modification methods have been applied to classical SPE adsorbents (such as silica (Shin and Choi 2009) and polymer (Qiao et al. 2012)) in order to increase the selectivity.

Room-temperature ionic liquids (RTILs) have several unique chemical and physical properties which make it useful for wide applications in organic chemistry, inorganic chemistry, electrochemistry, and analytical chemistry (Zhao 2006; Vidal et al. 2012). RTILs have good thermal stability, negligible vapor pressure, tunable viscosity and miscibility with water, high conductivity, and high heat capacity (Handy 2005; Koel 2009). In addition, extraction and separation techniques applying solid adsorbents modified with ionic liquids (ILs) have become very active fields in analytical chemistry (Anderson et al. 2006). ILs can be immobilized on the surface of solid supports for additional applications as solid phase extractors of metal ions from their matrices or aqueous solutions (Mahmoud and Al-Bishri 2011). They have been immobilized on multiwalled carbon nanotubes (Wang et al. 2008), nanosilica (Mahmoud 2011; Mahmoud and Al-Bishri 2011), and silica gel (Ayata et al. 2011; Liang and Peng 2010). Silica gel (SG) adsorbents, as an example of inorganic solid phases, afford several advantages over organic solid phases, such as high porosity and hydrophilicity and ease of surface modification (Ngeontae et al. 2009; Quang et al. 2012). However,

research studies were little in the abovementioned field of the applications of supported ionic liquid phases.

In accordance, a solid phase extractant (SG-N-PhenacylPyrNTf$_2$) was developed based on a hybrid combination of the hydrophobic character of newly synthesized ionic liquid with SG properties, without the need for partition treatment by chelating compounds. Both Fourier transform infrared (FT-IR) spectroscopy and scanning electron microscope (SEM) confirmed the formation of the resulted SG-N-PhenacylPyrNTf$_2$ adsorbent. The selectivity of SG-N-PhenacylPyrNTf$_2$ toward different metal ions, including Co(II), Fe(II), Fe(III), La(III), and Ni(II) was investigated. The uptake behavior of the new SG-N-PhenacylPyrNTf$_2$ adsorbent toward La(III) was evaluated under batch conditions. Adsorption isotherm data were well fit with the Langmuir adsorption model, strongly supporting that the adsorption process was mainly monolayer on a homogeneous adsorbent surface. Kinetic study also demonstrated that the adsorption of La(III) on the SG-N-PhenacylPyrNTf$_2$ phase obeyed the pseudo second-order kinetic model. The proposed method was ultimately applied to real water samples with satisfactory results.

Experimental details
Chemicals and reagents
All reagents used were of high purity and of analytical reagent grade, and doubly distilled deionized water was used throughout experiments. N-phenacylpyridinium bromide (N-PhenacylPyrBr), bis(trifluoromethane)sulfonimide lithium (LiNTf$_2$), ethyl alcohol (Et-OH), and diethyl ether were purchased from Sigma-Aldrich (Milwaukee, WI, USA). SG (SiO$_2$, particle size 10 to 20 nm) with purity of 99.5% was also obtained from Sigma-Aldrich. Lanthanum nitrate [La(NO$_3$)$_3$] and stock standard solutions of 1,000 mg L^{-1} of Co(II), Fe(II), Fe(III), and Ni(II) were purchased from Sigma-Aldrich.

Preparation of the new solid phase extractor
Preparation of N-PhenacylPyrNTf$_2$ ionic liquid
N-PhenacylPyrNTf$_2$ ionic liquid was prepared according to previously reported standard method by Marwani (Marwani 2013; 2010). Specifically, an amount of 2 g N-PhenacylPyrBr was separately weighed and dissolved in 18.2 MΩ·cm distilled deionized water. The N-PhenacylPyrBr solution was then mixed with an equimolar amount of LiNTf$_2$. The resultant reaction mixture was stirred for 2 h at room temperature, and the reaction resulted in two phases. The lower layer was separated and dried under vacuum overnight.

Activation of SG
SG powder (25.0 g) was first activated by refluxing and stirring with 200 mL of 50% (v/v) concentrated

hydrochloric acid solution for 8 h in order to remove metal oxide and nitrogenous impurity and to enhance the content of silanol groups on the SG surface. The activated SG powder was filtered, repeatedly washed with 18.2 MΩ·cm distilled deionized water until acid-free and oven dried at 120°C for 5 h to remove surface-adsorbed water.

Synthesis of SG-N-PhenacylPyrNTf$_2$

The preparation of SG-N-PhenacylPyrNTf$_2$ was based on the immobilization of ionic liquid (N-PhenacylPyrNTf$_2$) on the surface of activated SG by a hybridization process of the hydrophobic character of ionic liquid with SG properties. An amount of 5 g activated SG was suspended in 100 mL ethyl alcohol, and 1 g N-PhenacylPyrNTf$_2$ was weighed, completely dissolved by warming in 50 mL ethyl alcohol and added to the activated SG suspension. The reaction mixture was stirred at 60°C for 12 h. The newly modified SG-N-PhenacylPyrNTf$_2$ phase was filtered and washed with 50 mL ethyl alcohol on three portions followed by doubly distilled deionized water and diethyl ether. The SG-N-PhenacylPyrNTf$_2$ adsorbent was then allowed to dry in an oven at 80°C for 5 h and kept in a desiccator for further use. The synthetic route of SG-N-PhenacylPyrNTf$_2$ is shown in Scheme 1.

Batch procedure

In this study, the effect of solution pH, adsorption capacity determination, effect of contact time, and effect of coexisting ions were investigated under static conditions by batch mode. For the effect of pH on the selectivity of SG-N-PhenacylPyrNTf$_2$ toward selected metal ions, standard solutions of 2 mg L^{-1} of each metal ion were prepared and adjusted to pH values ranging from 1.0 to 9.0, except for Fe(II) and Fe(III), with a series of buffer solutions, 0.2 mol L^{-1} HCl/KCl for pH 1.0 and 2.0, 0.1 mol L^{-1} CH$_3$COOH/CH$_3$COONa for pH 3.0 to 6.0, and 0.1 mol L^{-1} Na$_2$HPO$_4$/HCl for pH 7.0 to 9.0. Both Fe(II) and Fe(III) were prepared at the same concentration as above but were only studied with buffer solutions at pH values ranging from 1.0 to 4.0 in order to avoid any precipitation with buffer solutions at pH 5.0 to 9.0. Each standard solution was individually mixed with 20 mg of dry SG-N-PhenacylPyrNTf$_2$ phase. All mixtures were shaken vigorously at room temperature for 1 h to facilitate adsorption of the metal ions onto the SG-N-PhenacylPyrNTf$_2$. The supernatant concentration of metal ions was determined directly by inductively coupled plasma-optical emission spectrometry (ICP-OES) after filtration. For the study of La(III) adsorption capacity, standard solutions of 0, 5, 10, 20, 30, 40, 60, 80, 100, 125, 150, 200, and 500 mg L^{-1} were prepared as above, adjusted to the optimum pH value of 6.0 with the buffered aqueous solution (0.1 mol L^{-1} CH$_3$COOH/

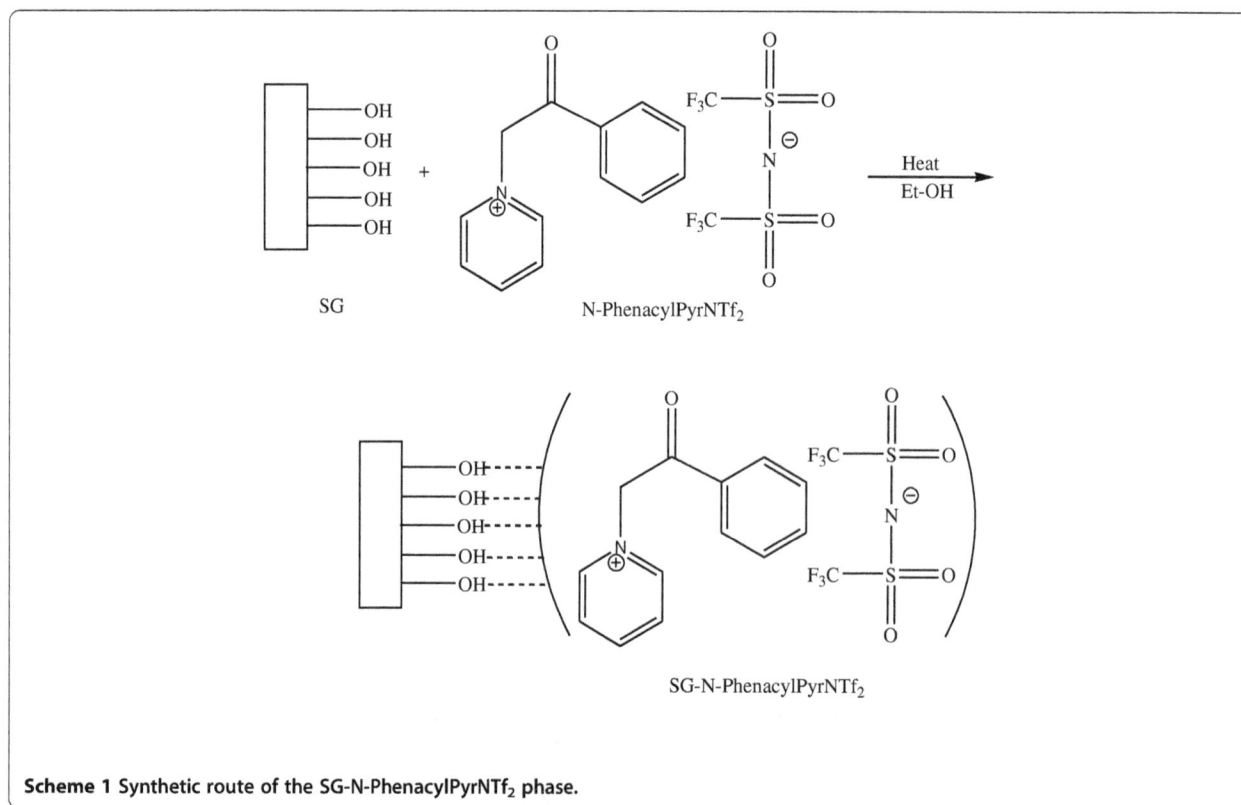

Scheme 1 Synthetic route of the SG-N-PhenacylPyrNTf$_2$ phase.

CH$_3$COONa) and individually mixed with 20 mg SG-N-PhenacylPyrNTf$_2$. The mixtures were mechanically shaken for 1 h at room temperature. In addition, the effect of shaking time on the La(III) uptake capacity was studied under the same batch conditions but at different equilibrium periods (2.5, 5, 10, 20, 30, 40, 50, and 60 min).

Methods

FT-IR spectra were recorded before and after modification of the SG phase on Perkin Elmer spectrum 100 series FT-IR spectrometer (Beaconsfield, Bucks, UK) in the range 4,000 to 600 cm^{-1}. A Jenway model 3505 laboratory pH meter (CamLab, Cambridgeshire, UK) was employed for the pH measurements and was calibrated with standard buffer solutions. Surface morphologies of SG before and after modification were investigated by SEM on a field emission scanning electron microscope (QUANT FEG 450, Amsterdam, Netherlands). The microscope was operated at an accelerating voltage of 15 kV. Thermolyne 47900 furnace was used to determine the millimoles per gram surface coverage value of SG-N-PhenacylPyrNTf$_2$ surface by thermal desorption analysis. ICP-OES measurements were acquired with the use of a Perkin Elmer ICP-OES model Optima 4100 DV, Shelton, CT, USA. The ICP-OES instrument was optimized daily before measurement and operated as recommended by the manufacturers. The ICP-OES spectrometer was used with the following parameters: FR power, 1,300 kW; frequency, 27.12 MHz; demountable quartz torch, Ar/Ar/Ar; plasma gas (Ar) flow, 15.0 L min^{-1}; auxiliary gas (Ar) flow, 0.2 L min^{-1}; nebulizer gas (Ar) flow, 0.8 L min^{-1}; nebulizer pressure, 2.4 bar; glass spray chamber according to Scott (Ryton), sample pump flow rate, 1.5 mL min^{-1}; integration time, 3 s; replicates, 3; and wavelength range of monochromator 165 to 460 nm. The wavelengths selected for the determination of Fe(II and III), Ni(II), Co(II), and La(III) were 238.204, 231.604, 228.616, and 348.902 nm, respectively.

Results and discussion

Determination of the surface coverage value of the SG-N-PhenacylPyrNTf$_2$ phase

An amount of 100 mg SG-N-PhenacylPyrNTf$_2$ adsorbent was weighed in a dry porcelain crucible. The weighed amount was then gradually heated into a furnace from 50°C to 700°C, and the ignited phase was kept at this temperature for 1 h. The remaining SG-N-PhenacylPyrNTf$_2$ phase was left to cool inside the furnace and then transferred to a desiccator. The weight loss of hydrophobic ionic liquid was determined by the difference in sample masses before and after the process of thermal desorption. Based on thermal desorption method, the concentration of N-PhenacylPyrNTf$_2$ was

determined to be 0.38 mmol g^{-1} on the surface of activated SG.

FT-IR and SEM characterization of SG-N-PhenacylPyrNTf$_2$

In order to emphasize the immobilization of the N-PhenacylPyrNTf$_2$ on activated SG surface, activated SG and SG-N-PhenacylPyrNTf$_2$ were evaluated by FT-IR spectroscopy. FT-IR spectrum of newly modified adsorbent shows spectral changes that are related to both N-PhenacylPyrNTf$_2$ and activated SG phases, confirming the formation of the new physically modified SG-N-PhenacylPyrNTf$_2$ phase. The band observed at 1,347 cm^{-1}, as displayed in Figure 1, was assigned to stretching vibrations of (NSO$_2$) bonds. Other characteristic bands of the SG-N-PhenacylPyrNTf$_2$ adsorbent appeared at the position of about 1,644 cm^{-1} for (C=C) and 1,713 cm^{-1} for (C=O). Two absorption peaks also appeared at 2,900 and 3,013 cm^{-1} which could be attributed to (–C–H) and (=C–H), respectively.

The formation of SG-N-PhenacylPyrNTf$_2$ phase was not only confirmed by FT-IR measurements but was also supported by taking SEM images of the activated silica gel and SG-N-PhenacylPyrNTf$_2$, as shown in Figure 2. Figure 2 displays a pronounced and characterized change of the surface morphology of activated SG as a result of the N-PhenacylPyrNTf$_2$ immobilization on the surface of activated SG. It can be clearly observed that the activated SG particles were collected in aggregate forms and completely covered with N-PhenacylPyrNTf$_2$. In addition, it is interesting to note that the particles of SG-N-PhenacylPyrNTf$_2$ (Figure 2B) are individually distributed in uniform and homogeneous shapes as compared to that of the activated SG (Figure 2A).

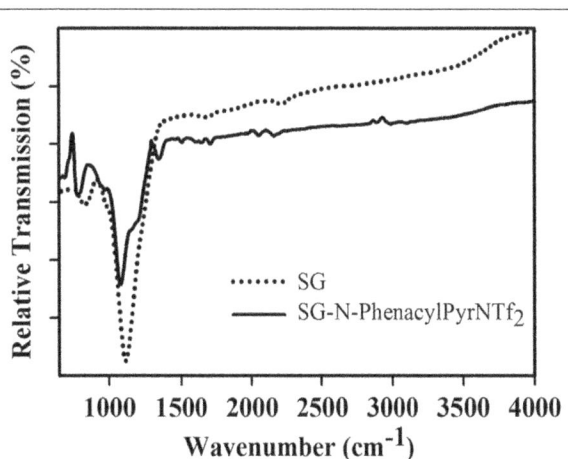

Figure 1 FT-IR of activated silica gel and SG-N-PhenacylPyrNTf$_2$ phases.

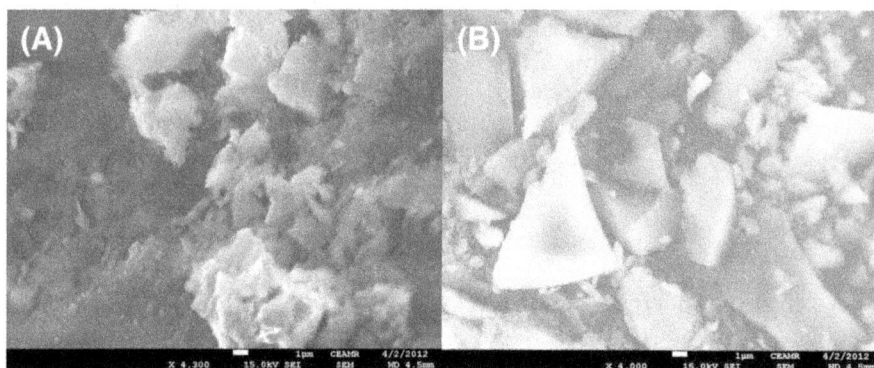

Figure 2 SEM images of (A) activated silica gel and (B) SG-N-PhenacylPyrNTf$_2$ phases.

Effect of pH and selectivity study

The acidity of solution plays an important role in the extraction of metal ions from different matrices. Therefore, the solution pH is the first parameter to be optimized. In order to evaluate the effect of pH on the adsorption of SG-N-PhenacylPyrNTf$_2$ toward Co(II), Fe(II), Fe(III), La(III), and Ni(II), pH values of the sample solution were studied in the range of 1.0 to 9.0 for all metal ions, except with Fe(II) and Fe(III) whose pH values were investigated in the range 1.0 to 4.0 in order to avoid any precipitation with buffer solutions at a pH value higher than 4.0. Selected metal ions of 2 mg L^{-1} were individually mixed with 20 mg SG-N-PhenacylPyrNTf$_2$ phase. All mixtures were mechanically shaken at room temperature for 1 h. Figure 3 depicts the effect of solution pH on the % extraction of selected metal ions. In general, it can be observed that there is an increase in % extraction of all metal ions with an increase in the pH. However, it is of interest to note that the highest % extraction is reached for La(III) among all metal ions included in this study. In addition, the selectivity of SG-

N-PhenacylPyrNTf$_2$ phase toward La(III) was found to be the most among all metal ions at pH value of 6.0.

The distribution coefficient was calculated for each metal ion at its optimum pH value for further confirmation of the selectivity of SG-N-PhenacylPyrNTf$_2$ phase toward La(III), as illustrated in Table 1. The distribution coefficient (K_d) corresponding to the character of a metal ion adsorbed by an adsorbent (mL g^{-1}) can be obtained from the following equation (Han et al. 2005):

$$K_d = \frac{(C_i - C_e)}{C_e} \times \frac{V}{m} \tag{1}$$

where C_i and C_e correspond to initial and final concentrations (mg L^{-1}), respectively, V donates the volume of solution (mL), and m refers to the mass of adsorbent (g). Results presented in Table 1 clearly indicated that La(III) had the greatest K_d value up to 2.50×10^6 mL g^{-1} on the SG-N-PhenacylPyrNTf$_2$ adsorbent among all other metal ions even at their optimum pH values. These results strongly supported the finding that the selectivity of SG-N-PhenacylPyrNTf$_2$ was the most toward La(III).

The low % extraction of La(III) in the acidic medium could be ascribed to the presence of H$^+$ ion competing with the La(III) ion for the adsorption sites of SG-N-PhenacylPyrNTf$_2$ phase. At high pH values, the negative charge produced on the surface of activated SG and incorporated donor atoms (N, O, and S) presented in the N-PhenacylPyrNTf$_2$, as a result of the N-PhenacylPyrNTf$_2$

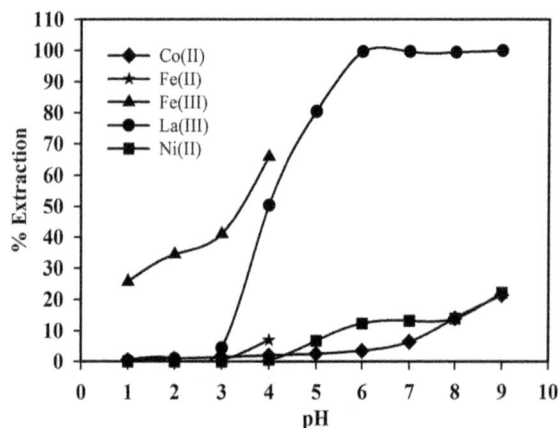

Figure 3 Effect of solution pH on the % extraction of selected metal ions.

Table 1 Selectivity study of 20 mg SG-N-PhenacylPyrNTf$_2$ toward different metal ions

Metal ion	Concentration (mg L^{-1})	q_e (mg g^{-1})	K_d (mL g^{-1})
Co(II)	2.00	0.54	340.33
Fe(II)	2.00	0.17	93.36
Fe(III)	2.00	1.65	2410.32
La(III)	2.00	2.50	2.50×10^6
Ni(II)	2.00	0.55	354.62

immobilization on the activated SG, strongly attained the selective adsorption of SG-N-PhenacylPyrNTf$_2$ toward La (III). Thus, the highest selectivity of the SG-N-PhenacylPyrNTf$_2$ phase toward La(III) may be attributed to electrostatic attraction or complex formation mechanism between SG-N-PhenacylPyrNTf$_2$ and La(III), as shown in Figure 4. Based on the above results, La(III) was selected among other metal ions for the study of other parameters controlling its maximum uptake on SG-N-PhenacylPyrNTf$_2$ under batch conditions and at the optimum pH value of 6.0.

Determination of La(III) adsorption capacity

To determine the loading capacity of SG-N-PhenacylPyrNTf$_2$, 25 mL aliquots of a series of La(III) concentrations (0 to 500 mg L^{-1}) were adjusted to pH 6.0, and the proposed separation procedure previously described above was applied. The amount of La(III) adsorbed at each concentration level was determined by ICP-OES. The adsorption profile of La(III) on 20 mg SG-N-PhenacylPyrNTf$_2$ was obtained by plotting the La(III)

concentration (mg L^{-1}) versus milligrams of La(III) adsorbed per gram SG-N-PhenacylPyrNTf$_2$ (Figure 5). From adsorption isotherm study, the adsorption capacity of SG-N-PhenacylPyrNTf$_2$ for La(III) was experimentally found to be 167.08 mg g^{-1}. The adsorption capacity of La(III) on the activated SG was also determined to be 85.06 mg g^{-1} under the same batch conditions as well as that of La(III) with SG-N-PhenacylPyrNTf$_2$ phase (Figure 5). These results indicated that the adsorption capacity for La(III) was increased by 96.43% with the newly modified SG-N-PhenacylPyrNTf$_2$ phase. The adsorption capacity of La(III) reported in the present study was also compared with those reported with SPE materials, as summarized in Table 2. As could be observed in Table 2, the adsorption capacity for La(III) obtained by SG-N-PhenacylPyrNTf$_2$ is comparable with those previously reported with other studies.

Adsorption isotherm models

In order to evaluate the adsorption of La(III) on SG-N-PhenacylPyrNTf$_2$ adsorbent, the adsorption isotherm model was evaluated using Langmuir and Freundlich isotherm models. The Freundlich isotherm model assumes that the adsorption occurs on heterogeneous surfaces. The Freundlich model is given by the following equation (Freundlich 1906):

$$\log q_e = \log K_f + 1/n \quad \log C_e \tag{2}$$

where K_f and n are the Freundlich constants and can be calculated from the intercept and slope, respectively, of the linear plot of $\log q_e$ versus $\log C_e$.

The Langmuir isotherm model assumes that the adsorption occurs at specific homogeneous adsorption sites within the adsorbent and intermolecular forces that rapidly decrease with the distance from the adsorption surface

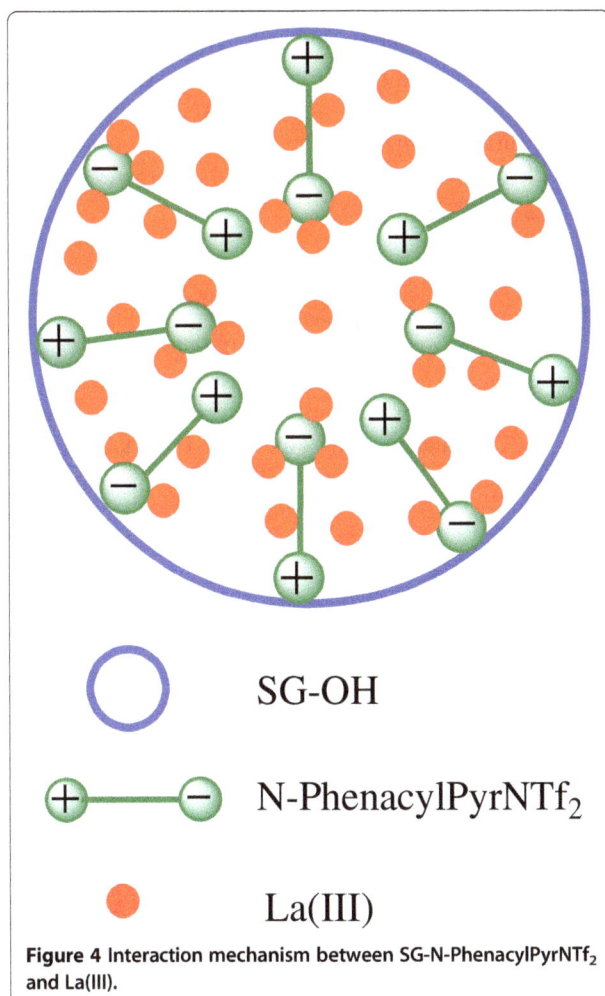

Figure 4 Interaction mechanism between SG-N-PhenacylPyrNTf$_2$ and La(III).

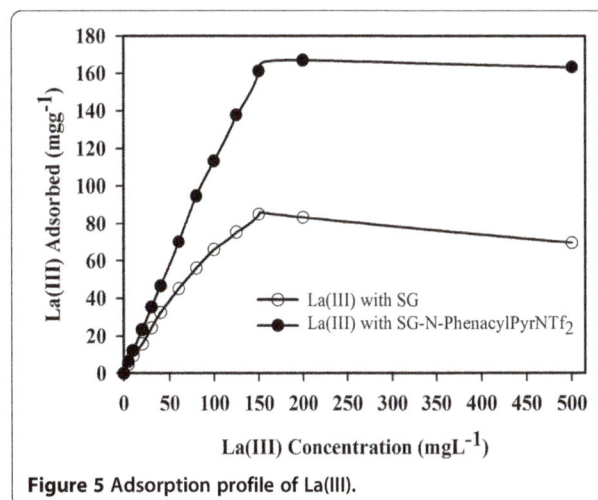

Figure 5 Adsorption profile of La(III).

Table 2 Comparison of SG-N-PhenacylPyrNTf$_2$ adsorption capacity for La(III) reported in the present study with other SPE materials

SPE material	Adsorption capacity (mg g^{-1})	Reference
SG-N-PhenacylPyrNTf$_2$	167.08	Present study
H,PEG400, PW[a]	220.80	(Zhang et al. 2009)
H,PEG400, PMo	214.40	(Zhang et al. 2009)
TA-MWCNTs[b]	5.35	(Tong et al. 2011)
MRH[c]	175.40	(Awwad et al. 2010)
Turbinaria conoides biomass	154.70	(Vijayaraghavan et al. 2010)
Powderized leaves of Platanus orientalis	28.65	(Sert et al. 2008)
MLTBC[d]	120.00	(Chen 2010)
XAD-4-OVSC[e]	2.30	(Jain et al. 2001)

[a]Polyethyleneglycol (PEG)-phosphomolybdic (PMo)/phosphotungstic (PW) heteropolyacids; [b]multiwalled carbon nanotube modified with tannic acid; [c]modified rice Husk activated carbon; [d]modified low-temperature bamboo charcoal; [e]amberlite XAD-4-o-vanillinsemicarbazone.

(Unlü and Ersoz 2006). The Langmuir model is described by the following equation (Langmuir 1916):

$$C_e/q_e = (C_e/Q_o) + 1/Q_o b \qquad (3)$$

where C_e corresponds to the equilibrium concentration of the metal ion in the supernatant (mg mL^{-1}) and q_e represents the amount of metal ion per gram of the adsorbent (mg g^{-1}). The symbols Q_o and b refer to Langmuir constants for SG-N-PhenacylPyrNTf$_2$ and are related to the maximum La(III) adsorption capacity (mg g^{-1}) and affinity parameter (L mg^{-1}), respectively. Langmuir constants can be obtained from a linear plot of C_e/q_e against C_e with a slope and intercept equal to $1/Q_o$ and $1/Q_o b$, respectively. In addition, the essential characteristics of the Langmuir adsorption isotherm can be represented in terms of a dimensionless constant separation factor or equilibrium parameter, R_L, which is defined as $R_L = 1/(1 + bC_o)$, where b is the Langmuir constant, indicating the nature of adsorption and the shape of the isotherm, and C_o is the initial concentration of the analyte of interest. The R_L value indicates the type of the isotherm, and R_L values lying between 0 and 1 indicates that the conditions were favorable for the adsorption process (McKay et al. 1982).

After evaluating both Freundlich and Langmuir isotherm models, it was found that adsorption isotherm data were well fit with the Langmuir model based on the least square fit. A close examination of Figure 6 reveals that a linear plot with correlation coefficient (R^2) value of 0.99 is obtained when plotting C_e/q_e against C_e. This result confirmed the validity of Langmuir adsorption isotherm model for the adsorption process of La(III) on SG-N-PhenacylPyrNTf$_2$. In consequence, adsorption

isotherm data indicated that the adsorption process was mainly monolayer on a homogeneous adsorbent surface.

The corresponding fitting parameters of Q_o and b of Langmuir isotherm model were also calculated and found to be 165.39 mg g^{-1} and 0.27 L mg^{-1}, respectively. The R_L value of La(III) adsorption on SG-N-PhenacylPyrNTf$_2$ was also determined to be 0.02, supporting a highly favorable adsorption process based on the Langmuir adsorption isotherm model. It is also of interest to notice that the La(III) adsorption capacity (165.39 mg g^{-1}) calculated from Langmuir equation was strongly consistent with that (167.08 mg g^{-1}) experimentally obtained from the adsorption isotherm study.

Effect of contact time

The influence of shaking time is an important factor for evaluating the affinity of SG-N-PhenacylPyrNTf$_2$ to La (III). The recommended static technique was carried out with a contact time varied from 2.5 to 60.0 min. Results of the effect of shaking time on the adsorption of La(III) on SG-N-PhenacylPyrNTf$_2$ phase provided that the SG-N-PhenacylPyrNTf$_2$ had rapid adsorption kinetics for La(III). As illustrated in Figure 7, over 152 mg g^{-1} La (III) was absorbed by the SG-N-PhenacylPyrNTf$_2$ phase after only 10 min of the equilibrium period. The loading capacity of La(III) was also raised up to more than 159 mg g^{-1} after 30 min until the maximum adsorption of SG-N-PhenacylPyrNTf$_2$ for La(III) was reached to 167.08 mg g^{-1} after 60 min.

Kinetic models

In order to analyze the uptake kinetic mechanism of La(III) adsorption on SG-N-PhenacylPyrNTf$_2$, several kinetic models were evaluated to find kinetic adsorption parameters correctly representing the nature of adsorption process. Conventionally, the kinetics of metal ion

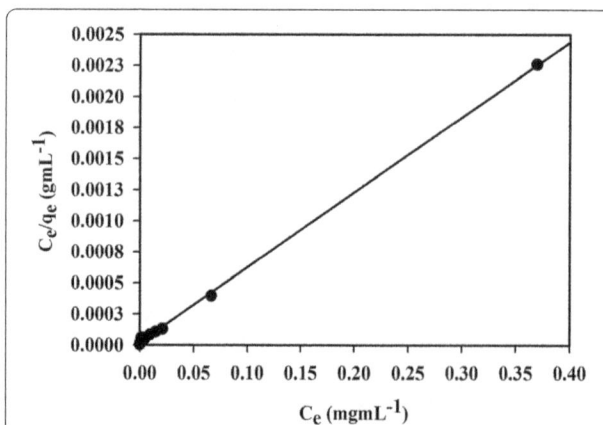

Figure 6 Langmuir adsorption isotherm model of La(III) adsorption on 20 mg SG-N-PhenacylPyrNTf$_2$ at pH 6.0 and 25°C.

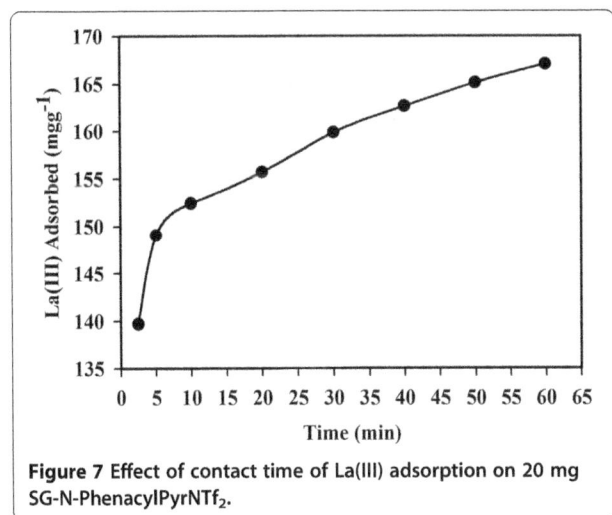

Figure 7 Effect of contact time of La(III) adsorption on 20 mg SG-N-PhenacylPyrNTf$_2$.

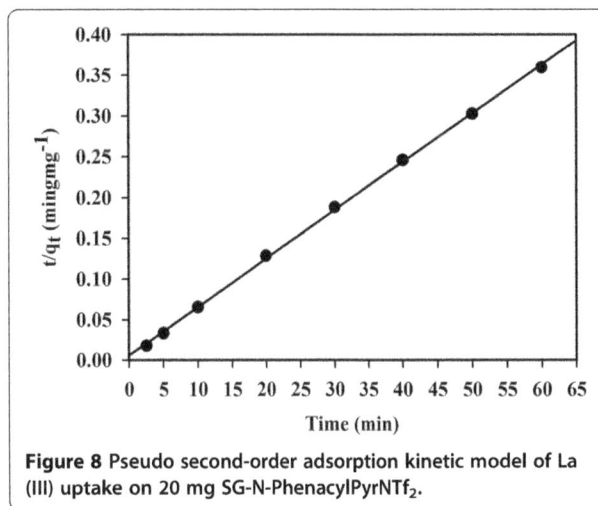

Figure 8 Pseudo second-order adsorption kinetic model of La (III) uptake on 20 mg SG-N-PhenacylPyrNTf$_2$.

adsorption is described following the expressions originally given by Lagergren, known as the pseudo first-order adsorption, which are special cases for the general Langmuir rate equation (Wu et al. 2001). The pseudo first-order equation can be given by the following equation:

$$\log(q_e - q_t) = \log q_e - (k_1/2.303)t \tag{4}$$

where q_e (mg g^{-1}) and q_t (mg g^{-1}) are the amount of adsorption at equilibrium and at time t (min), respectively, and k_1 denotes the adsorption rate constant of pseudo first-order adsorption (min^{-1}). The adsorption rate constant k_1 and adsorption capacity q_e can be calculated from the slope and intercepts of the plot of log($q_e - q_t$) against t.

In addition, the kinetics of La(III) adsorption on SG-N-PhenacylPyrNTf$_2$ was fit by the pseudo second-order kinetic model, which can be expressed as follows (Rao et al. 2009):

$$t/q_t = 1/v_o + (1/q_e)t \tag{5}$$

where $v_o = k_2 \, q_e^2$ is the initial adsorption rate (mg g^{-1} min^{-1}) and k_2 (g mg^{-1} min^{-1}) corresponds to the rate constant of the pseudo second-order adsorption; q_e (mg g^{-1}) is the amount of metal ion adsorbed at equilibrium, and q_t (mg g^{-1}) refers to the amount of metal ion on the adsorbent surface at any time t (min). Kinetic parameters of q_e and v_o can be obtained from the slope and intercept, respectively, of the linear plots of t/q_t versus t.

Adsorption kinetics data were well fit by the pseudo second-order model (Figure 8). The correlation coefficient (R^2) factor was found to be 0.99, indicating that the pseudo second-order adsorption is more reliable and accurate. Kinetic parameters of q_e and v_o were found to be 168.18 mg g^{-1} and 167.40 mg g^{-1} min^{-1}, respectively, and k_2 was determined to be 0.01 g mg^{-1} min^{-1} of La(III) adsorption

on the SG-N-PhenacylPyrNTf$_2$ phase. The La(III) adsorption capacity on SG-N-PhenacylPyrNTf$_2$ obtained from the pseudo second-order kinetic model (168.18 mg g^{-1}) was also closely related to those obtained from adsorption isotherm experiments (167.08 mg g^{-1}) and from the Langmuir isotherm model (165.39 mg g^{-1}), supporting the highest applicability of the pseudo second-order nature of the La(III) adsorption by SG-N-PhenacylPyrNTf$_2$ and the validity of Langmuir adsorption isotherm model.

Performance of method in analytical applications
Effect of interfering ions

The effect of coexisting ions on the % extraction of La (III) was studied under optimized conditions in order to evaluate the applicability of proposed method for analytical applications in analyzing real samples. Model standard solutions containing fixed amount of 1 mg L^{-1} La (III) with either individual or mixed matrix ions were treated according to the recommended procedure. The tolerance limit of coexisting ions is defined as the largest amount making the recovery of analyte less than 90%. Results shown in Table 3 displayed that the extraction of La(III) was not affected by the medium composition containing either individual or mixed ions. This may be due to the low adsorption capacity or rate for interfering ions toward the SG-N-PhenacylPyrNTf$_2$ phase. Thus, it can be clearly concluded that the newly modified SG-N-PhenacylPyrNTf$_2$ phase has high selectivity toward La(III) when compared to other interfering ions, and the proposed method can be implemented for the determination of La (III) in real samples.

Application of the proposed method

In order to evaluate the applicability of the proposed procedure for the determination of targeted metal ion, the method was applied for the determination of La(III)

Table 3 Effect of matrix interferences on the extraction of 1 mg L^{-1} La(III) on 20 mg SG-N-PhenacylPyrNTf$_2$ (N = 3)

Coexisting ions	Concentration (mg L^{-1})	% Extraction of La(III)
Na$^+$, K$^+$, NH$_4^+$	7,000	97.13
Ca^{2+}, Mg^{2+}	7,000	98.07
Cd^{2+}	600	97.43
Co^{2+}	600	96.04
Fe^{2+}	600	95.57
Ni^{2+}	600	98.30
Pb^{2+}	600	96.36
Al^{3+}	300	98.25
Cr^{3+}	300	97.86
Cl$^-$, F$^-$, NO$_3^-$	4,000	98.39
CO$_3^{2-}$, SO$_4^{2-}$	3,000	97.77

in real water samples. For the analysis of water samples, four different water samples, including drinking, lake, sea, and tap water, were collected from Jeddah in Saudi Arabia. Water samples were analyzed using the standard addition method under the same batch conditions as above. Results displayed in Table 4 demonstrated that the % extraction of La(III) was in the range of 94.85% to 98.66%. Thus, the proposed method promoted the proportionality of SG-N-PhenacylPyrNTf$_2$ for the determination of La(III) in real water samples.

Conclusions

In this study, the immobilization of N-PhenacylPyrNTf$_2$ on activated SG, as a new solid phase extractor (SG-N-PhenacylPyrNTf$_2$), was successfully accomplished via electrostatic interaction. The SG-N-PhenacylPyrNTf$_2$ phase attained a perfect selectivity for the extraction

and determination of La(III) in aqueous solution even in the presence of plentiful interfering ions. Results also demonstrated that adsorption isotherm data for La(III) adsorption on the SG-N-PhenacylPyrNTf$_2$ phase were well fit with the Langmuir classical adsorption isotherm model, providing that the formation of a monolayer over a homogeneous adsorbent surface. Moreover, kinetic isotherm data displayed that the adsorption of La (III) on the SG-N-PhenacylPyrNTf$_2$ phase obeyed a pseudo second-order kinetic reaction. Ultimately, the developed method can be applied and effectively utilized for the determination of La(III) in natural water samples with acceptable and reliable results.

Competing interests

The authors declare that they have no competing interests.

Authors' contributions

HMM designed the study and guided the research. AEA prepared sample solutions, carried out measurements, and drafted the manuscript. HMM modified the manuscript. Both authors read and approved the final manuscript.

Acknowledgements

The authors gratefully acknowledge the Department of Chemistry and Center of Excellence for Advanced Materials Research (CEAMR) at King Abdulaziz University for providing research facilities.

Table 4 Determination of La(III) at different concentrations in real water samples using 20 mg SG-N-PhenacylPyrNTf$_2$

Samples	Added (mg L^{-1})	Unadsorbed (mg L^{-1})	Extraction (%)
Tap water	1	0.02	98.00
	5	0.13	97.42
	10	0.39	96.15
Lake water	1	0.01	98.66
	5	0.14	97.22
	10	0.45	95.50
Seawater	1	0.03	97.40
	5	0.15	97.02
	10	0.52	94.85
Drinking water	1	0.02	98.46
	5	0.11	97.76
	10	0.36	96.45

References

Anderson JL, Armstrong DW, Wei G (2006) Ionic liquids in analytical chemistry. Anal Chem 78:2893–2902

Awwad NS, Gad HM, Ahmad MI, Aly HF (2010) Sorption of lanthanum and erbium from aqueous solution by activated carbon prepared from rice husk. Colloids Surf B 81:593–599

Ayata S, Bozkurt SS, Ocakoglu K (2011) Separation and preconcentration of Pb(II) using ionic liquid-modified silica and its determination by flame atomic absorption spectrometry. Talanta 84:212–215

Aydin FA, Soylak M (2007) A novel multi-element coprecipitation technique for separation and enrichment of metal ions in environmental samples. Talanta 73:134–141

Cai Y, Jiang G, Liu J, Zhou Q (2003) Multiwalled carbon nanotubes as a solid-phase extraction adsorbent for the determination of bisphenol A, 4-n-nonylphenol, and 4-tert-octylphenol. Anal Chem 75:2517–2521

Chen Q (2010) Study on the adsorption of lanthanum (III) from aqueous solution by bamboo charcoal. J Rare Earths 28:125–131

Cui Y, Chang X, Zhu X, Luo H, Hu Z, Zou X, He Q (2007) Chemically modified silica gel with p-dimethylaminobenzaldehyde for selective solid-phase extraction and preconcentration of Cr(III), Cu(II), Ni(II), Pb(II) and Zn(II) by ICP-OES. Microchem J 87:20–26

Dean JR (1998) Extraction methods for environmental analysis. Wiley, New York

Duran C, Gundogdu A, Bulut VN, Soylak M, Elci L, Sentürk HB, Tüfekci M (2007) Solid-phase extraction of Mn(II), Co(II), Ni(II), Cu(II), Cd(II) and Pb(II) ions from environmental samples by flame atomic absorption spectrometry (FAAS). J Hazard Mater 146:347–355

Farajzadeh MA, Bahram M, Zorita S, Mehr BG (2009) Optimization and application of homogeneous liquid-liquid extraction in preconcentration of copper (II) in a ternary solvent system. J Hazard Mater 161:1535–1543

Freundlich H (1906) Über die adsorption in lösungen (adsorption in solution). Z Phys Chem 57:384–470

Gaikwad AG, Damodaran AD (1993) Solvent extraction studies of holmium with acidic extractants. Sep Sci Technol 28:1019–1030

Han DM, Fang GZ, Yan XP (2005) Preparation and evaluation of a molecularly imprinted sol–gel material for on-line solid-phase extraction coupled with high performance liquid chromatography for the determination of trace pentachlorophenol in water samples. J Chromatogr A 1100:131–136

Handy ST (2005) Room temperature ionic liquids: different classes and physical properties. Curr Org Chem 9:959–988

Jain VK, Handa A, Sait SS, Shrivastav P, Agrawal YK (2001) Pre-concentration, separation and trace determination of lanthanum(III), cerium(III), thorium(IV) and uranium(VI) on polymer supported o-vanillinsemicarbazone. Anal Chim Acta 429:237–246

Jal PK, Patel S, Mishra BK (2004) Chemical modification of silica surface by immobilization of functional groups for extractive concentration of metal ions. Talanta 62:1005–1028

Khajeh M (2011) Response surface modelling of lead pre-concentration from food samples by miniaturised homogenous liquid-liquid solvent extraction: Box-behnken design. Food Chem 129:1832–1838

Koel M (2009) Ionic liquids in chemical analysis. CRC Press, Boca Raton

Komjarova I, Blust R (2006) Comparison of liquid-liquid extraction, solid-phase extraction and co-precipitation preconcentration methods for the determination of cadmium, copper, nickel, lead and zinc in seawater. Anal Chim Acta 576:221–228

Langmuir I (1916) The constitution and fundamental properties of solids and liquids. J Am Chem Soc 38:2221–2295

Liang P, Peng L (2010) Ionic liquid-modified silica as sorbent for preconcentration of cadmium prior to its determination by flame atomic absorption spectrometry in water samples. Talanta 81:673–677

Maanan M (2008) Heavy metal concentrations in marine molluscs from the Moroccan coastal region. Environ Pollut 153:176–183

Maestro P, Huguenin D (1995) Industrial applications of rare earths: which way for the end of the century. J Alloys Compd 225:520–528

Mahmoud ME (2011) Surface loaded 1-methyl-3-ethylimidazolium bis (trifluoromethylsulfonyl)imide [EMIM$^+$Tf$_2$N$^-$] hydrophobic ionic liquid on nano-silica sorbents for removal of lead from water samples. Desalination 266:119–127

Mahmoud ME, Al-Bishri HM (2011) Supported hydrophobic ionic liquid on nano-silica for adsorption of lead. Chem Eng J 166:157–167

Manzoori JL, Abdolmohammad-Zadeh H, Amjadi M (2007) Ultra-trace determination of silver in water samples by electrothermal atomic absorption spectrometry after preconcentration with a ligand-less cloud point extraction methodology. J Hazard Mater 144:458–463

Marahel F, Ghaedi M, Montazerozohori M, Nejati Biyareh M, Nasiri Kokhdan S, Soylak M (2011) Solid-phase extraction and determination of trace amount of some metal ions on duolite XAD 761 modified with a new Schiff base as chelating agent in some food samples. Food Chem Toxicol 49:208–214

Marwani HM (2010) Spectroscopic evaluation of chiral and achiral fluorescent ionic liquids. Cent Eur J Chem 8:946–952

Marwani HM (2013) Exploring spectroscopic and physicochemical properties of new fluorescent ionic liquids. J Fluoresc 23:251–257

McKay G, Blair HS, Gardner JR (1982) Adsorption of dyes on chitin. I. Equilibrium studies. J Appl Polym Sci 27:3043–3057

Ngeontae W, Aeungmaitrepirom W, Tuntulani T, Imyim A (2009) Highly selective preconcentration of Cu(II) from seawater and water samples using amidoamidoxime silica. Talanta 78:1004–1010

Palmieri MC, Volesky B, Garcia O Jr (2002) Biosorption of lanthanum using sargassum fluitans in batch system. Hydrometallurgy 67:31–36

Qiao R, Zhang R, Zhu W, Gong P (2012) Lab simulation of profile modification and enhanced oil recovery with a quaternary ammonium cationic polymer. J Ind Eng Chem 18:111–115

Quang DV, Kim JK, Sarawade PB, Tuan DH, Kim HT (2012) Preparation of amino-functionalized silica for copper removal from an aqueous solution. J Ind Eng Chem 18:83–87

Rao MM, Kumar Reddy DHK, Venkateswarlu P, Seshaiah K (2009) Removal of mercury from aqueous solutions using activated carbon prepared from agricultural by-product/waste. J Environ Manage 90:634–643

Safavi A, Abdollahi H, Hormozi Nezhad MR, Kamali R (2004) Cloud point extraction, preconcentration and simultaneous spectrophotometric determination of nickel and cobalt in water samples. Spectrochim Acta Part A 60:2897–2901

Saracoglu S, Soylak M, Kacar Peker DS, Elci L, dos Santos WNL, Lemos VA, Ferreira SLC (2006) A pre-concentration procedure using coprecipitation for determination of lead and iron in several samples using flame atomic absorption spectrometry. Anal Chim Acta 575:133–137

Sert S, Kütahyali C, Inan S, Talip Z, Cetinkaya B, Eral M (2008) Biosorption of lanthanum and cerium from aqueous solutions by platanus orientalis leaf powder. Hydrometallurgy 90:13–18

Shin EM, Choi HS (2009) Column preconcentration and determination of cobalt (II) using silica gel loaded with 1-nitroso-2-naphthol. Bulletin of the Korean Chemical Society 30:1516–1520

Simpson NJK (2000) Solid phase extraction: principles, strategies and applications. Marcel Dekker, New York

Soylak M, Erdogan ND (2006) Copper(II)-rubeanic acid coprecipitation system for separation-preconcentration of trace metal ions in environmental samples for their flame atomic absorption spectrometric determinations. J Hazard Mater 137:1035–1041

Tao GH, Fang Z (1998) Dual stage preconcentration system for flame atomic absorption spectrometry using flow injection on-line ion-exchange followed by solvent extraction. J Anal Chem 360:156–160

Tong S, Zhao S, Zhou W, Li R, Jia Q (2011) Modification of multi-walled carbon nanotubes with tannic acid for the adsorption of La, Tb and Lu ions. Microchim Acta 174:257–264

Unlü N, Ersoz M (2006) Adsorption characteristics of heavy metal ions onto a low cost biopolymeric sorbent from aqueous solutions. J Hazard Mater 136:272–280

Vidal L, Riekkola M-L, Canals A (2012) Ionic liquid-modified materials for solid-phase extraction and separation: a review. Anal Chim Acta 715:19–41

Vijayaraghavan K, Sathishkumar M, Balasubramanian R (2010) Biosorption of lanthanum, cerium, europium, and ytterbium by a brown marine alga, turbinaria conoides. Ind Eng Chem Res 49:4405–4411

Wang Z, Zhang Q, Kuehner D, Xu X, Ivaska A, Niua L (2008) The synthesis of ionic-liquid-functionalized multiwalled carbon nanotubes decorated with highly dispersed Au nanoparticles and their use in oxygen reduction by electrocatalysis. Carbon 46:1687–1692

Wu F-C, Tseng R-L, Juang R-S (2001) Kinetic modeling of liquid-phase adsorption of reactive dyes and metal ions on chitosan. Water Res 35:613–618

Zang Z, Li Z, Zhang L, Li R, Hu Z, Chang X, Cui Y (2010) Chemically modified attapulgite with asparagine for selective solid-phase extraction and preconcentration of Fe(III) from environmental samples. Anal Chim Acta 663:213–217

Zhang L, Ding S-D, Yang T, Zheng G-C (2009) Adsorption behavior of rare earth elements using polyethyleneglycol (phosphomolybdate and tungstate) heteropolyacid sorbents in nitric solution. Hydrometallurgy 99:109–114

Zhang N, Peng H, Hu B (2012) Light-induced pH change and its application to solid phase extraction of trace heavy metals by high-magnetization Fe$_3$O$_4$@SiO$_2$@TiO$_2$ nanoparticles followed by inductively coupled plasma mass spectrometry detection. Talanta 94:278–283

Zhao H (2006) Innovative applications of ionic liquids as "green" engineering liquids. Chem Eng Commun 193:1660–1677

12

Selective spectrofluorimetric method for the determination of perindopril erbumine in bulk and tablets through derivatization with dansyl chloride

Amir Alhaj Sakur[1], Tamim Chalati[2] and Hanan Fael[1*]

Abstract

Background: Perindopril erbumine is an antihypertensive, which belongs to the category of angiotensin-converting enzyme inhibitors (ACE inhibitors) that inhibit the conversion of angiotensin I to angiotensin II.

Methods: A new, selective, and sensitive spectrofluorimetric method was developed for the determination of perindopril erbumine based on the reaction with dansyl chloride in alkaline medium to give a highly fluorescent derivative which was measured at 496 nm after excitation at 340 nm in dichloromethane. The reaction conditions were studied and optimized.

Results: Under the optimum conditions, the fluorescence intensity was linear over a concentration range of 1.0 to 21.0 µg/mL ($R^2 = 0.9997$) with a detection limit of 0.242 µg/mL. In order to validate the method, the results were compared with those obtained by a high performance liquid chromatography method.

Conclusions: The proposed method was successfully applied to the analysis of perindopril erbumine in pure form and tablets with good precision and accuracy as revealed by t- and F tests. The mechanism of the reaction has also been discussed.

Keywords: Perindopril erbumine; Dansyl chloride; Derivatization; Spectrofluorimetry

Background

Perindopril erbumine (PDE) is the tert-butylamine salt of perindopril, which is the ethyl ester prodrug of the angiotensin-converting enzyme (ACE) inhibitor, perindoprilat. Perindopril erbumine is chemically described as 2-methylpropan-2-amine (2S,3aS,7aS)-1-[(2S)-2-[[(1S)-1-(ethoxycarbonyl) butyl] amino] propanoyl]octahydro-1H-indole-2-carboxylate, Figure 1. Its empirical formula is $C_{19}H_{32}N_2O_5C_4H_{11}N$.

Perindopril erbumine belongs to the category of angiotensin-converting enzyme inhibitors (ACE inhibitors) that inhibit the conversion of angiotensin I to angiotensin II. Perindopril erbumine is indicated for the treatment of hypertension; this effect appears to result primarily from

the inhibition of circulating and tissue ACE activity thereby reducing angiotensin II formation and decreasing vasoconstriction. Perindopril erbumine is also indicated for patients with congestive heart failure [British National Formulary BNF 2014].

Literature reported only few analytical methods for the determination of PDE in its bulk, dosage forms and human plasma, such as high performance liquid chromatography (Raju and Rao 2011; Zaazaa et al. 2013; Riyaz et al. 2012; Chaudhary et al. 2010; Jogia et al. 2010; Joseph et al. 2011; Prajapati et al. 2011a), HPLC-MS (Jaina et al. 2006 and Nirogi et al. 2006), high performance thin layer chromatography (Dewani et al. 2011), and spectrophotometry (Neelam et al. 2012; Rahman et al. 2012; Prajapati et al. 2011b). However, the chromatographic methods were found to have certain drawbacks, such as the expensive instrumentation and high analysis cost. Spectrophotometric methods, on the other

* Correspondence: hananfael@hotmail.com
[1]Department of Analytical Chemistry, Faculty of Pharmacy, University of Aleppo, Aleppo, Syria
Full list of author information is available at the end of the article

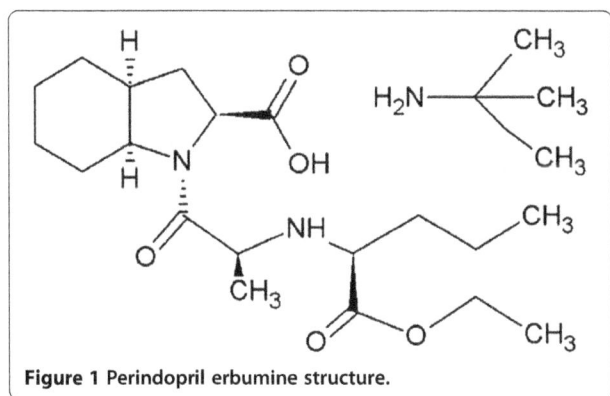

Figure 1 Perindopril erbumine structure.

hand, are not such sensitive methods in spite of being simple and economic technique. Therefore, it is still significant to develop a new, simple and sensitive method for the determination of perindopril erbumine.

There seems to be no reports on determination of such important drug, perindopril erbumine, using spectrofluorimetry, which shows several advantages such as high sensitivity, low detection limit, ease of use, and less time consumption comparing with other analytical methods.

Dansyl chloride (DNS) is known to react with primary and secondary amines, phenolic and alcoholic hydroxyl groups, and carboxylic acid groups (Bartzatt 2003). DNS has been used as a fluorogenic reagent for the determination of many pharmaceutical compounds (Aydoğmuş et al. 2012; Abd El Ghaffar et al. 2011; Abdel Fattah et al. 2010; Ulu 2011; Karasakal and Ulu 2013).

This paper describes, for the first time, the derivatization of PDE with dansyl chloride. The proposed method is sensitive, accurate, simple, and selective. It was applied for the determination of PDE in bulk and as well as in pharmaceutical preparations.

Methods

Chemicals and materials

All reagents and solvents were of analytical grade.

Perindopril erbumine (ROLABO outsourcing S.L., Spain) stock standard solution of 1.0 mg/mL was prepared in deionized (DI) water. This solution was freshly prepared at time of study. A series of working standard solutions were prepared by diluting aliquots of stock standard solution with DI water. Dansyl chloride (5-dimethylaminonaphthalene-1-sulphonyl chloride) was purchased from Merck, Germany. Solution of DNS was freshly prepared at 1.0 mg/mL in acetonitrile. Bicarbonate buffer (0.1 M) solution was prepared in DI water and adjusted to pH 9.5 with 0.1 M sodium hydroxide. Bicarbonate buffer solution was kept in refrigerator and used within about 5 days.

Perindopril erbumine tablets, Revosyl® (Ibn Alhaytham Pharma. Industries Co., Syria) and Neomeril® (Oubari Pharma, Syria) containing 4 and 8 mg, were purchased from local medical stores.

Instrumentation

Fluorescence spectra and measurements were obtained using fluorescence spectrophotometer F-2700 (Hitachi, Japan) equipped with xenon lamp. Excitation and emission wavelengths were set at 340 and 496 nm, respectively. The slit widths for excitation and emission monochromators were fixed at 5 nm. All measurements were performed in 1-cm quartz cell at room temperature.

Chromatographic (HPLC) analysis was performed on (Agilent 1200 series, Agilent Technologies, Germany) apparatus equipped with UV detector, autosampler, and column oven. Chromatographic separation was achieved on C18 column (5 µm, 100×4.6 mm).

Derivatization procedure

A 100 µL of PDE working standard solutions equivalent to a final concentration of 1.0 to 21.0 µg/mL was transferred into a series of 2-mL micro tubes that contain 100 µL of pH 9.5 bicarbonate buffer solution. A 300 µL of dansyl chloride solution was then added, and solution was mixed vigorously; then, tubes were kept in dry block heater at 40°C for 30 min. The tubes were then cooled, and the dansyl derivative was extracted three times with 1.5 mL of dichloromethane by a vortex mean. The organic layer was separated after centrifuging at 5,000 rpm for 1 min to ensure separation of organic-aqueous layers. The combined dichloromethane extracts were adjusted to 5 mL with the same solvent. The fluorescence intensity of the resulting solution was measured at 496 nm after excitation at 340 nm against reagent blank that had been treated similarly.

Determination of stoichiometric relationship

The composition ratio of the derivative product was determined using Job's continuous variation method and molar ratio method. In Job's method, equimolar solutions (2.26×10^{-3} M) of perindopril erbumine and dansyl chloride were mixed in which the total moles of reactants were kept at 4.53×10^{-7} moles. The volume of reaction phase was kept constant at 300 µL; then, steps were completed as described under the derivatization procedure. A plot of fluorescence intensities against the mole fraction of reagent was then constructed.

On the other hand, the molar ratio method was carried out. Increasing volumes of dansyl chloride were added to a fixed volume of drug solution. The obtained fluorescence intensities were then plotted against reagent molar ratio.

Procedure for pharmaceutical samples

Ten individual tablets were weighed and pulverized carefully. An accurately weighed amount of the powder equivalent to 8 mg of PDE was transferred into 25-mL volumetric flask and dissolved in 20 mL of bicarbonate buffer. The content of the flask was sonicated for 20 min then diluted to volume with bicarbonate buffer. Portion of this solution was centrifuged at 5,000 rpm for 10 min. Suitable aliquot of the supernatant was then transferred into micro tubes that contain 100 µL of DI water. A 300 µL of dansyl chloride solution was then added, and procedure was continued as mentioned above.

Results and discussion

Fluorescence spectra

Perindopril erbumine contains two amino groups and can therefore react with dansyl chloride in alkaline medium to give a strongly fluorescent product. On contrast, a reagent blank gave a negligible fluorescence signal at the chosen excitation and emission wavelengths. Under the described experimental conditions, the excitation spectra was obtained showing two maximum excitation wavelength at 260 and 340 nm, respectively. The excitation wavelength of 340 was employed, and emission spectra were obtained showing emission wavelength maxima at 496 nm (Figure 2).

Optimization of reaction conditions

Effect of pH

Effect of pH on the derivatization reaction was investigated using three different buffers in the alkaline region. Bicarbonate, phosphate, and borate buffers were studied. Buffers with amino groups such as tris and triethylamine were excluded, since they react with DNS reagent. The reaction was carried out initially at lab temperature for 30 min. The highest fluorescence intensity was obtained using pH 9.5 bicarbonate and borate buffer (Figure 3).

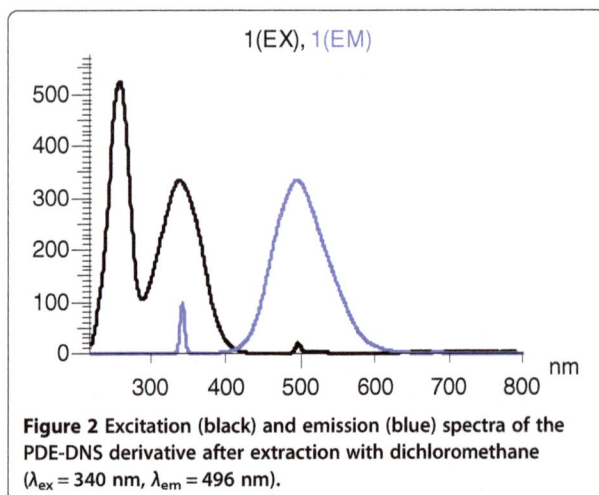

Figure 2 Excitation (black) and emission (blue) spectra of the PDE-DNS derivative after extraction with dichloromethane (λ_{ex} = 340 nm, λ_{em} = 496 nm).

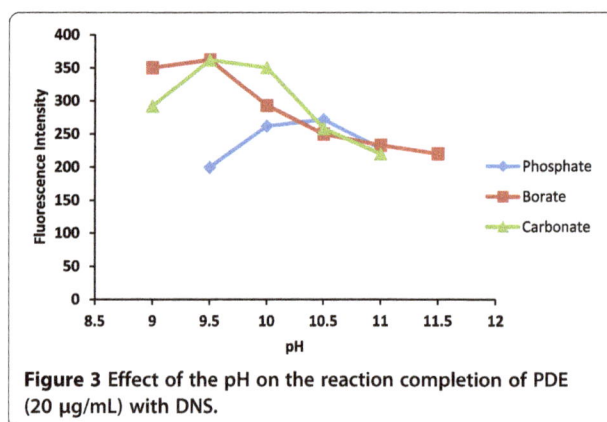

Figure 3 Effect of the pH on the reaction completion of PDE (20 µg/mL) with DNS.

Following that, in the study of temperature effect, bicarbonate and borate buffer were tested to find out which buffer is more appropriate.

Effect of time and temperature

In this study, the reaction between PDE and dansyl chloride was performed using pH 9.5 bicarbonate buffer at different temperatures (20°C, 30°C, 40°C, and 50°C) for various time intervals (10, 20, 30, 45, and 60 min). As it is seen in Figure 4, the derivatization reaction was found to be completed after 30 min at 40°C. Subsequently, borate buffer was tested at 40°C for 30 min and bicarbonate buffer was preferred over it.

Effect of buffer volume and concentration

Under the above described experimental conditions, the volume required of 0.1 M bicarbonate buffer (pH 9.5) was tested. As shown in Figure 5, a volume of 100 µL has given a maximum fluorescence intensity; thus, it was chosen to proceed the reaction. In addition, the buffer concentration was investigated at three different molarities (0.05, 0.1, and 0.2 M). It was found that 0.1 M has given the best results; thus, it was used for the next experiments.

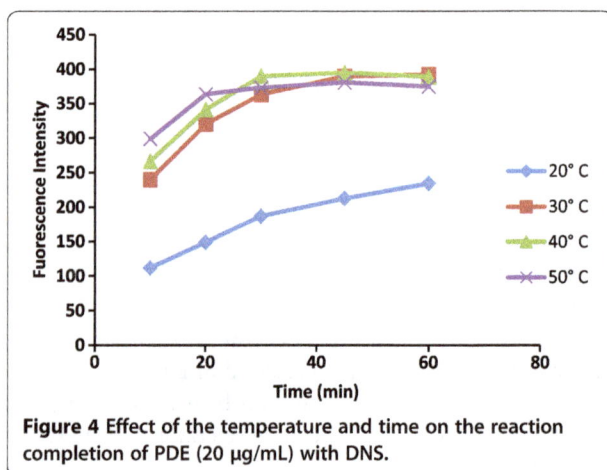

Figure 4 Effect of the temperature and time on the reaction completion of PDE (20 µg/mL) with DNS.

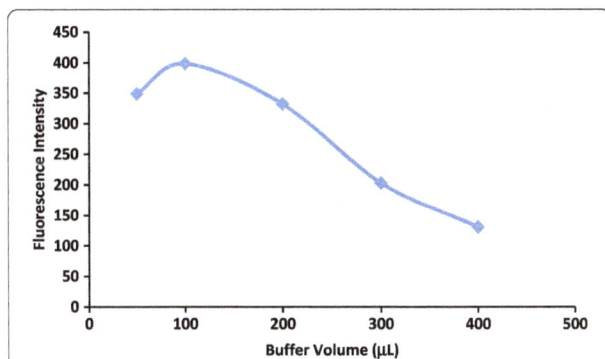

Figure 5 Effect of the volume added of 0.1 M bicarbonate buffer at pH 9.5 on the derivatization reaction of PDE (20 µg/mL).

Table 1 The maximum excitation and emission wavelengths of the PDE-DNS derivatization product and its fluorescence intensities in different organic extraction solvents

Extraction solvent	$\lambda_{ex}/\lambda_{em}$ (nm)	Fluorescence intensity[a]	
		Sample	Blank
Dichloromethane	340/496	540.3	3.6
Chloroform	337/494	432.7	3.5
Diethyl ether	330/489	391.5	3.0
Ethyl acetate	323/459	876.9	636.3

[a]PDE concentration = 20 µg/mL.

Effect of dansyl chloride volume

The influence of the volume of dansyl chloride solution was examined by addition of different volumes of 0.1% w/v reagent in the range of 50 to 500 µL (Figure 6). A maximum and steady fluorescence intensity was obtained when more than 200 µL of dansyl chloride solution was utilized. Thus, a fixed volume of 300 µL was used in the optimal procedure

Effect of extraction solvent

The aqueous reaction medium contains, in addition to the derivatization product, a highly fluorescent secondary product: dansyl hydroxide (Bartzatt 2003). In order to avoid the interference of this compound, an extraction step has been performed, so that the polar dansyl hydroxide remained in the aqueous phase and derivatization product moved to the immiscible organic solvent. For this purpose, different solvents including dichloromethane, chloroform, diethyl ether, and ethyl acetate were tested.

Ethyl acetate was rejected, since the blank value was very high when it was employed as an extractant. However, the highest fluorescence was obtained upon using dichloromethane (Table 1). The emission and excitation

spectra of derivatization product of perindopril erbumine in dichloromethane are shown in Figure 2.

Stoichiometric relationship of the reaction

Under the described conditions, the stoichiometry of the reaction between the drug and DNS was studied by Job's method of continuous variation and molar ratio method. As shown in Figures 7 and 8, the stoichiometry of the reaction was found to be 2:1 ratio (DNS/drug), confirming that one molecule of PDE reacts with two molecules of DNS. Perindopril erbumine contains a secondary amine in the perindopril moiety and a primary aliphatic amine in the erbumine molecule. In alkaline medium, these amine groups become more basic, and thus the electron pairs on the nitrogen atoms are free and could be involved easily in nucleophilic reactions. The reaction may be illustrated by the attack of these nucleophilic groups into the sulfonyl chloride group of DNS. A schematic proposal of the reaction pathway is given in Scheme 1.

Validation of the proposed method
Linearity

Under the optimum experimental conditions, standard calibration curve was constructed at eight concentration levels ($n = 5$). The correlation coefficient was 0.9997, indicating good linearity over the concentration range of 1.0 to 21.0 µg/mL. The intercept, slope, limit of

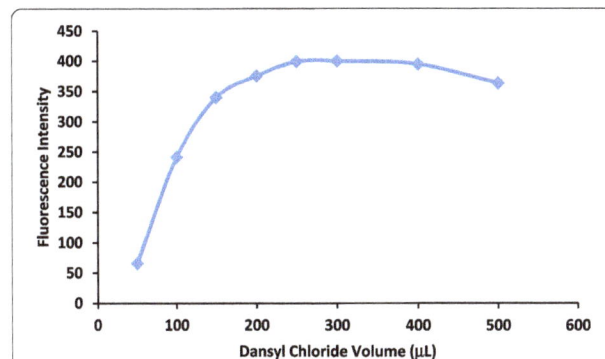

Figure 6 Effect of the volume added of 0.1% w/w dansyl chloride on the derivatization reaction of PDE (20 µg/mL).

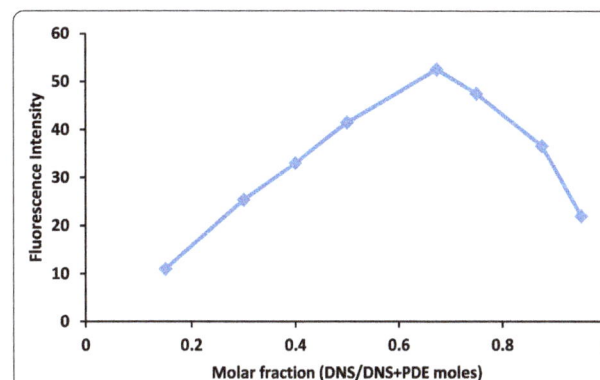

Figure 7 Job's plot of continuous variation for the stoichiometry of reaction between PDE and DNS.

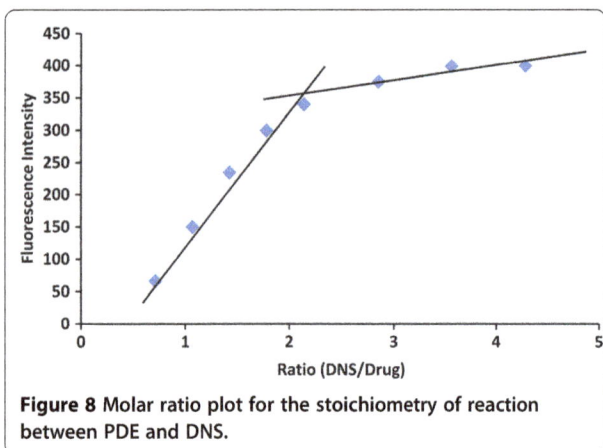

Figure 8 Molar ratio plot for the stoichiometry of reaction between PDE and DNS.

Table 2 Statistics and analytical parameters of PDE determination

Parameter	Result
$\lambda_{ex}/\lambda_{em}$ (nm)	340/496
Linear range (µg/mL)	1.0 to 21.0
Slope	27.164
Standard deviation in the slope	0.178
Intercept	4.5958
Standard deviation in the intercept	1.992
Correlation coefficient	0.9997
Limit of detection (µg/mL)	0.242
Limit of quantification (µg/mL)	0.733

detection (LOD), and limit of quantitation (LOQ) are summarized in Table 2. LOD and LOQ values were calculated according to ICH Q2B using the following equations:

$$LOQ = 10\,\sigma/S$$

$$LOD = 3.3\,\sigma/S$$

where σ is the standard deviation of intercept of regression line and S is the slope of the calibration curve (Table 2).

Selectivity

The effects of some common excipients used in pharmaceutical preparations were studied by analyzing solutions containing suggested amounts of each excipient. Frequently encountered excipients or additives were studied such as lactose, microcrystalline cellulose (Avicel), soluble starch, polyvinylpyrrolidone (PVP k30), talc, and magnesium stearate. None of the studied excipients has given any fluorescent product. So, the proposed method is suitable for analysis of perindopril erbumine in its dosage forms and application in quality control laboratories.

Precision

The repeatability of proposed method was estimated by measuring five replicate samples of each concentration of perindopril erbumine prepared in one laboratory on the same day. The precision expressed as the relative standard deviation (RSD%) ranged from 0.61% to 4.92% for the smallest concentration, indicating good precision (Table 3).

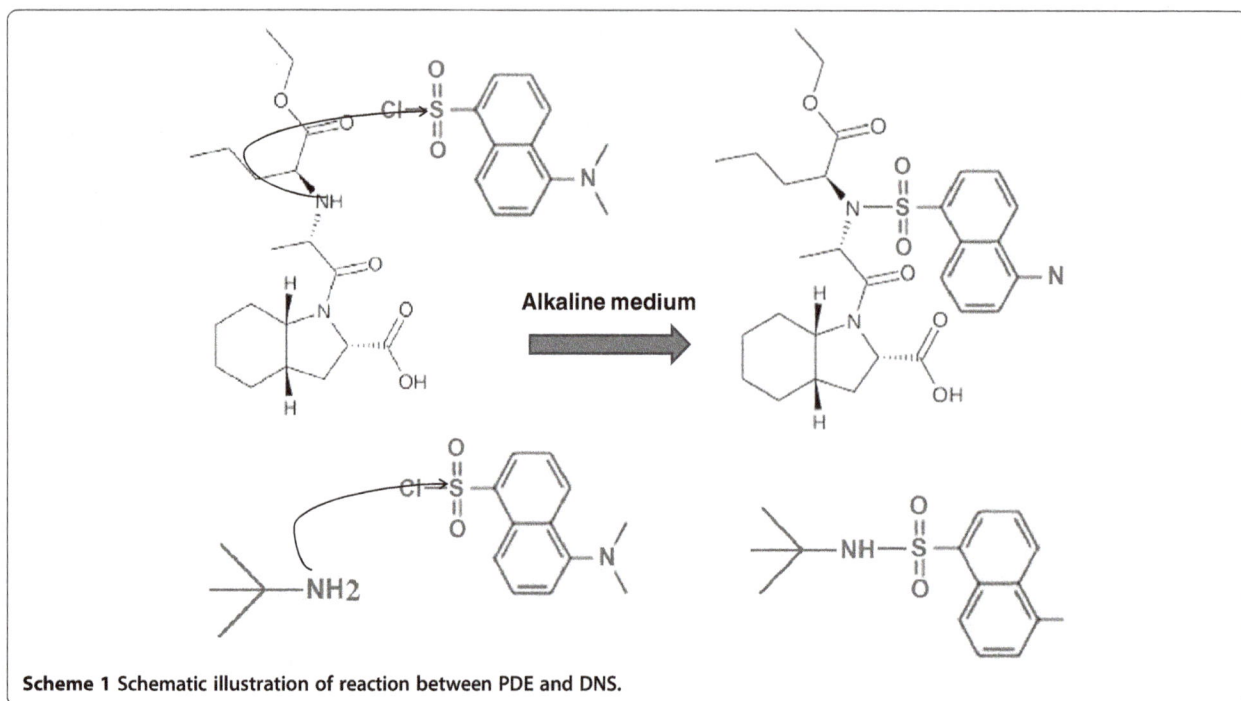

Scheme 1 Schematic illustration of reaction between PDE and DNS.

Table 3 Precision and accuracy for determination of PDE in pure form

Perindopril erbumine (µg/mL)		SD	RSD%	Recovery %	t-test[b]
Taken	Found[a]				
1.00	0.976 ± 0.059	0.048	4.92	97.60	1.118
2.20	2.195 ± 0.074	0.060	2.73	99.77	0.186
4.50	4.590 ± 0.104	0.084	1.83	102.00	2.395
6.70	6.733 ± 0.118	0.095	1.41	100.49	0.776
8.70	8.770 ± 0.156	0.126	1.44	100.80	1.242
11.20	11.169 ± 0.125	0.101	0.90	99.72	0.686
16.80	16.940 ± 0.182	0.147	0.86	100.83	2.129
21.00	20.930 ± 0.160	0.129	0.61	99.66	1.213

[a]Average of five determination ± confidence limit.
[b]The tabulated t-value at 95% confidence limit for 4 degrees of freedom ($n = 5$) is 2.78.

Accuracy

The proposed method was applied on the available commercial tablets that contain PDE, and recoveries are mentioned in Table 4. However, the method's accuracy is judged by (1) determining the average amount of PDE in pure form at several levels and using a significance test to compare it with actual amount μ (Harvey 2009]):

$$t = \frac{|\bar{X} - \mu|}{SD}\sqrt{n}$$

As shown in Table 3, the calculated t-value is less than tabulated $t\,(0.05, 4)$ value (2.78), and thus there are no significant differences between the taken and found concentration at 95% confidence level. Accuracy was indicated as well by analyzing the recoveries of known different amounts of PDE (Table 3) which varied from 97.60% to 102.00%. (2) The method's accuracy is also judged by comparing the results obtained from the presently proposed method with those obtained from a reference method such as high performance liquid chromatography (HPLC) (Raju and Rao 2011). The obtained results were statistically compared with each other (Table 4) using

t- and F-tests. t_{exp} was calculated using the following equation (Harvey 2009):

$$t_{exp} = \frac{|\bar{X}_A - \bar{X}_B|}{\sqrt{(S_A^2/n_A) + (S_B^2/n_B)}}$$

Where $\bar{X}_A$ and $\bar{X}_B$ are PDE mean values in each pharmaceutical product using the proposed and reference methods, respectively. S and n are the standard deviation and the number of replicate trials conducted on samples, respectively. With respect to t- and F tests, no significant differences were found between the calculated values of both the proposed and the reported methods at 95% confidence level.

Robustness

Robustness was investigated by evaluating the influence of minute variations in the experimental conditions such as volume of reagent (±10 µL), volume of bicarbonate solution (±5 µL), and reaction time (±5 min). These minor changes that may happen during the analysis did not have any significant effect on fluorescence intensity of the reaction product.

Application to tablets

The proposed method was successfully applied to analysis of two different commercial tablets (Revosyl® and Neomeril® tablets) were labeled to contain 4 and 8 mg of PDE. The mean recovery values were ranged from 96.50 to 104.25, which were identical to the recoveries recorded by the reference method (HPLC) as revealed by t- and F test (Table 4).

Comparison with reported analytical methods

The analytical methods reported in the literature suffered from one or more disadvantages like poor sensitivity, use of expensive chemicals, and/or complicated instruments, as can be seen from Table 5. However, the proposed method was found to be more sensitive than spectrophotometric and chromatographic methods (except for LC-MS);

Table 4 Precision and accuracy for determination of PDE in tablets

Tablets	Labeled amount of PDE	Average PDE found (mg/tablet) ± SD[a] (recovery %)[b]		t- and F test[c]
		Proposed method	Reference method[d]	
Revosyl	4 mg	4.10 ± 0.036 (102.50)	4.06 ± 0.024 (101.50)	1.734, 2.207
	8 mg	8.34 ± 0.064 (104.25)	8.44 ± 0.040 (105.50)	2.464, 2.612
Neomeril	4 mg	3.86 ± 0.035 (96.50)	3.90 ± 0.026 (97.50)	1.604, 1.830
	8 mg	7.77 ± 0.075 (97.12)	7.87 ± 0.042 (98.37)	2.299, 3.196

[a]Average and standard deviation of five determinations for the proposed method and three determinations for the reference method.
[b]Recoveries were calculated considering the labeled amount reported by the manufacturer.
[c]The tabulated t-value at 95% confidence limit for 4 degrees of freedom ($n = 5$) is 2.78 and the tabulated F value at 95% confidence limit for (4, 2) degrees of freedom for the proposed and reference methods, respectively, is 6.944.
[d]HPLC (Raju and Rao 2011.

Table 5 Performance characteristics of the existing methods used for the determination of PDE

No	Method	Medium	Application	Linear range	Reference
1	HPLC	Phosphate buffer: acetonitrile (65:35)	Tablets	20 to 100 µg/mL	Raju and Rao 2011
2	HPLC	Phosphate buffer: acetonitrile: Tetrahydrofuran (60:40:0.1)	Tablets (combination with amlodipine)	10 to 100 µg/mL	Zaazaa et al. 2013
3	HPLC	Phosphate buffer: acetonitrile (55:45)	Tablets (combination with amlodipine)	16 to 96 µg/mL	Riyaz et al. 2012
4	HPLC	Acetonitrile: acidic water (50:50)	Tablets (combination with losartan potassium)	1 to 30 µg/mL	Chaudhary et al. 2010
5	HPLC	Phosphate buffer: acetonitrile (75:25)	Dosage forms (combination with indapamide)	24 to 56 µg/mL	Jogia et al. 2010
6	HPLC	Phosphate buffer: acetonitrile (60:40)	Dosage forms (combination with indapamide)	8 to 24 µg/mL	Joseph et al. (2011)
7	HPLC	Phosphate buffer: acetonitrile (65:35)	Tablets (combination with amlodipine)	8 to 60 µg/mL	Prajapati et al. 2011a
8	LC-MS/MS	-	Human plasma	0.5 to 350 ng/mL	Jaina et al. 2006
9	LC/MS	-	Human plasma	0.1 to 100 ng/mL	Nirogi et al. [2006]
10	HPTLC	Dichloromethane: methanol: glacial acetic acid (9.5:0.5:0.1)	Dosage forms (combination with indapamide)	1 to 5 µg/band	Dewani et al. 2011
11	Spectrophotometry	Chloroform	Tablets	5 to 125 µg/mL	Neelam et al. 2012
12	Spectrophotometry	Dimethylsulfoxide	Tablets	2.5 to 25 µg/mL	Rahman et al. 2012
13	Spectrophotometry	Methanol	Tablets (combination with amlodipine)	4 to 12 µg/mL	Prajapati et al. 2011b
14	Spectrofluorimetry	Dichloromethane	Tablets	1 to 21 µg/mL	This work

in addition to less time-consuming compared with HPLC methods.

Conclusion

New, simple, and sensitive spectrofluorimetric method for the determination of PDE has been successfully developed and validated. The method involved the formation of a fluorescent derivatization product resulted from the reaction of PDE with DNS in alkaline medium. The proposed method was specific, precise, and accurate with a comparable low detection limit value of 0.242 µg/mL. The method was effectively applied for determining PDE in pure form and in tablets without any interference with the excipients. Therefore, the developed method can be suitable for routine analysis of PDE in quality control laboratories.

Competing interests

The authors declare that they have no competing interests.

Authors' contributions

HF has performed the experimental and analytical work and prepared the draft of the manuscript. The guidelines and supervision of this work was provided by AAS. AAS and TC read and modified the manuscript. All authors read and approved the final manuscript.

Author details

[1]Department of Analytical Chemistry, Faculty of Pharmacy, University of Aleppo, Aleppo, Syria. [2]Department of Pharmaceutics, Faculty of Pharmacy, University of Aleppo, Aleppo, Syria.

References

Abd El Ghaffar ME, El Wasseef DR, El Sherbiny DT, El Ashry SM (2011) Spectrofluorimetric determination of two β agonist drugs in bulk and pharmaceutical dosage forms via derivatization with dansyl chloride. J Anal Chem 66:476–481

Abdel Fattah LS, Mohamed TA, Taha EA (2010) Spectrofluorimetric determination of carvedilol in dosage form and spiked human plasma through derivatization with 1-dimethylaminonaphthalene-5-sulphonyl chloride. Chem Ind Chem Eng Q 16:31–38

Aydoğmuş Z, Sarı F, Ulu ST (2012) Spectrofluorimetric determination of aliskiren in tablets and spiked human plasma through derivatization with dansyl chloride. J Fluoresc 22:549–556

Bartzatt R (2003) Dansylation of aromatic, aliphatic and medicinal carboxylic acid compounds in 1 M Na_2CO_3 buffer. Anal Chim Acta 488:203–209

Joint Formulary Committee (2014) British National Formulary, 67th edition. British Medical Association and Royal Pharmaceutical Society of Great Britain, London

Chaudhary AB, Patel RK, Chaudhary SA (2010) Determination of losartan potassium and perindopril erbumine in tablet formulations by reversed-phase HPLC. International Journal of ChemTech Research 2:1141–1146

Dewani MG, Bothara KG, Madgulkar AR, Damle MC (2011) Simultaneous estimation of perindopril erbumine and indapamide in bulk drug and tablet dosage form by HPTLC. International Journal of Comprehensive Pharmacy 2:1–4

Harvey D (2009). Modern analytical chemistry. Second ed., David Harvey.

Jaina DS, Subbaiah G, Sanya M, Pande UC, Shrivastav P (2006) First LC-MS/MS electrospray ionization validated method for the quantification of perindopril and its metabolite perindoprilat in human plasma and its application to bioequivalence study. J Chromatogr B 837:92–100

Jogia H, Khandelwal U, Gandhi T, Singh S, Modi D (2010) Development and validation of a stability-indicating assay method for simultaneous determination of perindopril and indapamide in combined dosage form by reversed-phase high-performance liquid chromatography. J AOAC Int 93:108–115

Joseph J, Philip B, Sundarapandian M (2011) Method development and validation for simultaneous estimation of perindopril erbumine and indapamide by RP-HPLC in pharmaceutical dosage forms. International Journal of Pharmacy and Pharmaceutical Sciences 3:288–293

Karasakal A, Ulu ST (2013) New spectrofluorimetric method for the determination of nizatidine in bulk form and in pharmaceutical preparations. Opt Spectrosc 115:306–309

Neelam S, Gopisetti J, Chandra BS (2012) Spectrophotometric analysis of perindopril erbumine in bulk and tablets using bromophenol blue. Der Pharmacia Lettre 4:159–169

Nirogi RVS, Kandikere VN, Shukla M, Mudigonda K, Maurya S, Komarneni P (2006) High-throughput quantification of perindopril in human plasma by liquid chromatography/tandem mass spectrometry: application to a bioequivalence study. Rapid Commun Mass Spectrom 20:1864–1870

Prajapati J, Patel A, Patel MB, Prajapati N, Prajapati R (2011a) Analytical method development and validation of amlodipine besylate and perindopril

erbuminee in combine dosage form by RP-HPLC. International Journal of
      PharmTech Research 3:801–808
Prajapati J, Patel MB, Prajapati N, Prajapati R (2011b) Simultaneous determination
      of perindopril erbumine and amlodipine besylate by absorption factor
      method. Int J Appl Biol Pharmaceut Tech 2:230–233
Rahman N, Rahman H, Khatoon A (2012) Development of spectrophotometric
      method for the determination of perindopril erbumine in pharmaceutical
      formulations using 2, 4 dinitrofluorobenzene. J Chil Chem Soc 57:1069–1073
Raju VB, Rao AL (2011) Development and validation of new HPLC method for the
      estimation of perindopril in tablet dosage forms. Rasayan J Chem 4:113–116
Riyaz SMD, Vasanth PM, Ramesh M, Ramesh R, Ramesh T (2012) A sensitive RP-HPLC
      method development and validation for the simultaneous estimation of
      perindopril erbumine and amlodipine besilate in tablet dosage form.
      International journal of chemical and life science 1:1033–1038
Ulu ST (2011) Sensitive spectrofluorimetric determination of tizanidine in
      pharmaceutical preparations, human plasma and urine through derivatization
      with dansyl chloride. Luminescence: The Journal of Biological and Chemical
      Luminescence. doi:10.1002/bio.1367
Zaazaa HE, Abbas SS, Essam HA, El Bardicy MG (2013) Validated chromatographic
      methods for determination of perindopril and amlodipine in pharmaceutical
      formulation in the presence of their degradation products. J Chromatogr Sci
      51:533–543

13

Coronary stent as a tubular flow heater in magnetic resonance imaging

Stanislav Vrtnik[1,2], Magdalena Wencka[3], Andreja Jelen[1,2], Hae Jin Kim[4] and Janez Dolinšek[1,2*]

Abstract

Background: A coronary stent is an artificial metallic tube, inserted into a blocked coronary artery to keep it open. In magnetic resonance imaging (MRI), a stented person is irradiated by the radio-frequency electromagnetic pulses, which induce eddy currents in the stent that produce Joule (resistive) heating. The stent in the vessel is acting like a tubular flow heater that increases the temperature of the vessel wall and the blood that flows through it, representing a potential hazard for the stented patient.

Methods: Heating of a metallic coronary stent in MRI was studied theoretically and experimentally. An analytical theoretical model of the stent as a tubular flow heater, based on the thermodynamic law of heat conduction, was developed. The model enables to calculate the time-dependent stent's temperature during the MRI examination, the increase of the blood temperature passing through the stent and the distribution of the temperature in the vessel wall surrounding the stent. The model was tested experimentally by performing laboratory magnetic resonance heating experiments on a non-inserted stainless-steel coronary stent in the absence of blood flow through it. The model was then used to predict the temperature increase of the stainless-steel coronary stent embedded in a coronary artery in the presence of blood flow under realistic MRI conditions.

Results: The increase of the stent's temperature and the blood temperature were found minute, of the order of several tenths of a degree, because the blood flow efficiently cools the stent due to a much larger heat capacity of the blood as compared to the heat capacity of the stent. However, should the stent in the vessel become partially re-occluded due to the restenosis problem, where the blood flow through the stent is reduced, the stent's temperature may become dangerously high.

Conclusions: In the normal situation of a fully open (unoccluded) stent, the increase of the stent temperature and the blood temperature exiting the stent were found minute, of less than 1°C, so that the blood flow efficiently cools the stent. However, should the problem of restenosis occur, where the blood flow through the stent is reduced, there is a risk of hazardous heating.

Keywords: Coronary stent; Magnetic resonance imaging; Radiofrequency field heating effect; Modeling biomedical systems; MRI safety

Background

In medicine, a *stent* is an artificial "tube" inserted into a natural passage/conduit in the body to prevent, or counteract, a disease-induced, localized flow constriction. The most widely known stent use is in the coronary arteries (Hubner 1998), by employing a bare-metal stent, a drug-eluting stent or occasionally a covered stent. Coronary stents are inserted during a percutaneous coronary intervention (PCI) procedure to keep the blocked coronary arteries open. Stents are also applied to the urinary tract (Yachia 1998), where ureteral stents are used to ensure patency of a ureter, which may be compromised, for example, by a kidney stone. Prostatic stents (Yachia 1998) are needed if a man is unable to urinate due to an enlarged prostate. Stents are also used in a variety of vessels aside from the coronary arteries and as a component of peripheral artery angioplasty.

* Correspondence: jani.dolinsek@ijs.si
[1]Jožef Stefan Institute, Jamova 39, SI-1000 Ljubljana, Slovenia
[2]Faculty of Mathematics and Physics, University of Ljubljana, Jadranska 19, SI-1000 Ljubljana, Slovenia
Full list of author information is available at the end of the article

A coronary stent is a tubular metal mesh, attached initially in its collapsed form onto the outside of a balloon catheter. In the angioplasty procedure, the physician threads the stent through the lesion in the vessel and expands the balloon that deforms the stent to its expandable size by matching the undeformed vessel diameter. After removal of the deflated balloon, the framework of the stent remains in direct contact with the vessel wall (Figure 1), where it is overgrown by the endothelial tissue in the course of subsequent months. The coronary stent remains permanently inserted in the vessel, representing a metallic object firmly incorporated into the human body for life.

Stents can be assembled from a range of metallic alloys, including stainless steel, nitinol (nickel–titanium) and cobalt–chromium. The presence of a metallic object in the body brings up several safety issues in Magnetic Resonance Imaging (MRI) diagnostics. The two most important are the influence of magnetic forces on the implanted stent (Ahmed and Shellock 2001; Jost and Kumar 1998; Scott and Pettigrew 1994; Shellock and Shellock 1999; Strohm et al. 1999; Kagetsu and Litt 1991; Woods 2007; Lopič et al. 2013) and the stent heating by the radio-frequency (rf) electromagnetic pulses (Shellock and Morisoli 1994; Nyenhuis et al. 2005; Shellock 2011). In MRI, a stented person is irradiated by the rf pulses, which induce eddy currents in the stent that produce Joule (resistive) heating of the stent and its surroundings. During the MRI, the stent in the vessel is acting much like a tubular flow heater that increases the temperature of the vessel wall and the blood that flows through it. Due to the possible heat-induced protein coagulation and the formation of blood clots, stent heating in MRI deserves careful attention. In this paper, we present an analytical theoretical model of the stent as a tubular flow heater in the MRI examination. The model is based on the thermodynamic law of heat conduction and enables us to calculate the time-dependent stent temperature during the MRI examination, the increase of the blood temperature passing through the stent and the distribution of the temperature in the vessel wall surrounding the stent. We have tested the model experimentally by performing laboratory magnetic resonance rf

heating experiments on a non-inserted stainless-steel coronary stent in the absence of blood flow through it and good matching to the theory was found. The model was then used to predict the temperature increase of the stainless-steel coronary stent embedded in a coronary artery in the presence of blood flow through it under realistic MRI conditions. The results indicate that the increase of the stent's temperature and the blood temperature are minute, of the order of several tenths of a degree, because the blood flow efficiently cools the stent due to a much larger heat capacity of the blood as compared to the heat capacity of the stent. However, should the problem of restenosis occur, where the stent in the vessel becomes partially re-occluded and the flow reduces, there is a risk of hazardous heating and the stent's temperature may become dangerously high.

Methods
Stent description and characterization
Our experiments were performed on a commercial balloon-expandable coronary stent (HORUSS HDS 1625, International Biomedical Systems, Trieste). The stent was fabricated of a surgical stainless steel, having the nominal length of 16 mm, the nominal diameter of 2.5 mm and the nominal pressure for the expansion of 8 atm. A small part of the stent was cut away for the physical property determination of the material, whereas the large part (12 mm length) was used for the rf heating experiments. The photograph of the employed stent is shown in Figure 2a.

The stent's material was surgical stainless steel type 316LVM (where "L" stands for Low Carbon and "VM" denotes Vacuum Melted), using a wire of 200–μm diameter (Figure 2b). The 316LVM is an austenitic steel, which is widely used for implants because it never develops surface rust and shows superior resistance to constant salt water exposure. According to the international standards (ASM International Handbook Committee 1990), the elemental composition of 316LVM is in the range 0.03 wt.% C, up to 2.0% Mn, 2.0 – 3.0% Mo, up to 1.0% Si, 16.0 – 18.0% Cr, 10.0 – 14.0% Ni, up to max. 0.16% N, and about 65% Fe as the majority element. We have determined the particular chemical composition of our investigated stent by the energy-dispersive X-ray spectrometer (EDS) using a scanning electron microscope (SEM) Supra VP 35 Zeiss (Carl Zeiss AG, Oberkochen, Germany). The resulting chemical composition (in weight %) is displayed as a histogram in Figure 2c. The too high carbon concentration (2.94%) is artificial; it originates from the contamination of the SEM by the hydrocarbons (a known problem in SEM microscopy). Apart from the carbon, other elements are within the specifications for the 316LVM steel.

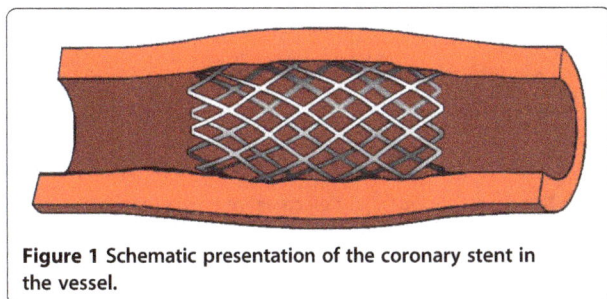

Figure 1 Schematic presentation of the coronary stent in the vessel.

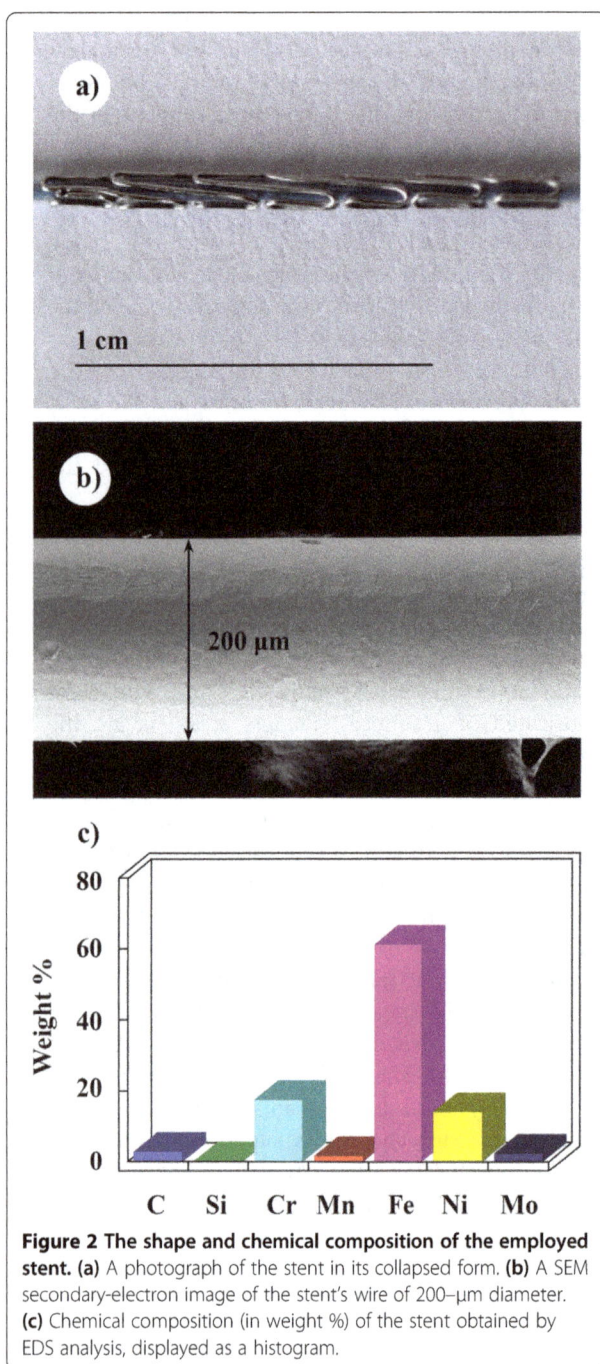

Figure 2 The shape and chemical composition of the employed stent. (a) A photograph of the stent in its collapsed form. **(b)** A SEM secondary-electron image of the stent's wire of 200–μm diameter. **(c)** Chemical composition (in weight %) of the stent obtained by EDS analysis, displayed as a histogram.

Since the induction of the eddy currents by the rf field is strong in metallic alloys of low electrical resistivity, we have measured the electrical resistivity ρ of the stent's wire. The direct current (dc) resistivity was determined in the temperature interval from 2 to 360 K by a standard four-contact method using a Quantum Design PPMS (Physical Property Measurement System). The dc resistivity is usually good approximation to the frequency-dependent (ac) resistivity $\rho(\omega)$ up to the microwave frequencies, so that it is considered valid also in the radio-frequency range of the MRI experiments. The result is shown in Figure 3, where it is evident that $\rho(T)$ exhibits a positive temperature coefficient at the values in the range $\rho \approx 100 - 150\mu\Omega cm$, typical of moderately electrically conducting alloys. At the body temperature of 37°C, the resistivity amounts $\rho_{37^{\circ}C} = 146\mu\Omega cm$, which is low enough that a significant induction-heating effect may be expected under the rf-pulse irradiation.

To verify the analytical model of the stent as a tubular flow heater presented in this paper, the specific heat c_s of the stent must be known. We have determined c_s experimentally by using a Quantum Design PPMS. The graph of the temperature-dependent c_s in the interval from 2 to 370 K is presented in Figure 4, showing that at 37°C, c_s = 0.46 J/gK.

Rf heating experiments

Rf heating experiments of the stent were conducted in a standard 4.7 T vertical-bore NMR spectrometer operating at the proton resonance frequency ν_0 (^{1}H) = 200 MHz. An AMT 300 W rf power transmitter was used. To monitor the temperature of the stent, a platinum Pt100 resistor was glued to its outer surface by a thermally conducting varnish (GE/IMI 7031). The stent with the sensor was wrapped up into a Teflon foil of 1.0 mm total thickness. The output of the sensor was connected to a data logger (PT-104 PT 100 Converter, Pico Technology, Cambridgeshire, UK) that has digitized the signal and enabled us to follow the time-dependent increase of the stent's temperature under the rf irradiation.

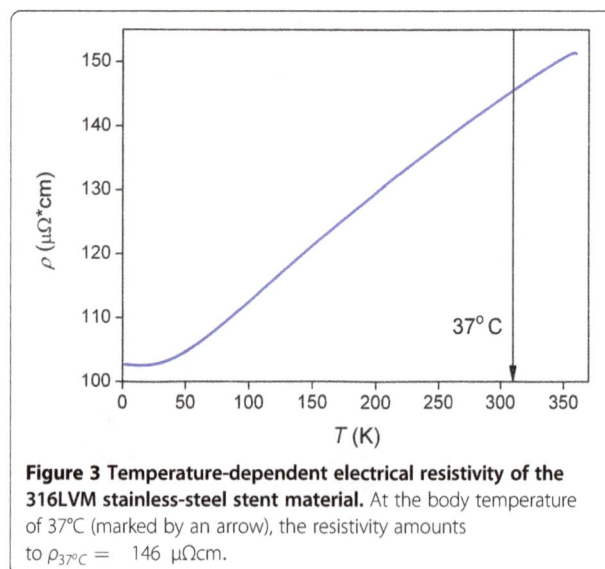

Figure 3 Temperature-dependent electrical resistivity of the 316LVM stainless-steel stent material. At the body temperature of 37°C (marked by an arrow), the resistivity amounts to $\rho_{37^{\circ}C} = 146 \mu\Omega cm$.

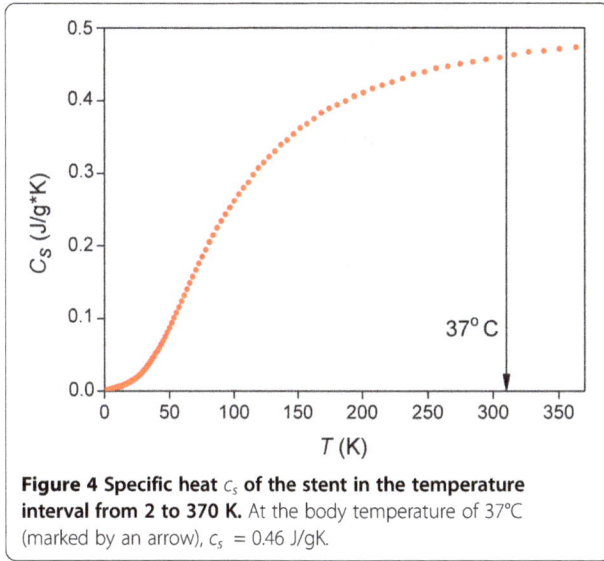

Figure 4 Specific heat c_s of the stent in the temperature interval from 2 to 370 K. At the body temperature of 37°C (marked by an arrow), c_s = 0.46 J/gK.

Results and discussion

Analytical model of the stent as a tubular flow heater in MRI

We approximate the actual stent's geometry of a cylindrical metal mesh by a homogeneous thin cylinder of the length l and the radius R (Figure 5). The mass of the stent is m_s and its specific heat at constant pressure is c_s. The stent is surrounded by the vessel wall of cylindrical shape with the wall thickness d and the thermal conductivity λ. The stent's temperature is T_s, whereas the temperature at the outer surface of the vessel is T_0 (taken roughly as the body temperature 37°C). The blood mass flow $\Phi_b = dm_b/dt$ (where m_b is the mass of the blood) enters the stent at the body temperature T_0

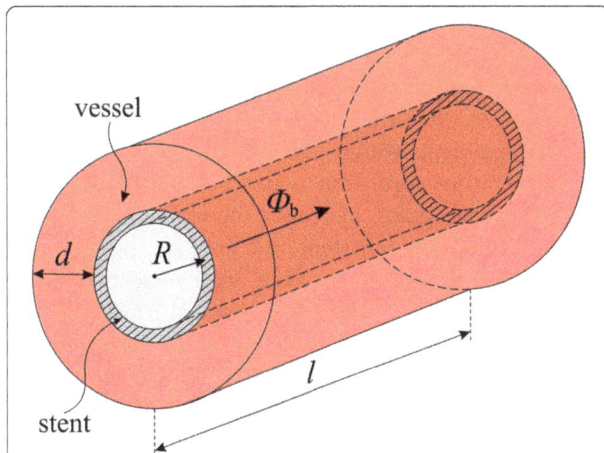

Figure 5 Schematic presentation of the stent as a tubular flow heater in the MRI examination. In the model, the cylindrical metal mesh geometry of the stent is approximated by a thin homogeneous cylinder of the radius R and length l. The surrounding vessel wall of the thickness d is assumed to be cylindrical as well. A blood flow Φ_b is passing through the stent.

and exits at an elevated temperature T_b. Due to the heart pulsing, the blood flow is pulsed, but we approximate it by a stationary flow $\Phi_b = \rho_b S_s \bar{v}_b$, where ρ_b is the blood density, $S_s = \pi R^2$ is the stent's cross section and $\bar{v}_b$ is the average blood velocity through the stent. The specific heat at constant pressure of the blood is c_b.

The rf electromagnetic pulses during the MRI examination supply the stent with the rf power P_{rf}, which transforms into the heat $dQ = P_{rf}dt$ via the Joule heating by the induced eddy currents. A part of this heat is released through the vessel wall. For a cylindrical vessel, the thermal power (heat flow) P_v through the wall amounts (Halliday et al. 2005)

$$P_v = \frac{\lambda 2\pi l}{\ln(1 + d/R)}(T_s - T_0). \tag{1}$$

The blood flow through the stent takes away the thermal power

$$P_b = \Phi_b c_b (T_b - T_0). \tag{2}$$

The heat imbalance $(P_{rf} - P_v - P_b)\,dt$ increases the stent's temperature by dT_s,

$$(P_{rf} - P_v - P_b)\,dt = m_s c_s dT_s. \tag{3}$$

Using Equations 1 and 2, we rewrite Equation 3 in the form

$$P_{rf} - \frac{\lambda 2\pi l}{\ln(1 + d/R)}(T_s - T_0) - \Phi_b c_b (T_b - T_0)$$
$$= m_s c_s \frac{dT_s}{dt}, \tag{4}$$

which contains two unknown variables, $T_s(t)$ and $T_b(t)$. To proceed, we assume that the time-dependence of the blood temperature T_b follows the time-dependence of the stent's temperature T_s, though T_b may be lower than T_s,

$$T_b - T_0 = \varepsilon(T_s - T_0), \tag{5}$$

with $0 \le \varepsilon \le 1$. Equation 4 is then cast into the form

$$\frac{dT_s}{dt} + \alpha(T_s - T_0) = \frac{P_{rf}}{m_s c_s}, \tag{6}$$

where

$$\alpha = \frac{1}{m_s c_s}\left(\frac{\lambda 2\pi l}{\ln(1 + d/R)} + \varepsilon \Phi_b c_b\right). \tag{7}$$

The solution of Equation 6 is

$$T_s = T_0 + \Delta T(1 - e^{-\alpha t}), \tag{8}$$

where $\Delta T = P_{rf}/\alpha\, m_s c_s$. The stent reaches the new steady-state temperature $T_s(t \to \infty) = T_0 + \Delta T$ exponentially with the time constant α^{-1} after the start of the rf pulsing in the MRI examination. Using the definition of α, the increase of the stent's temperature can also be written in the form

$$\Delta T = \frac{P_{rf}}{\frac{\lambda 2\pi l}{\ln(1+d/R)} + \varepsilon \Phi_b c_b}. \tag{9}$$

The time-dependent stent's temperature given by Equation 8 is shown in Figure 6a.

According to the above model, the blood temperature $T_b(t)$ follows the stent's temperature $T_s(t)$, as expressed by Equation 5. The efficiency of the heat transfer from the stent to the blood is given by the empirical factor ε, which assumes a value between 1 and 0, depending on the details of the vessel and the blood flow through it. ε should be determined experimentally for a particular vessel and the type of inserted stent. The time-dependent blood temperature obeys the equation $T_b(t) = T_0 + \varepsilon (T_s(t) - T_0)$, where $T_s(t)$ is given by Equation 8.

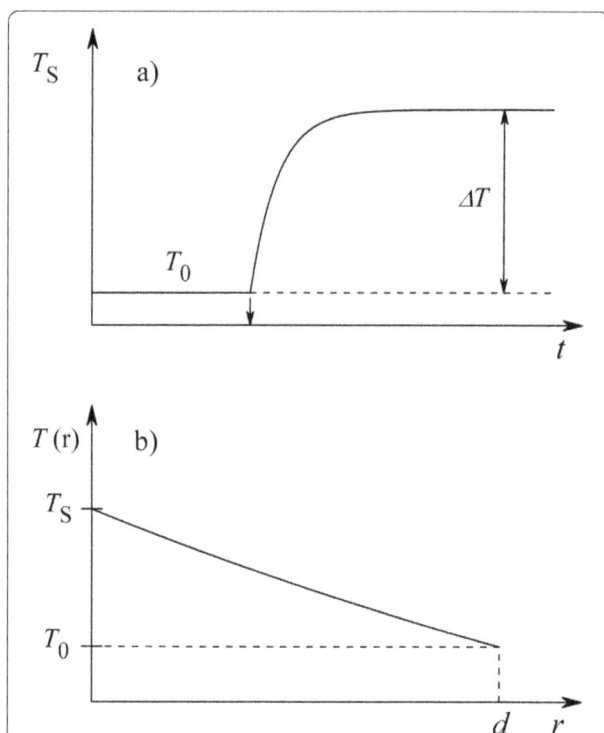

Figure 6 Theoretical stent's temperature in the MRI examination. (a) The time-dependent stent's temperature $T_s(t)$ given by Equation 8. The start of the rf irradiation is marked by an arrow on the time axis. The time-dependent blood temperature $T_b(t)$ exiting the stent has the same form, except that the steady-state temperature increase is reduced to $\varepsilon \Delta T$ with $0 \le \varepsilon \le 1$. **(b)** Radial distribution of the temperature $T(r)$ within the vessel wall surrounding the stent ($0 \le r \le d$) in the steady state, as given by Equation 11. At the contact surface to the stent, the vessel wall heats up to the stent temperature, $T(r=0) = T_s$, whereas at the vessel's outer surface, the temperature drops to the body temperature, $T(r=d) = T_0$, via a $\ln(1 + r/R)$ radial dependence.

The $T_s(t)$ curve shown in Figure 6a, scaled by a factor ε, is thus valid for the blood temperature $T_b(t)$ as well. After the steady-state is reached during the irradiation, the increase of the blood temperature passing the stent is $\varepsilon \Delta T$ with ΔT given by Equation 9.

The radial distribution of the temperature $T(r)$ within the vessel wall surrounding the stent ($0 \le r \le d$) in the steady state is obtained by assuming a stationary radial heat flow through the wall, so that P_v as given by Equation 1 is constant at any radial distance r from the stent. The condition

$$P_v = \frac{\lambda 2\pi l (T_s - T(r))}{\ln(1 + r/R)} = const. \tag{10}$$

yields the $T(r)$ dependence

$$T(r) = T_s - \frac{P_v \ln(1 + r/R)}{\lambda 2\pi l}, \tag{11}$$

which is shown in Figure 6b. At the contact surface to the stent, the vessel wall heats up to the stent temperature, $T(r=0) = T_s$, whereas at the vessel's outer surface, the temperature drops to the body temperature, $T(r=d) = T_0$, via a $\ln(1 + r/R)$ radial dependence.

In the above analytical model of the stent as a tubular flow heater, some simplifications were used mostly to ensure mathematical tractability of the calculation. Two of them deserve to be discussed in more detail. In the model, the vessel wall surrounding the stent is considered to be cylindrical of the thickness d, where the temperature at the contact surface to the stent is assumed to equal the stent temperature T_s, whereas at the outer surface it equals the body temperature T_0. The vessel wall thickness was not specified, but for the coronary arteries and the coronary stents it is reasonable to assume the inequality $d < R$, where R is the radius of the stent. This approximation assumes a very powerful cooling process in the body and an excessive temperature gradient within the vessel wall. In fact human temperature regulation is not powerful enough to justify this assumption. In reality, the temperature in the tissue surrounding the stent will drop to the body temperature over the distance of the order of several R, thus considerably larger than the vessel wall thickness. In the case where the vessel and the tissue behind it have similar thermal conductivity λ values (a reasonable assumption), this discrepancy can be removed by simply taking larger d value in Equations 1 to 9. Since d always appears in a logarithmic function of the form $\ln(1 + d/R)$, which is located in the denominator of the expression for ΔT (Equation 9), larger d will reduce the heat flow P_v through the vessel wall. Due to the logarithmic dependence on d, the changes are relatively weak (e.g., for a thickness increase from

$d = R$ to $d = 10R$, the function $\ln(1 + d/R)$ increases by a factor 3.4 only). Smaller P_v will increase the stent's steady-state temperature ΔT, thus subjecting the inner side of the vessel to higher temperatures and also heating stronger the blood flowing through the stent. The heating effect is thus increased under the assumption that the temperature of the tissue surrounding the stent drops to the "unperturbed" body temperature at a distance considerably larger than the stent's diameter R.

The second simplification is the assumption that the blood temperature follows the stent temperature, as expressed by Equation 5. This assumption has enabled the elimination of one unknown variable (the blood temperature $T_b(t)$) from the calculation and kept the model simple and analytically tractable. The assumption required the introduction of the empirical "heat-transfer efficiency factor" ε (with $0 \leq \varepsilon \leq 1$,) describing the efficiency of the heat transfer from the stent to the blood. While it is intuitively plausible to relate the blood temperature to the stent temperature by the Equation 5, the factor ε is not well-defined as the stent-to-blood heat transfer efficiency will depend on the details of the vessel, the type and geometry of the inserted stent and the blood flow through it. Weaker heat transfer ($\varepsilon \rightarrow 0$) will increase the risk of high temperatures developed in the stent, as the stent is not giving up the heat to the blood. Good heat transfer can generally be expected for longer stents and lower blood velocity.

Rf heating experiments on a coronary stent in the absence of blood flow

In our experimental study of the temperature increase of the stainless-steel coronary stent subjected to irradiation by the rf pulses, the stent with the attached Pt100 thermometer was placed into the rf coil of the NMR probe head and inserted into the magnet. A typical MRI rf pulse sequence contains one or more pulses that are usually shaped in the time domain, where a truncated sinc and a Gaussian shape are most commonly employed (Callaghan 1991). Instead of using shaped pulses, our pulse sequence was composed of a train of

50 rectangular pulses of $\tau = 20$ μs length each (1 ms total pulse duration), separated by 5 μs and repeated with the repetition rate $t_0 = 100$ ms (Figure 7), yielding the duty cycle $\delta_D = 0.01$. A shaped rf pulse in a realistic MRI experiment has a similar duration and repetition rate. The power of the rf pulses has been varied during the experiment and the temperature raise of the stent was monitored at different power levels. Here it is worth mentioning that the actual shape of the rf pulses is relatively unimportant for the heating effect; what matters is the average rf power delivered by the pulses to the stent.

The irradiation of the stent started by switching on the pulse sequence of Figure 7 at a given moment of time and then continuously repeating it at a selected transmitter rf output power level. This resulted in rapid initial growth of the stent temperature, which has saturated to a constant plateau after some time when the balance between the incoming rf energy and the outgoing heat due to the thermal conduction was achieved. In order to minimize heat losses by thermal conduction to the surrounding air, the rf probe head with the stent was placed into an Oxford continuous-flow cryostat CF 1200 (Oxford Instruments, Abingdon, Oxfordshire, UK), where the air could be evacuated to a pressure down to 0.2 bar. After a steady-state temperature was reached with time at a given rf power level, the transmitter power was increased and the new stent's temperature was recorded. In the following we present the stent's temperature increase as a function of the average rf power over the pulse sequence repetition time t_0, defined as $\bar{P} = (1/t_0) \int_0^{t_0} P(t) \, dt = \delta_D P_{tr}$, where P_{tr} is the transmitter power (e.g., $\bar{P} = 3$ W for the full transmitter power $P_{tr} = 300$ W and the duty cycle $\delta_D = 0.01$). The time-dependent stent's temperature under the rf irradiation at different average power levels $\bar{P} = 0.1$, 0.3, 1, and 3 W is shown in Figure 8a. The initial stent's temperature was 19.5°C. We observe that at each power level, the rapid initial increase of the temperature slows down with time and reaches a steady state in about 100 s. For the highest average rf power of $\bar{P} = 3$ W, the stent has reached an astonishingly high temperature

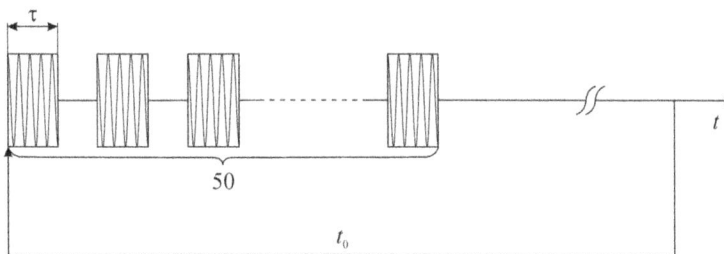

Figure 7 The rf pulse sequence used in the stent heating experiment. A train of 50 rectangular rf pulses of $\tau = 20$μs duration each, separated by 5 μs was continuously repeated with the repetition rate of $t_0 = 100$ ms.

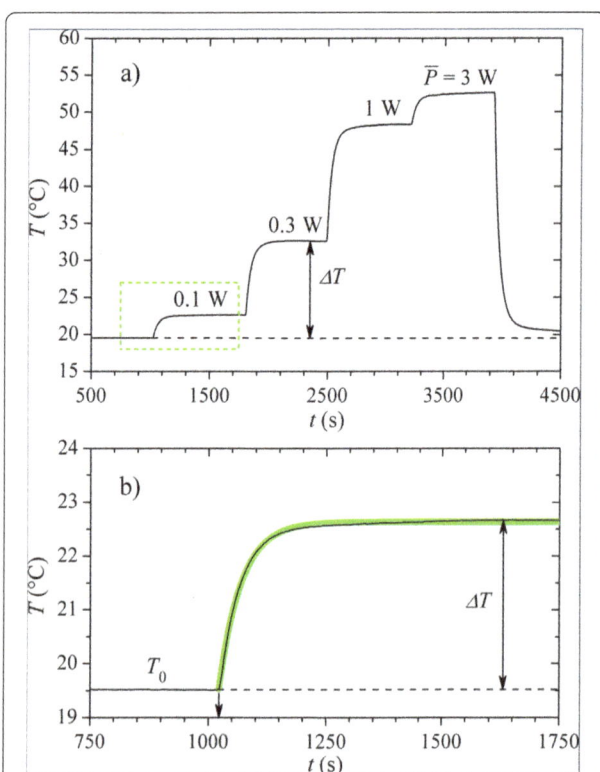

Figure 8 Experimental stent's temperature under the rf irradiation. (a) The time-dependent stent's temperature under irradiation at different average power levels $\bar{P}$ = 0.1, 0.3, 1, and 3 W (denoted on the graph). The initial stent temperature was 19.5°C. At each higher power level, the temperature has reached a new steady-state temperature ΔT higher than the initial temperature. The dashed box encloses the time-dependent temperature increase of the stent for the initial average power $\bar{P}$ = 0.1 W and is shown expanded in panel **(b)**. The experimental data in the panel (b) (thin black curve) were reproduced theoretically by the exponential function of Equation 8 (thick green curve) with the fit parameters given in the text. The irradiation by the rf pulses on the time axis began at the point marked by an arrow.

of 52.5°C (yielding an increase by as much as ΔT = 33°C from the initial temperature before the irradiation). The values of the steady-state temperature increase ΔT, as a function of $\bar{P}$, are given in Table 1. The detailed shape of the stent's time-dependent temperature $T(t)$ under irradiation by the rf pulses for the initial power level of

Table 1 The temperature increase ΔT of the stent as a function of the rf power $\bar{P}$

$\bar{P}$ (W)	ΔT (°C)
0.1	3.1
0.3	13.0
1	28.8
3	33.0

$\bar{P}$ = 0.1 W (enclosed in a dashed box in Figure 8a), is shown expanded in Figure 8b, where an exponential increase is obvious. We have also checked the increase of the stent's temperature in the air environment at the ambient pressure of 1 bar, where the stent's heat supplied by the rf irradiation is taken away more efficiently by the thermal convection to the surrounding air. The highest temperature of the stent in the 1 bar air atmosphere for $\bar{P}$ = 3 W has dropped to 48°C, as compared to 52.5°C in an identical experiment in the reduced 0.2 bar atmosphere, showing that the thermal convection to the air takes away considerable amount of the heat from the stent.

The above results indicate the possibility of hazardous heating of the stent in the MRI examination by as much as $\Delta T \approx 30$°C. It is, however, important to emphasize that this conclusion is based on experiments with no blood flow through the stent. We shall discuss in the following how does this conclusion change under the blood flow condition.

Comparison between the theory and experiment

The stent's temperature $T_s(t)$ in our rf heating experiment of Figure 8b was reproduced theoretically by the Equation 8. Excellent fit (thick green curve in Figure 8b) was obtained using the parameters ΔT = 3.1°C and the time constant α^{-1} = 45 s, confirming that T_s reaches the new steady-state value exponentially in time. The experimental ΔT and α^{-1} values were compared to the theoretical values, calculated from Equations 9 and 7. In the absence of the blood flow, $\Delta T = P_{rf}/[\lambda 2\pi l/\ln(1 + d/R)]$. The role of the vessel wall in the experiment was played by the Teflon jacket of the thickness d = 1 mm and the thermal conductivity (at 25°C) λ = 0.25 W/mK around the stent. Taking the employed $P_{rf} = \bar{P} = 0.1$ W, and using the stent's geometrical parameters l = 12 mm and R = 1.25 mm, we obtain ΔT = 3.1°C, a value that matches perfectly the experimental one. The parameter $\alpha = [\lambda 2\pi l/\ln(1 + d/R)]/m_s c_s$ was calculated by using the stent mass m_s = 21.7 mg and the specific heat value at 37°C c_s = 0.46 J/gK, yielding α^{-1} = 0.3 s. The theoretical time constant α^{-1} is a factor 150 smaller than the experimental one, so that the theory predicts a much faster increase of the stent temperature than observed experimentally. This discrepancy can be understood by noticing that in our experiment, a Pt100 sensor was rigidly attached to the stent and was heated up together with it. The thermal conductivity of the Pt100 ceramic housing is much lower than that of the metallic stent, so that the combined stent–Pt100 system has reached the new steady state temperature in a considerably longer time that it would be reached by the metallic stent alone.

Application of the model to the coronary stent in the presence of blood flow

In order to predict the temperature increase of the stainless-steel coronary stent embedded in a coronary artery *in vivo* in a realistic MRI examination, we calculate the parameter ΔT for our investigated stent in the presence of the blood flow. We take the geometrical parameters of the as-fabricated stent $l = 16$ mm and $R = 1.25$ mm. For the coronary artery, we take the following order-of-magnitude estimated parameters: the wall thickness $d = 1$ mm and the thermal conductivity $\lambda = 1$ W/mK (this value was estimated from the reported thermal conductivity of the human skin plus fat that amounts to 0.73 W/mK at 36°C and the thermal conductivity of muscles that amounts to 1.91 W/mK at 36°C (Ducharme and Tikuisis 1991)). For the blood flow through the stent we take a typical volume flow through a coronary artery $\Phi_{bV} = 2$ ml/s (Spaan 1991). Since the blood density is $\rho_b = 1.06$ g/cm^3, this yields the blood mass flow $\Phi_b = \rho_b \Phi_{bV} = 2$ g/s. 2 g/s. The specific heat of the blood is $c_b = 3.78$ J/gK. For the stent-to-blood heat transfer efficiency parameter we take an *ad hoc* value $\varepsilon = 0.5$. P_{rf} is taken arbitrary as 3 W (recall that at this rf power, the stent has heated up by as much as $\Delta T = 33$°C in the absence of the blood flow, as shown in Figure 8a).

Using the above parameter values, the increase of the stent's temperature was calculated from Equation 9 to amount $\Delta T = 0.8$°C only, whereas the blood temperature increase is by $\varepsilon \Delta T = 0.4$°C. This ΔT value is minute as compared to the case where there is no blood flow through the stent. In the absence of the blood flow (setting $\Phi_b = 0$ in Equation 9), the increase of the stent's temperature would be considerable, $\Delta T = 17.6$°C. The reason for the smallness of the ΔT value in the presence of the blood flow becomes evident by inspecting the denominator of Equation 9 that contains two terms. The first term $\lambda 2\pi l / \ln(1 + d/R) = 0.17$ W/K originates from the heat flow through the vessel wall, whereas the second term $\varepsilon \Phi_b c_b = 3.78$ W/K originates from the heat taken away by the blood flow. The second term is much larger than the first one, $\varepsilon \Phi_b c_b / [\lambda 2\pi l / \ln(1 + d/R)] = 22$, so that the blood flow efficiently cools the stent in the MRI examination, owing to the much larger heat capacity of the blood, $C_b = m_b c_b$, as compared to the heat capacity of the stent, $C_s = m_s c_s$ (where the ratio of the specific heats is $c_b / c_s = 8.2$). The estimated increase of the stainless-steel coronary stent temperature by $\Delta T = 0.8$°C during MRI *in vivo* is thus small enough to be considered harmless to the human body.

The problem of restenosis

The above result of a minute increase of the stent's temperature due to the efficient cooling by the blood flow applies to the normal situation, where the stent's cross section is large enough to enable the rated (unrestricted) blood flow through a coronary vessel, i.e., the stent is fully "open". However, the problem of restenosis is sometimes encountered after the stent insertion in the course of months or years, where the stent becomes partially re-occluded and the flow reduces. Consequently, the reduced flow is no more capable of efficiently cooling the stent in the MRI examination of a patient with a partially re-occluded stent and there may appear a risk of hazardous heating of the stent's surroundings. Defining the blood flow reduction factor $x = \left(1 - \Phi_b / \Phi_b^0\right) \times 100$ (in %) with Φ_b^0 denoting the unrestricted flow, we are able to predict from Equation 9 the temperature increase of the stent ΔT for an arbitrary reduced blood flow. The $x = 0\%$ value corresponds to the fully open stent (no flow reduction), whereas $x = 100\%$ corresponds to the fully blocked stent (100% flow reduction). For the calculation we took the same stent and vessel parameters as before (recall that for these parameters, the model yielded $\Delta T = 0.8$°C for the fully open stent, whereas $\Delta T = 17.6$°C for the fully blocked stent). The graph of the stent's temperature in the body, $T_s = 37$°C $+ \Delta T$, as a function of the blood flow reduction, is shown in Figure 9. We observe that for the flow reduction between 0 and 90%, the stent's temperature increase is relatively small (T_s increases from 37.8°C at 0% reduction to 42.5°C at 90%), whereas T_s increases drastically for the high flow reduction between 90% and 100% (from 42.5°C at 90% to 54.6°C at 100% reduction). This

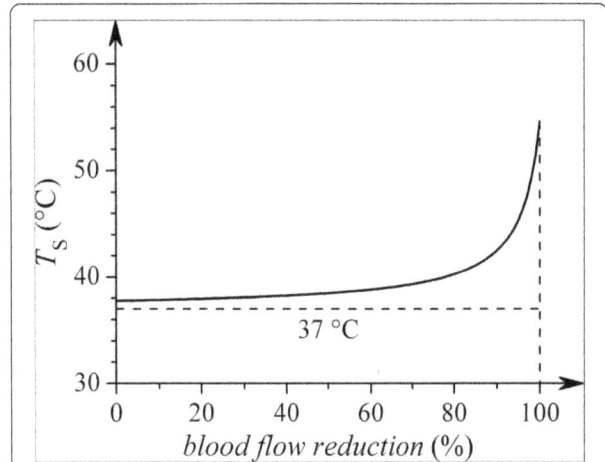

Figure 9 The problem of restenosis in MRI. Theoretical stent's steady-state temperature in the body, $T_s = 37$°C $+ \Delta T$, under the rf irradiation is presented as a function of the blood flow reduction due to restenosis, where ΔT was calculated from Equation 9 (see text). The *blood flow reduction* is defined as $x = \left(1 - \Phi_b / \Phi_b^0\right) \times 100$ (in %) with Φ_b^0 denoting the unrestricted flow. The $x = 0$ % value corresponds to the fully open stent (no flow reduction), whereas $x = 100$ % corresponds to the fully blocked stent (100 % flow reduction).

behavior is again a consequence of the much larger heat capacity of the blood as compared to the stent, demonstrating that even a substantially diminished blood flow through the stent is still able to cool it efficiently. In contrast, dangerously high temperatures are developed in the body for the stent occlusion close to 100%.

In the MRI examination, the patient is irradiated by the rf pulses typically for a time of about 20 – 30 minutes, which represents the time during which the stent "heater" is switched on. The long heater switch-on time and the high enough temperature for the heat-induced protein coagulation and the formation of blood clots represent a risk of hazardous heating in the stent's surroundings during the MRI of a stented patient with a high stent occlusion between 90% and 100%. Restenosis thus represents a potentially hazardous heating problem in MRI.

Conclusions

We have investigated the heating of a metallic coronary stent in a MRI examination. The experimental results presented in this paper are valid for the particular geometrical parameters (length and diameter) of the employed stent, the 316LVM stainless steel material, the proton resonance frequency of 200 MHz (corresponding to the 4.7 T magnetic field) and the average rf irradiation power up to 3 W. For the highest average rf power of 3 W employed in our experiments on the stent in the absence of the blood flow through it, the stent has heated up by as much as $\Delta T = 33°C$ from the initial temperature before the irradiation. The experimental and theoretical methodologies applied in this study are, however, suitable to investigate other types of stents with different geometries, fabricated of different metallic alloys, e.g., nickel–titanium and cobalt–chromium and other rf irradiation strengths.

The metallic coronary stent acting as a tubular flow heater in the MRI examination was also modeled theoretically, by considering that the stent receives the energy from the rf electromagnetic field and heats up the surrounding vessel and the blood flowing through it. The analytical model has successfully reproduced the exponential increase of the stent's temperature during our rf heating experiments in the absence of blood flow through the stent. The model was then used to predict the increase of the temperature of the stainless-steel coronary stent embedded in a coronary artery in the presence of blood flow through it, mimicking an *in vivo* realistic MRI examination. In the normal situation of a fully open (unoccluded) stent, the increase of the stent's temperature as well as the increase of the blood temperature exiting the stent were found minute, of less than 1°C, so that the blood flow efficiently cools the stent. This is a consequence of the much larger heat capacity of the blood as compared to the heat capacity of the stent. However, should the problem of restenosis occur with time after the stent insertion, where the stent in the vessel becomes partially re-occluded and the flow reduces, there is a risk of hazardous heating. The temperature of the occluded stent may become dangerously high to enable protein coagulation and the formation of blood clots in the stent's surroundings.

Competing interests
The authors declare that they have no competing interests.

Authors' contributions
SV carried out the stent heating experiments. MW carried out the physical-property measurements of the stent's material. AJ carried out the scanning electron microscopy experiments and the EDS compositional analysis. HJK participated in the application of the theoretical model to the experimental data. JD conceived of the study, developed the analytical model of a stent as a tubular flow heater, and performed the coordination. All authors read and approved the final manuscript.

Author details
[1]Jožef Stefan Institute, Jamova 39, SI-1000 Ljubljana, Slovenia. [2]Faculty of Mathematics and Physics, University of Ljubljana, Jadranska 19, SI-1000 Ljubljana, Slovenia. [3]Institute of Molecular Physics, Polish Academy of Sciences, Smoluchowskiego 17, PL-60-179 Poznań, Poland. [4]Division of Materials Science, Korea Basic Science Institute, Daejeon 305-333, Republic of Korea.

References
Ahmed S, Shellock FG (2001) Magnetic resonance imaging safety: implications for cardiovascular patients. J Cardiovasc Magn Reson 3:171–182
ASM International Handbook Committee (1990) Metals handbook, vol 1, 10th edn. ASM International Handbook Committee, Ohio Park
Callaghan PT (1991) Principles of nuclear magnetic resonance microscopy. Clarendon Press, Oxford, p 100
Ducharme MB, Tikuisis P (1991) In vivo thermal conductivity of the human forearm tissues. J Appl Physiol 70:2682–2690
Halliday D, Resnick R, Walker J (2005) Fundamentals of Physics, 7th edn. John Wiley & Sons, New York, p 493
Hubner PJB (1998) Guide to coronary angioplasty and stenting. Harwood Academic Publishers, Amsterdam
Jost C, Kumar V (1998) Are current cardiovascular stents MRI safe? J Invas Cardiol 10:477–479
Kagetsu ND, Litt AW (1991) Important considerations in measurement of attractive forces on metallic implants in MR imaging. Radiology 179:505–508
Lopič N, Jelen A, Vrtnik S, Jagličić Z, Wencka M, Starc R, Blinc A, Dolinšek J (2013) Quantitative determination of magnetic force on a coronary stent in MRI. J Magn Reson Imaging 37:391–397
Nyenhuis JA, Park SM, Kamondetdacha R, Amjad A, Shellock FG, Rezai A (2005) MRI and implanted medical devices: basic interactions withan emphasis on heating. IEEE Trans Device Mat Rel 5:467–474
Scott NA, Pettigrew RI (1994) Absence of movement of coronary stents after placement in a magnetic resonance imaging field. Am J Cardiol 73:900–901
Shellock FG (2011) Reference manual for magnetic resonance safety, implants and devices. Biomedical Research Publishing Group, Los Angeles, pp 246–251
Shellock FG, Morisoli SM (1994) Ex vivo evaluation of ferromagnetism, heating, and artifacts for heart valve prostheses exposed to a 1.5 Tesla MR system. J Magn Reson Imaging 4:756–758
Shellock FG, Shellock VJ (1999) Metallic stents: evaluation of MR imaging safety. Am J Roentgenol 173:543–547
Spaan JAE (1991) Coronary blood flow: mechanics, distribution and control. Kluwer Academic Publishers, Dordrecht

Strohm O, Kivelitz D, Gross W, Schulz-Menger J, Liu X, Hamm B, Dietz D, Friedrich MG
    (1999) Safety of implantable coronary stents during 1H-magnetic resonance
    imaging at 1.0 and 1.5 T. J Cardiovasc Magn Reson 1:239–245
Woods TO (2007) Standards for medical devices in MRI: present and future.
    J Magn Reson Imaging 26:1186–1189
Yachia D (1998) Stenting the urinary system. Isis Medical Media, Oxford

14

Bioanalytical method for quantification of Solifenacin in rat plasma by LC-MS/MS and its application to pharmacokinetic study

Srinivasa Babu Puttagunta[1], Rihana Parveen Shaik[1,2]*, Chandrasekhar Kothapalli Bannoth[2], Bala Sekhara Reddy Challa[3] and Bahlul Zayed Sh Awen[4]

Abstract

Background: Solifenacin succinate is a competitive muscarinic acetylcholine receptor antagonist used in the treatment of overactive bladder with or without urge incontinence.

Methods: Liquid chromatography–tandem mass spectrometry method was used for quantification of Solifenacin (SF) in rat plasma. Solifenacin-d5 (SFD5) used as an internal standard. Chromatographic separation was performed Gemini-NX C18, 50 × 4.6 mm, 5 μm, 110 Å column. Mobile phase composed of 5 mM Ammonium formate, pH 3.0: methanol (20:80 v/v), with 0.4 mL/min flow-rate. Drug and IS were extracted by Liquid- liquid extraction method. SF and SFD5 were detected with proton adducts at m/z 363.2®193.2 and 368.2®198.2 in multiple reaction monitoring (MRM) positive mode respectively. The method was validated with the correlation coefficients of (r2) ≥ 0.9975 over a linear concentration range of 0.1-100.0 ng/mL.

Results: This method demonstrated intra and inter-day precision within 1.09 to 4.84 and 1.75 to 7.68 % and accuracy within 101.21 to 106.67 and 97.94 to 104.79 % for SF.

Conclusions: This method is successfully applied in the Pharmacokinetic study of rat plasma.

Keywords: Mass spectrometry; Solifenacin; Rat plasma; Pharmacokinetics

Background

Solifenacin succinate is a competitive muscarinic acetylcholine receptor antagonist used in the treatment of overactive bladder with or without urge incontinence. Chemically, it is 1-azabicyclo[2.2.2]oct-8-yl(1S)-1-phenyl-3,4-dihydro-1H-isoquinoline-2-carboxylate.

The molecular formula of Solifenacin succinate is $C_{23}H_{26}N_2O_2$ with its molecular weight 362.46. Solifenacin is extensively metabolized in the liver. One pharmacologically active metabolite (4R-hydroxy Solifenacin) occurs at low concentrations and three pharmacologically inactive metabolites (N-glucuronide and the N-oxide and 4R-hydroxy-N-oxide of Solifenacin) in human plasma after oral dosing. After oral administration of vesicare to healthy

volunteers, peak plasma levels (C_{max}) of Solifenacin reached within 3 to 8 h after administration and at steady state ranged from 32.3 to 62.9 ng/mL for the 5 and 10 mg vesicare tablets, respectively. The terminal elimination half-life of Solifenacin (SF) is approximately 45 to 68 h. Solifenacin is approximately 98% (*in vivo*) bound to human plasma proteins, principally to alpha1-acid glycoprotein (Morales-Olivas and Estan 2010; Doroshyenko and Fuhr 2009; Hoffstetter and Leong 2009; Kuipers et al. 2004; Leone Roberti Maggiore et al. 2012; Uchida et al. 2004; Yamada et al. 2012; Maruyama et al. 2008; Kuipers et al. 2006; Callegari et al. 2011).

Literature survey reveals that quantification of Solifenacin in human plasma (Macek et al. 2010; Mistri et al. 2008), rat plasma (Yanagihara et al. 2007), pharmaceutical compounds (Krishna et al. 2010; Desai et al. 2012; Rami Reddy et al. 2013; Desai et al. 2011), and industrial waste streams (Ann-Marie et al. 2011) were reported. These

* Correspondence: rihanaparveen@gmail.com
[1]Vignan Colllege of pharmacy, Vadlamudi, Guntur, Andhra Pradesh 522213, India
[2]Jawaharlal Nehru Technological University, Anantapur, Andhra Pradesh 515002, India
Full list of author information is available at the end of the article

methods were reported by using liquid chromatography-electrospray ionization-tandem mass spectrometry (LC-MS/MS) (Macek et al. 2010; Mistri et al. 2008; Ann-Marie et al. 2011), high-performance liquid chromatography (HPLC) (Yanagihara et al. 2007; Krishna et al. 2010; Desai et al. 2012; Rami Reddy et al. 2013), and HPTLC (Desai et al. 2011). Among all, quantification of Solifenacin by LC-MS/MS in biological matrices (Macek et al. 2010; Mistri et al. 2008; Yanagihara et al. 2007) was proved best results.

Macek et al. 2010 reported with the linearity range of 0.47 to 42 ng/mL and used PPT method for extraction of drug and internal standard (IS). They used 250 μL of plasma sample for extraction procedure and obtained good chromatography within 3 min run time. They used Solifenacin d5 as an internal standard. Mistri et al. (2008) reported with the linearity range of 0.6 to 60 ng/mL and used liquid-liquid extraction (LLE) method for extraction of drug and IS. They used 500 μL of plasma sample for extraction procedure and obtained good chromatography with in 3 min run time. They used propranolol as an internal standard. (Yanagihara et al. 2007) reported with the linearity range of 2.0 to 2,000.00 ng/mL and used LLE method for extraction of drug and IS. They used 1,000 μL of plasma sample for extraction procedure and obtained good chromatography within 25 min run time. They used ((−)-[(1R or 1S),3_R]-quinuclidin-3_-yl 1-benzyl-1,2,3,4-tetrahydroisoquinoline-2-carboxylate monohydrochloride as an internal standard.

The reported methods have some drawbacks in terms of large amount of plasma sample usage, lower sensitivity (Macek et al. 2010; Mistri et al. 2008; Yanagihara et al. 2007), long run analysis time, and internal standard usage (Yanagihara et al. 2007). The main goal of the present study is to develop and validate the novel simple, higher sensitive, selective, rapid, rugged, and reproducible bioanalytical method for quantitative determination of SF in rat plasma by LC-MS/MS with a small amount of sample volume. The developed method would be applied in the pharmacokinetic study of rat plasma.

Methods
Chemicals and reagents
Solifenacin succinate, Solifenacin d5 hydrochloride obtained from Hetero Drugs, Hyderabad, India (Figure 1). HPLC grade methanol was purchased from Jt. Baker Mallinckrodt Baker, Inc., Phillipsburg, NJ, USA. Formic acid was purchased from S.D. Fine Chemicals, Mumbai, India. Diethyl ether was purchased from Merck Speciality Private Limited, Worli, Mumbai, India. Ultrapure water from Milli-Q system (Millipore, Bedford, MA, USA) was used through the study. All other chemicals in this study were of analytical grade. Rats were obtained from Bioneeds, Bangalore, Karnataka, India.

Instrumentation
HPLC system (1200 Series Agilent Technologies, Deutschland, Germany) connected with triple quadrupole mass spectrometer instrument (API 4000, Toronto, Canada). Data processing was performed with the Analyst 1.5.1 software package (SCIEX, Framingham, MA 01701, USA). Ionization was performed by electrospray positive mode with unit resolution.

Detection
Mass parameters were optimized to get the product ions of m/z, 193.2 and m/z, 198.2 from its respective precursor ions of SF $[M + H]^+$ (m/z, 363.2) and SFD5 $[M + H]^+$ (m/z, 368.2) with source temperature 500°C, ion spray voltage 5,500 V, heater gas, nebulizer gas 35 psi each, curtain gas 20 psi, CAD gas 5 psi (all gas channels with nitrogen), source flow rate 400 μL/min without split, entrance potential 10 V, declustering potential 55 V for analyte and 65 V for internal standard, collision energy 25 V for both analyte and internal standard, and collision cell exit potential 13 V for analyte and 12 V for internal standard.

Chromatographic conditions
Chromatography was performed using Gemini-NX C18, 50 × 4.6 mm, 5 μm, 110 Å analytical column at 30°C, with 5 mM ammonium formate, pH 3.0/methanol (20:80 v/v) as

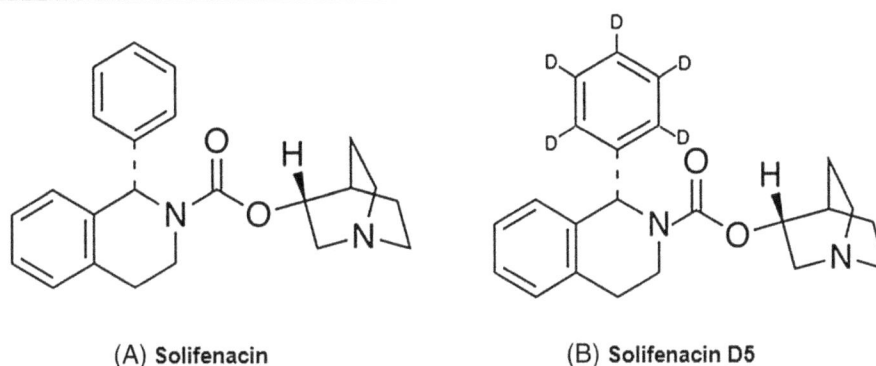

Figure 1 Chemical structures of Solifenacin (A) and Solifenacin d5 (B).

mobile phase at a flow rate of 0.4 mL/min. SFD5 was used as an internal standard in terms of chromatography and extractability. The drug and internal standard was eluted at 1.2 ± 0.2 min with 2 min total run time.

Preparation of standards and quality control samples

Standard stock solutions of SF (50.0 μg/mL) and SFD5 (50.0 μg/mL) was prepared in methanol. The internal standard spiking solution (50.0 ng/mL) was prepared in water from SFD5 standard stock solution (50.0 μg/mL). Standard stock solutions and internal standard spiking solutions were stored in refrigerator conditions (2°C to 8°C) until analysis. Standard stock solution of SF was added to screened drug-free rat plasma to obtain concentration levels of 0.1, 0.2, 1.0, 5.0, 10.0, 40.0, 60.0, 80.0, and 100.0 ng/mL for analytical standards and 0.1, 0.3, 50.0, 75.0 ng/mL for quality control (QC) standards and stored in a –30°C freezer until analysis. Respective aqueous standards were prepared in reconstitution solution (5 mM ammonium formate pH 3.0/methanol (20:80) and stored in refrigerator conditions 2°C to 8°C until analysis.

Sample preparation

Liquid-liquid extraction was used to isolate drug and IS from rat plasma. For this purpose, 50 μL of IS (40.0 ng/mL) and 100 μL of plasma sample (respective concentration) was added into labeled polypropylene tubes and vortexed briefly. Followed by 2.5 mL of extraction solvent (diethyl ether) was added and vortexed for 10 min. Then, the samples were centrifuged at 4,000 rpm for 10 min at 20°C temperature. Subsequently, the supernatant from each sample was transferred into respective polypropylene tubes. After that, all the samples were kept for evaporation under nitrogen at 40°C. The dried residue was reconstituted with 1,000 μL of reconstitution solution (5 mM ammonium formate pH 3.0/methanol (20:80)) and vortexed briefly. Finally, the extracted sample was transferred into auto sampler vials and injected into LC-MS/MS.

Selectivity and specificity

The selectivity of the method was determined by six different rat blank plasma samples, which were pretreated and analyzed to test the potential interferences of endogenous

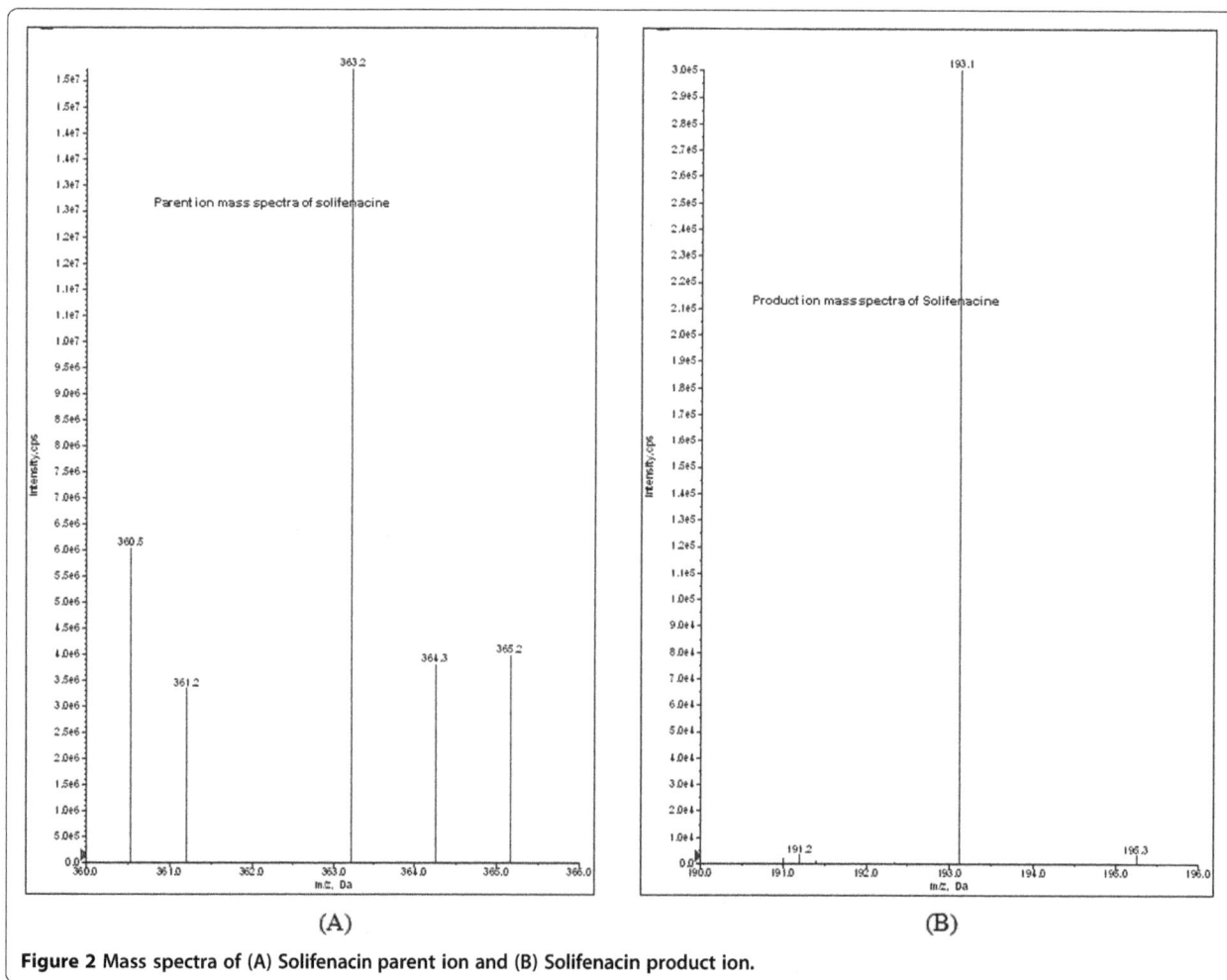

Figure 2 Mass spectra of (A) Solifenacin parent ion and (B) Solifenacin product ion.

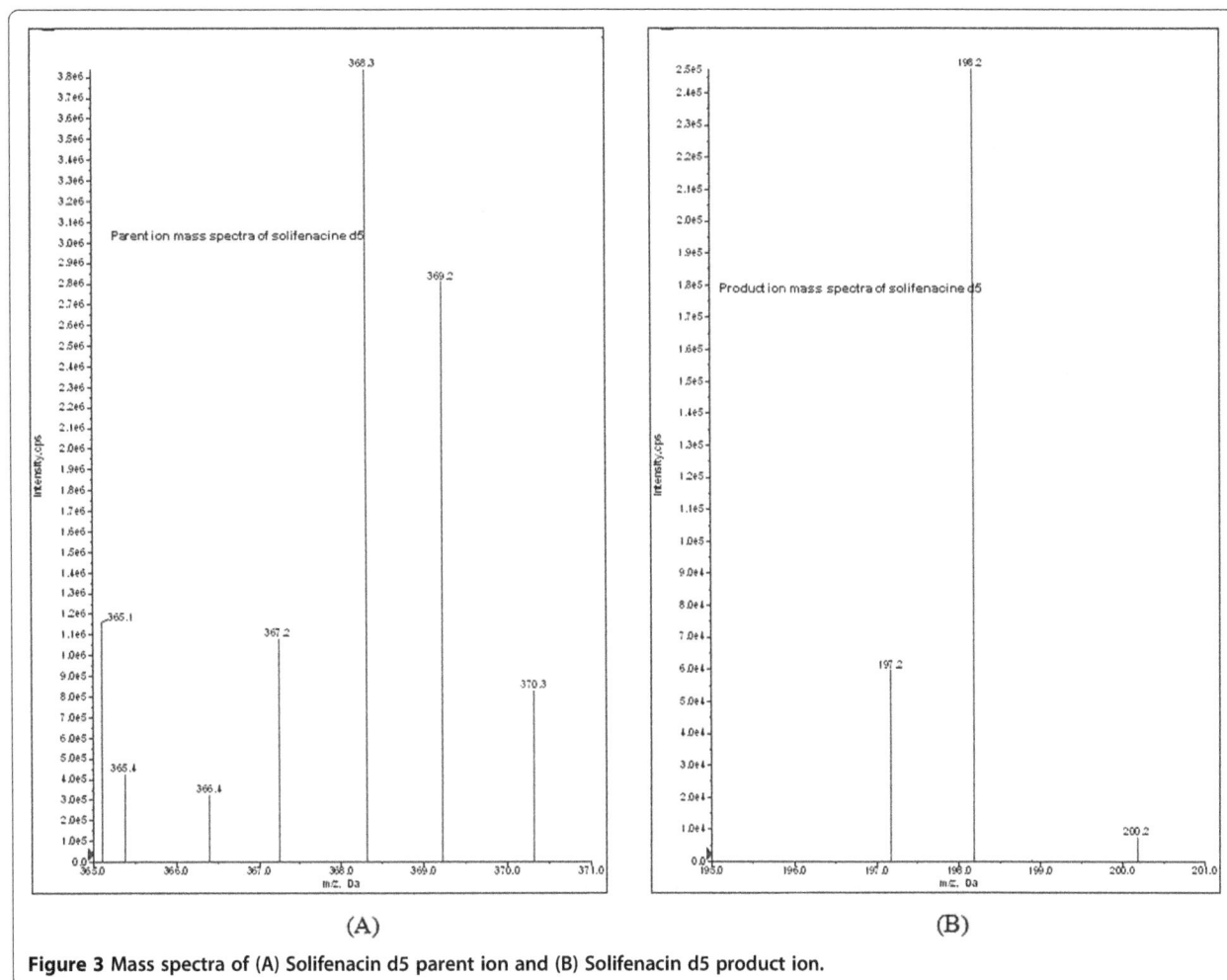

Figure 3 Mass spectra of (A) Solifenacin d5 parent ion and (B) Solifenacin d5 product ion.

compounds co-eluting with analyte and IS. Chromatographic peaks of analyte and IS were identified based on their retention times and multiple reaction monitoring (MRM) responses. The peak area of SF at the respective retention time in blank samples should not be more than 20% of the mean peak area of limit of quantification (LOQ) of SF. Similarly, the peak area of SFD5 at the respective retention time in blank samples should not be more than 5% of the mean peak area of LOQ of SFD5.

Recovery

The extraction recovery of SF and SFD5 from rat plasma was determined by analyzing quality control samples. Recovery at three concentrations (1.5, 25.0, and 35.0 ng/mL) was determined by comparing peak areas obtained from the plasma sample and the standard solution spiked with the blank plasma residue. A recovery of more than 85% was considered adequate to obtain required recovery.

Limit of detection and limit of quantification

The limit of detection (LOD) is a parameter that provides the lowest concentration in a sample that can be detected from background noise but not quantitated. LOD was determined using the signal-to-noise ratio (S/N) of 3:1 by comparing test results from samples with known concentrations of analytes with blank samples.

The LOQ is defined as the lowest concentration of analyte that can be determined with acceptable precision and accuracy. The LOQ was found by analyzing a set of mobile phase and plasma standards with a known concentration of SF.

Matrix effect

To predict the variability of matrix effects in samples from individual subjects, matrix effect was quantified by determining the matrix factor, which was calculated as follows:

$$\text{Matrix factor} = \frac{\text{Peak response ratio in presence of extracted matrix (post extracted)}}{\text{Peak response ratio in aqueous standards}}$$

Six lots of blank biological matrices were extracted each in triplicates and postspiked with the aqueous standard at the low and high QC level and compared with aqueous standards of same concentration. The overall precision of the matrix factor is expressed as coefficient of variation (%CV) and %CV should be <15%.

Calibration curve, precision, and accuracy

The calibration curve was constructed using values ranging from 0.1 to 100.0 ng/mL of SF in rat plasma. Calibration curve was obtained by linear model with weighted $1/x^2$ regression analysis. The ratio of SF/SFD5 peak area was plotted against the ratio of SF concentration in ng/mL. Calibration curve standard samples and quality control samples were prepared in replicates (n = 6) for analysis. Precision and accuracy for the back-calculated concentrations of the calibration points, should be within ≤15 and ± 15% of their nominal values. However, for LLOQ, the precision and accuracy should be within ≤20 and ±20%.

Stability (freeze - thaw, auto sampler, bench top, long-term) of SF in plasma

Low-quality control and high-quality control samples (n = 6) were retrieved from a deep freezer after three freeze-thaw cycles according to the clinical protocol. Samples were stored at –30°C in three cycles of 24, 36 and 48 h. In addition, the long-term stability of SF in quality control samples was also evaluated by analysis after 45 days of storage at –30°C. Autosampler stability was studied following 61.5-h storage period in the autosampler tray with control concentrations. Bench top stability was studied for 25-h period with control concentrations. Stability samples were processed and extracted along with the freshly spiked calibration curve standards. The precision and accuracy for the stability samples must be ≤15 and ±15%, respectively, of their nominal concentrations.

Application to pharmacokinetic study

The developed LC-MS/MS method was successfully applied to a pharmacokinetic study by administration of SF to six male Sprague-Dawley rats by oral route using BD syringe attached with oral gavage needle (size 18) at the dose of 4 mg/200 g body weight. Required quantity of test item (4 mg SF) was accurately weighed and transferred to a mortar and triturated with 2% (w/w) Tween 80 using a pestle to make a smooth paste. Then, 0.5% (w/w) carboxymethyl cellulose (CMC) was gradually added and suspended to make a required concentration (1 mg/mL of SF). The final suspension was kept under

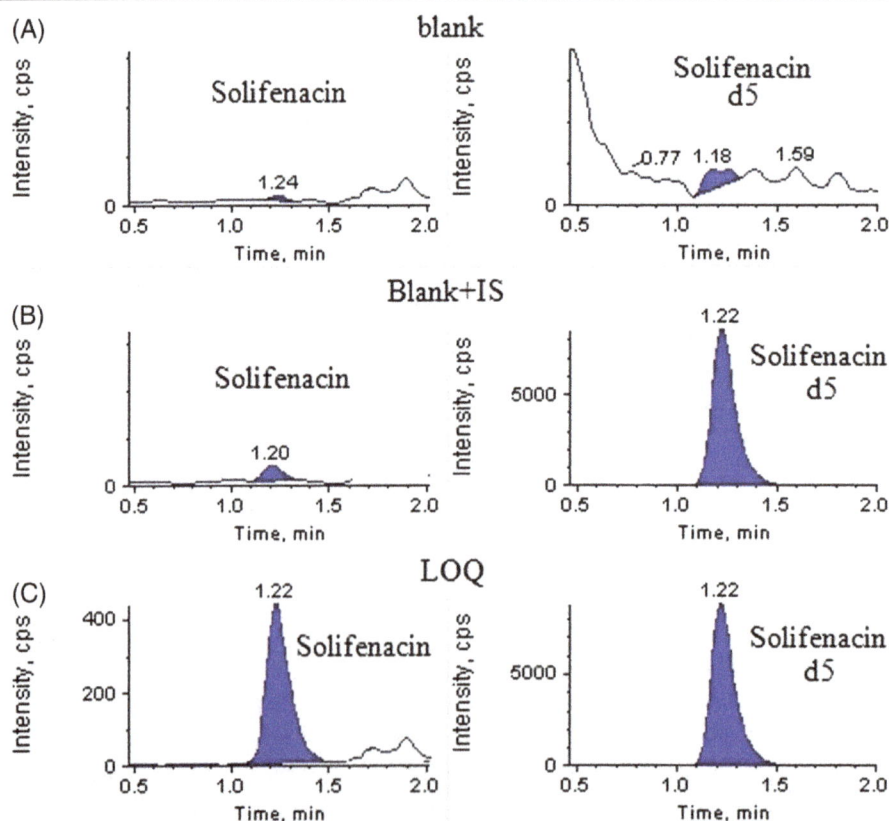

Figure 4 Chromatogram of Solifenacin and Solifenacin d5 in blank plasma (A), blank + IS (B), and LOQ (C).

Table 1 Calibration curves details

Spiked plasma concentration (ng/mL)	Mean concentration (ng/mL) ± S.D.	S.D.	(CV %) (n = 5)	Accuracy (%)
0.10	0.11	0.01	6.46	110.40
0.20	0.19	0.01	4.78	95.40
1.00	0.97	0.01	1.33	97.10
5.00	5.12	0.16	3.17	102.32
10.00	10.10	0.09	0.94	101.00
40.00	39.68	0.39	0.98	99.19
60.00	59.89	0.63	1.05	99.82
80.00	80.74	0.68	0.84	100.92
100.00	99.55	0.35	0.35	99.55

continuous stirring till the dose administration. Approximately, 0.2 mL of blood samples from each anesthetized (isoflurane) rat at pre-determined time intervals was collected from the retro-orbital plexus using a capillary tube into pre-labeled eppendorf tubes containing 10% of K_2EDTA anticoagulant (20 μL). The time intervals for the sample collection were 0 (predose), 0.5, 1, 2, 3, 4, 5, 6, 8, 16, 24, 36, 48, and 72 h (postdose). The total blood volume collected from each rat was approximately 1.9 to 2.2 mL which does not exceed the maximal recommended blood volume of 20% (2.0 mL for a 200 g body weight rat). Plasma was obtained by centrifuging blood samples at 3,000 rpm for 10 min. The obtained plasma samples were transferred into pre-labeled microcentrifuge tubes and stored at –30°C. All the samples were analyzed by the developed method. Pharmacokinetic parameters were calculated by non-compartmental analysis by using Win Nonlin® 5.1 software. Concentrations obtained from the above bio-analytical method were compiled (FDA 2002; FDA 2003).

Results and discussion

Method development and method validation
LC-MS/MS has been used as one of the most powerful analytical tools in clinical pharmacokinetics for its selectivity, sensitivity, and reproducibility. The goal of this work is to develop and validate a simple, sensitive, rapid, rugged, and reproducible assay method for the quantitative determination of SF from rat plasma samples.

Chromatographic conditions, especially the composition and nature of the mobile phase, usage of different columns, and different extraction methods such as solid phase, precipitation, and liquid-liquid extraction methods were optimized through several trials to achieve the best resolution and increase the signal of SF and SFD5. The MS optimization was performed by direct infusion of solutions of both SF and SFD5 into the ESI source of the mass spectrometer. The critical parameters in the ESI source that include the needle (ESI) voltage, capillary voltage, source temperature, and other parameters such as nebulizer gas, heater gas, and desolvation gasses were optimized to obtain a better spray shape, resulting in better ionization of the protonated ionic SF and SFD5 molecules. Product ion spectrum for SF and SFD5 yielded high-abundance fragment ions of m/z 193.2 and m/z 198.2, respectively (Figures 2 and 3). After mass spectrometer parameters optimized, chromatographic conditions such as mobile phase optimization, column optimization, and extraction method optimization was performed to obtain a fast and selective LC method.

A good separation and elution were achieved using 5 mM ammonium formate, pH 3.0/methanol (20:80 v/v) as the mobile phase at a flow rate of 0.4 mL/min and injection volume of 5 μL. Gemini-NX C18, 50 × 4.6 mm, 5 μm, 110 Å column, and liquid-liquid extraction method was optimized for the best chromatography (Figure 4).

The developed method was validated over a linear concentration range 0.1 to 100.0 ng/ml. The validation parameters that include selectivity and specificity, LOD and LOQ, matrix effect, precision and accuracy, recovery, stability (freeze - thaw, auto sampler, bench top, long-term) were evaluated under validation section (FDA 2001).

Selectivity and specificity
The analysis of SF and SFD5 using MRM function was highly selective with no interfering compounds. Chromatograms obtained from plasma spiked with SF (0.1 ng/mL) and SFD5 (50.0 ng/mL) are shown in Figure 4.

Limit of detection and quantification
The limit of detection was used to determine the instrument detection levels for SF even at low concentrations.

Table 2 Precision and accuracy

Spiked plasma con (ng/mL)	Intraday			Interday		
	Concentration measured (n = 6) (ng/mL) (mean ± S.D)	(CV %)	Accuracy (%)	Concentration measured (n = 30) (ng/mL) (mean ± S.D.)	(CV %)	Accuracy (%)
0.10	0.11 ± 0.01	4.84	106.67	0.10 ± 0.01	7.68	98.53
0.30	0.32 ± 0.01	2.58	105.56	0.29 ± 0.04	3.60	97.94
50.00	50.61 ± 0.55	1.09	101.21	50.84 ± 0.75	1.48	101.67
75.00	79.20 ± 1.18	1.49	105.60	78.59 ± 1.38	1.75	104.79

Five microliters of a 0.5-pg/mL solution was injected, and estimated LOD was 3.2 fg with S/N values ≥3 to 5. The limit of quantification for this method was proven as the lowest concentration of the calibration curve which was proven as 0.1 ng/ml.

Matrix effect

Six lots of blank biological matrices were extracted each in triplicates and postspiked with the aqueous standard at the mid-QC level and compared with neat standards of the same concentration in alternate injections. The overall precision of the matrix factor is 3.45 for Solifenacin. There was no ion suppression and ion enhancement effect observed due to IS and analyte at respective retention time.

Precision and accuracy

Calibration curves were plotted as the peak area ratio (SF/SFD5) versus (SF) concentration. Precision and accuracy of calibration curve standards and quality control standards are represented in Tables 1 and 2.

Stability (freeze - thaw, auto sampler, bench top, long-term)

Quantification of the SF in plasma subjected to three freeze-thaw cycles (−30°C to room temperature), autosampler, room temperature (benchtop), and long-term stability details was shown in Table 3.

Recovery

The recovery following the sample preparation using liquid-liquid extraction with diethyl ether was calculated by comparing the peak area of SF in plasma samples with the peak area of solvent samples and was estimated at control levels of SF. The recovery of SF was determined at three different concentrations; 1.5, 25.0, and 50.0 ng/mL were found as 82.05%, 80.94%, and 83.33%, respectively. The overall average recovery of SF and SFD5 were found to be 82.11% and 78.86%, respectively.

Table 3 Stability of the samples

Stability	Spiked plasma concentration (ng/mL)	Concentration measured (ng/mL) (mean ± SD; $n = 6$)	(CV %) ($n = 6$)	
Room temperature stability (25.0 h)	0.30	0.32	0.01	3.54
	75.00	77.30	1.28	1.66
Processed sample stability (61.5 h)	0.30	0.30	0.01	2.08
	75.00	78.83	0.67	0.84
Long term stability (45 days)	0.30	0.32	0.02	6.08
	75.00	71.93	2.90	4.03
Freeze-thaw stability (cycle 3, 48 h)	0.30	0.32	0.01	3.51
	75.00	77.65	0.59	0.76

Table 4 Mean pharmacokinetic parameters of Solifenacin in rat plasma after oral administration of 4 mg/200 g male rat

Pharmacokinetic Parameter	Solifenacin values
AUC_{0-t} (ng·h/mL)	1,029.81
C_{max} (ng/mL)	17.98
$AUC_{0-\infty}$ (ng·h/mL)	1,540.77
K_{el} (h/1)	0.01433
T_{max} (h)	18
$T_{1/2}$ (h)	48.37

$AUC_{0-\infty}$, area under the curve extrapolated to infinity; AUC_{0-t}, area under the curve up to the last sampling time; C_{max}, the maximum plasma concentration; T_{max}, the time to reach peak concentration; K_{el}, the apparent elimination rate constant.

Pharmacokinetics and statistical analysis

The validated method has been successfully applied to quantify SF concentrations into a single dose (4 mg/ 200 g body weight of rat) in rats. The pharmacokinetic parameters evaluated were C_{max} (maximum observed drug concentration during the study), $AUC_{0 \text{ to } 72}$ (area under the plasma concentration-time curve measured 24 h, using the trapezoidal rule), T_{max} (time to observe maximum drug concentration), Kel (apparent first-order terminal rate constant calculated from a semi-log plot of the plasma concentration versus time curve, using the method of least square regression), and $T_{1/2}$ (terminal half-life as determined by quotient 0.693/Kel). Pharmacokinetic details are shown in Table 4. The mean concentration versus time profile of SF in rat plasma is shown in Figure 5 FDA (2002), FDA (2003) Guidence.

Conclusions

The method described in this manuscript has been developed and validated over the concentration range of 0.1 to 100.0 ng/mL in rat plasma. The intrabatch precision was less than 4.84% and accuracy ranged from 101.21% to 106.67%. The interbatch precision was less

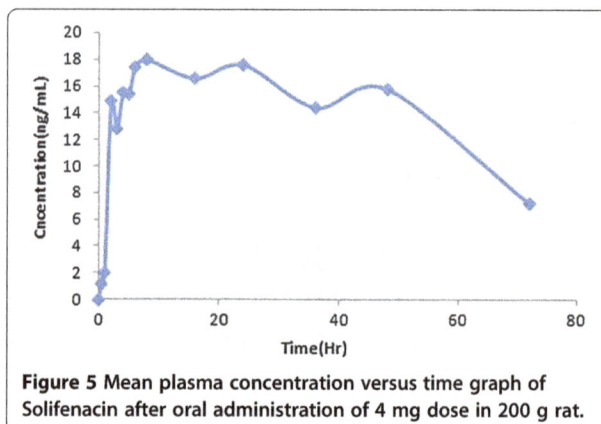

Figure 5 Mean plasma concentration versus time graph of Solifenacin after oral administration of 4 mg dose in 200 g rat.

than 7.68% and accuracy ranged from 97.94% to 104.79%. The selectivity, sensitivity, precision, and accuracy obtained with this method make it suitable for the purpose of the present study. The simplicity of the method, and using rapid liquid-liquid extraction and sample turnover rate of 2.0 min per sample, makes it an attractive procedure in high-throughput bioanalysis of Solifenacin. The validated method was successfully applied in the pharmacokinetic study of rats by oral administration of 4 mg/200 g in six healthy rats.

Abbreviations
LC-MS/MS: liquid chromatography-electrospray ionization-tandem mass spectrometry; MRM: multiple reaction monitoring; SF: Solifenacin; SFD5: Solifenacin d5; LLOQ: lower limit of quantification; LOQ: limit of quantification; IS: internal standard; CAD: collisionally activated dissociation.

Competing interests
The authors declare that they have no competing interests.

Authors' contributions
SBP carried out the Protocol writing,design of the study, RPS and BRC participated in the Bioanalysis and Pharmacokinetic study, CKB drafted the manuscript and participate the technical guidence of the manuscript. All authors read and approved the final manuscript.

Acknowledgements
The authors wish to thank the support received from Indian Institute of Chemical Technology (IICT), Hyderabad, India, for providing literature survey and Anthem Bioscience Pvt., Ltd., Banglore, India, for carrying out this research work.

Author details
[1]Vignan Colllege of pharmacy, Vadlamudi, Guntur, Andhra Pradesh 522213, India. [2]Jawaharlal Nehru Technological University, Anantapur, Andhra Pradesh 515002, India. [3]Vaagdevi College of Pharmacy, Gurazala, Guntur, Andhra Pradesh 522415, India. [4]Faculty of Pharmacy, Tripoli University, Tripoli 13610, Libya.

References
Ann-Marie D, Mark C, Michael O, Kieran N, John T, Anne M (2011) A SPE-LC-MS/MS Method for the Detection of Low Concentrations of Pharmaceuticals in Industrial Waste Streams. Anal Lett 44(17):2808–2820

Callegari E, Malhotra B, Bungay PJ, Webster R, Fenner KS, Kempshall S, LaPerle JL, Michel MC, Kay GG (2011) A comprehensive non-clinical evaluation of the CNS penetration of antimuscarinic agents for the treatment of overactive bladder. Br J Clin Pharmacol 72(2):235–46

Desai DJ, Patel G, Ruikar D, Jain RA, Rajput SJ (2011) Development and validation of stability-indicating HPTLC method of solifenacin succinate. Asian J Phar Biol Res 1(3):310–316

Desai D, Patel G, Shukla N, Rajput S (2012) Development and validation of stability-indicating HPLC method for solifenacin succinate: Isolation and identification of major base degradation product. Acta Chromatogr 24(3):399–418. http://www.akademiai.com/content/48123rm7t8085531/

Doroshyenko O, Fuhr U (2009) Clinical pharmacokinetics and pharmacodynamics of solifenacin. Clin Pharmacokinet 48(5):281–302

FDA (2001) Guidance for industry: bioanalytical method validation, U.S. Department of Health and Human Services, Food and Drug Administration, Center for Drug Evaluation and Research (CDER), Center for Biologics Evaluation and Research (CBER).

FDA (2002) Guidance for industry: Food- effect bio availability and Fed Bio equivalence studies. U.S. Department of Health and Human services Food and Drug Administration Centre for Drug Evaluation and research (CDER).

FDA (2003) Guidance for industry Bio availability and Fed Bio equivalence Studies for Orally Administered Drug Products-General considerations U.S.

Department of Health and Human services Food and Drug Administration Centre for Drug Evaluation and research (CDER).

Hoffstetter S, Leong FC (2009) Solifenacin succinate for the treatment of overactive bladder. Expert Opin Drug Metab Toxicol 5(3):345–50

Krishna SR, Rao BM, Rao NS (2010) A validated rapid stability-indicating method for the determination of related substances in solifenacin succinate by ultra-fast liquid chromatography. J Chromatogr Sci 48(10):807–10

Kuipers ME, Krauwinkel WJ, Mulder H, Visser N (2004) Solifenacin demonstrates high absolute bioavailability in healthy men. Drugs R D 5(2):73–81

Kuipers M, Smulders R, Krauwinkel W, Hoon T (2006) Open-label study of the safety and pharmacokinetics of solifenacin in subjects with hepatic impairment. J Pharmacol Sci 102(4):405–12

Leone Roberti Maggiore U, Salvatore S, Alessandri F, Remorgida V, Origoni M, Candiani M, Venturini PL, Ferrero S (2012) Pharmacokinetics and toxicity of antimuscarinic drugs for overactive bladder treatment in females. Expert Opin Drug Metab Toxicol 8(11):1387–408

Macek J, Ptacek P, Klima J (2010) Determination of solifenacin in human plasma by liquid chromatography-tandem mass spectrometry. J Chromatogr B Analyt Technol Biomed Life Sci 878(31):3327–30

Maruyama S, Tsukada H, Nishiyama S, Kakiuchi T, Fukumoto D, Oku N, Yamada S (2008) In vivo quantitative autoradiographic analysis of brain muscarinic receptor occupancy by antimuscarinic agents for overactive bladder treatment. J Pharmacol Exp Ther 325(3):774–81

Mistri HN, Jangid AG, Pudage A, Rathod DM, Shrivastav PS (2008) Highly sensitive and rapid LC-ESI-MS/MS method for the simultaneous quantification of uroselective alpha1-blocker, alfuzosin and an antimuscarinic agent, solifenacin in human plasma. J Chromatogr B Analyt Technol Biomed Life Sci 876(2):236–44. http://www.ncbi.nlm.nih.gov/pubmed/19010093

Morales-Olivas FJ, Estan L (2010) Solifenacin pharmacology. Arch Esp Urol 63(1):43–52

Rami Reddy BV, Srinivasa Reddy B, Raman NVVSS, Reddy KS, Rambabu C (2013) Development and Validation of a Specific Stability Indicating High Performance Liquid Chromatographic Methods for Related Compounds and Assay of Solifenacin Succinate. J Chem. http://dx.doi.org/10.1155/2013/412353

Uchida T, Krauwinkel WJ, Mulder H, Smulders RA (2004) Food does not affect the pharmacokinetics of solifenacin, a new muscarinic receptor antagonist: results of a randomized crossover trial. Br J Clin Pharmacol 58(1):4–7. http://www.ncbi.nlm.nih.gov/pubmed/15206986

Yamada S, Kuraoka S, Osano A, Ito Y (2012) Characterization of bladder selectivity of antimuscarinic agents on the basis of in vivo drug-receptor binding. Int Neurourol J 16(3):107–15

Yanagihara T, Aoki T, Soeishi Y, Iwatsubo T, Kamimura H (2007) Determination of solifenacin succinate, a novel muscarinic receptor antagonist, and its major metabolite in rat plasma by semi-micro high performance liquid chromatography. J Chromatogr B Analyt Technol Biomed Life Sci 859(2):241–5

15

Influence of decomposition time and H$_2$ pressure on properties of unsupported ammonium tetrathiomolybdate-derived MoS$_2$ catalysts

Jamie Whelan[1,2], Ionut Banu[3], Gisha E Luckachan[1], Nicoleta Doriana Banu[1,4], Samuel Stephen[1], Anjana Tharalekshmy[1], Saleh Al Hashimi[1], Radu V Vladea[1], Marios S Katsiotis[1] and Saeed M Alhassan[1*]

Abstract

Background: Molybdenum sulfide (MoS$_2$) catalysts to be used for hydrodesulfurization (HDS) processes were prepared via the reductive thermal decomposition of ammonium tetrathiomolybdate at fixed temperature (653 K) by varying decomposition times and H$_2$ pressures. Both parameters were found to strongly influence textural and catalytic properties of the resulting MoS$_2$ catalysts.

Methods: Nitrogen sorption, FT-IR, and XRD analyses revealed the effect of varying decomposition times (3 to 7 h) and H$_2$ pressure (20 to 1,000 psig) on the morphology and structure of the catalysts. Dibenzothiophene (DBT) was used to assess catalytic efficiency for HDS reactions.

Results: The influence of time on specific surface was minimal at low pressures but increased at higher decomposition pressures. Vibrational energies of Mo-S bonds in FT-IR indicate that MoS$_2$ catalysts prepared at higher pressures exhibit weaker Mo-S bonds. Analysis of XRD patterns point towards an increase in stacking and crystallite size with increasing pressure; interlayer rotation about both the *a*- and *c*-axes of the stacks was also observed. Catalytic testing results show that conversion increases at higher values of decomposition time and pressure. Partially hydrogenated products were also observed at higher pressures, and the ratio of partially to fully hydrogenated DBT was calculated as an additional measure of catalytic efficiency.

Conclusions: Decomposition time and H$_2$ pressure during ammonium tetrathiomolybdate (ATM) thermal decomposition have a significant impact on the morphological and catalytic properties of the derived MoS$_2$ catalysts. Samples prepared for 5 h at 1,000 psig exhibited the highest conversion of DBT and the lowest ratio of partially to fully hydrogenated products.

Keywords: Ammonium tetrathiomolybdate; MoS$_2$; Hydrodesulfurization; Reductive decomposition pressure

Background

With environmental concerns continually on the rise, greater demand for fuels with low-sulfur content has increased the focus on hydrotreating (HDT) catalysts (Topsøe et al. 1996). Molybdenum sulfide (MoS$_2$)-based catalysts, varyingly promoted with cobalt or nickel, are one of the most common metal sulfides used in HDT, with a strong emphasis on hydrodesulfurization (HDS) reactions (Brunet et al. 2005; Egorova and Prins 2006;

Álvarez et al. 2008; Breysse et al. 2008; Chianelli et al. 2009; Klimov et al. 2010). There are several common methods to synthesize this catalyst such as the direct sulfidation of molybdenum oxide, hydrothermal and sono-chemical synthesis, and the relatively simple procedure of thermally decomposing ammonium tetrathiomolybdate (ATM) (Camacho-Bragado et al. 2005; Devers et al. 2002; Mdleleni et al. 1998; Afanasiev 2008; Polyakov et al. 2008).

Thermal decomposition of ATM is generally a solid-state reaction and, like similar reactions, can be influenced by a number of different experimental parameters such as temperature, gaseous environment, time, and pressure. The proposed reaction mechanism is a two-step process,

* Correspondence: salhassan@pi.ac.ae
[1]Department of Chemical Engineering, The Petroleum Institute, P.O. Box 2533, Abu Dhabi, United Arab Emirates
Full list of author information is available at the end of the article

as can be shown below as Reactions 1 and 2 (Walton et al. 1998):

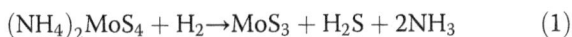

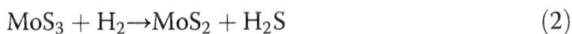

$$(NH_4)_2MoS_4 + H_2 \rightarrow MoS_3 + H_2S + 2NH_3 \quad (1)$$

$$MoS_3 + H_2 \rightarrow MoS_2 + H_2S \quad (2)$$

While several studies of note have already examined the effect of pre-treatment of ATM and the correlation between MoS_2 HDS activity by varying gaseous environment (e.g., H_2S/H_2) and Mo precursors as well as reducing and sulfiding conditions, little work has focused on the influence of decomposition pressure (Liang et al. 1986; Zhang and Vasudevan 1995; Alonso et al. 1998; Afanasiev 2010). As a general rule, pressure increases are known to decrease the rate of thermal decomposition; however, other influences have been observed. In their study of nitramine compounds, Piermarini et al. found a change in decomposition mechanism above a certain pressure (Piermarini et al. 1987). In addition, Criado et al. studied the decomposition of $CaCO_3$ and observed a shift towards higher decomposition temperatures with increasing CO_2 pressure (Criado et al. 1995).

Though some examples in literature report pressure-induced effects on MoS_2 properties such as electrical conductivity and critical current density, little is known regarding the pressure effects on decomposition of ATM and HDS activity of unsupported MoS_2 catalyst (Sánchez et al. 2006; Alekseevskii et al. 1977). While it could be argued that the impact of decomposition may be small relative to other 'stronger' experimental parameters, clearly, the studies on decomposition of nitramine compounds and $CaCO_3$ show it to be a potentially fruitful exercise. Thus, the present study focuses on pressure and time effects on reductive thermal decomposition of ATM and the catalytic activity of the resulting MoS_2. It is shown that by varying the decomposition parameters, resulting structural and chemical differences prove insightful towards designing an economical catalyst for the effective removal of sulfur. The degree of influence these experimental parameters have on the morphology and activity of MoS_2 catalysts is described below.

Methods
Reagents and solutions
The following chemicals were used as purchased: ATM (Aldrich, Dorset UK, 99.97%), dibenzothiophene (DBT) (Aldrich, 98%), hexadecane (Aldrich, 99%), hydrogen gas (Air Products, 99.992%), and nitrogen gas (Air Products, Allentown, PA, USA; 99.995%).

Catalyst preparation
Ammonium tetrathiomolybdate was weighted on an aluminum boat and placed into a 300-cm^3 batch reactor at room temperature. The reactor was sealed, flushed with N_2 and H_2, and then heated to 623 K (10 K min^{-1}). Upon reaching the reaction temperature, H_2 was injected into the reactor at the required pressure, taken as time zero. After the chosen heating duration was completed, heating would be stopped and the reactor would be allowed to cool naturally while maintaining a reductive (H_2) atmosphere. Upon reaching room temperature, the reactor was degassed, flushed with N_2, opened, and the resulting product (MoS_2) was removed and weighted. Immediately afterwards, the specimen was ground using a pestle and mortar and used for characterization and HDS testing. MoS_2 specimens prepared by this method were named as follows: number (time in hours)-number (hydrogen pressure, psig); decomposition times were 3, 5, and 7 h and H_2 pressures were 20 (0.138 MPa), 500 (3.447 MPa), and 1,000 psig (6.895 MPa). For example, 3-1,000 implies MoS_2 prepared from ATM thermally decomposed at 623 K for 3 h at 1,000 psig H_2.

Characterization
Textural characterization was carried out on all catalysts with N_2 sorption at 77 K with a Quantachrome Autosorb-1 (Quantachrome Instruments, Boynton Beach, FL, USA). Prior to analysis, each sample was degassed under vacuum at 573 K for 2 h; the BET surface area (S_{BET}) was determined from the resulting isotherm. FT-IR spectra were obtained using diffuse reflectance infrared Fourier transform (DRIFT) spectroscopy on a Bruker Vertex 70 (Bruker AXS, Inc., Madison, WI, USA). The dark-colored catalysts were mixed with KBr at a ratio MoS_2:KBr = 1:100 to improve infrared transmission; spectra were collected in the 4,000 to 350-cm^{-1} range. Samples for XRD were mounted on a zero background holder, and spectra were collected with a X'Pert PRO Panalytical Powder diffractometer (PANalytical, Almelo, The Netherlands), using Cu Kα radiation (45 kV and 40 mA) in the 2-theta range 10° to 80° with a step time of 0.01 s. Temperature-programmed reduction (TPR) analyses were carried out under continuous H_2 flow (5% H_2 in He) in a quartz cell at 10 K min^{-1} using a Quantachrome ChemBET 3000 (Quantachrome Instruments, Boynton Beach, FL, USA) coupled with a Hiden Analytical HPR 20 QIC mass spectrometry detector (Hiden Analytical, Warrington, UK). It should be mentioned that in no case was any specimen exposed to air for more than 2 min, thus avoiding oxidation of the sulfide catalysts.

Activity measurements
Freshly synthesized and ground MoS_2 (0.050 g, 3.1 × 10^{-4} mol) was added to a 100-cm^3 batch reactor. Feedstock used was 1% DBT in hexadecane (25 cm^3). The reactor was sealed, flushed with N_2, and then heated to 573 K under stirring (1,000 rpm). Upon reaching the reaction temperature, H_2 (500 psig) was injected

into the reactor (time zero). Heating and stirring would be stopped after 3 h, and the reactor would be left to cool naturally, while retaining a reductive (H_2) atmosphere. Upon reaching room temperature, the reactor was degassed and a sample of the reaction mixture was removed, centrifuged, and the supernatant diluted and analyzed on a gas chromatograph coupled with a sulfur chemiluminescence detector (GC-SCD - Agilent 6C 6980 and SCD 335 (Agilent Technologies, Inc., Santa Clara, CA, USA)). The column was 100% dimethylpolysiloxane, 30 m × 0.32 mm × 1 μm, with a maximum temperature of 598 K. In this study, conversion of DBT was calculated based on the decrease in DBT signal (and increase in partially hydrogenated DBT (HYD)) from the GC-SCD compared to the initial concentration following calibration.

Results and discussion

TPR-MS experiments (Figure 1) show two peaks for the reductive thermal decomposition of ATM in H_2, supporting the proposed ATM decomposition mechanism. Thus, the peak at 475 K is assigned to Reaction (1), the release of H_2S and NH_3 (m/z peaks followed were 16, 17, 32, 33, and 34 amu; for display purposes, only molecular ion peaks are shown), while the peak at 613 K is assigned to Reaction (2), i.e., the release of the second molecule of H_2S.

According to the reaction mechanism, for every mole of ATM that decomposes, four moles of gaseous products are produced ($2NH_3$ and $2H_2S$). Based on the starting concentration of ATM, it was calculated that there was a pressure increase of approximately 15 psig above the H_2 injected upon reaching decomposition temperature; no attempt was made to correct for this during catalyst preparation. In general, throughout this paper, the H_2 decomposition pressures applied are termed as low

(20 psig), medium (500 psig), and high (1,000 psig), and it is only against the pressure trend that meaningful conclusions are obtained, not the actual value itself. It should be noted that the actual pressure 'felt' by the ATM is not exactly the same pressure as mentioned above; variation of pressure around the decomposition reaction zone lead to different values than the set point of the external pressure regulator.

Textural characterization

Textural characterization of the catalysts shows a change in S_{BET} (Figure 2) and total pore volume (TPV) (Figure 3) as a function of decomposition time and pressure, respectively. In general, catalysts prepared at low pressure (20 psig) and low decomposition time (<5 h) exhibited little change in morphology; however, with an increase in pressure, the influence of heating time also increased. Within each time series, increasing pressure resulted in increasing S_{BET} and TPV with the largest changes observed for the 5-h series.

XRD characterization

All samples display the typical diffraction profile for poorly crystalline MoS_2, namely the diffraction peaks of (002), (100), (103), (105), and (110). For the sake of article space, only spectra from specimens prepared at 1,000 psig are shown in Figure 4; all spectra can be found in the Additional file 1. Using the Debye-Scherrer equation applied to the broadening of the (110) diffraction peak, it was found that over time there was an increase in crystalline order along the basal direction, likewise with increasing pressure as shown in Table 1 (Daage and Chianelli 1994). Calculations of d-spacing yield no discernible pattern across the samples (average of 6.30 Å). Using previously reported intensity ratio analysis (e.g., I_{110}:I_{002}), it was found that stacking was affected by a

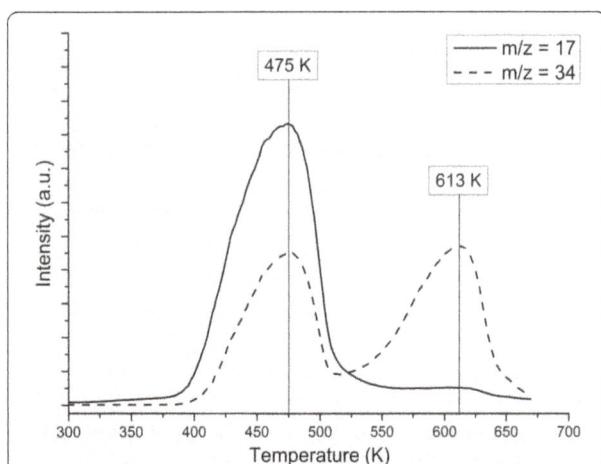

Figure 1 TPR-MS of reductive thermal decomposition of ATM.
TPR-MS of reductive thermal decomposition of ATM under H_2 (5% H_2/He) showing evolution of NH_3 (m/z = 17) and H_2S (m/z = 34).

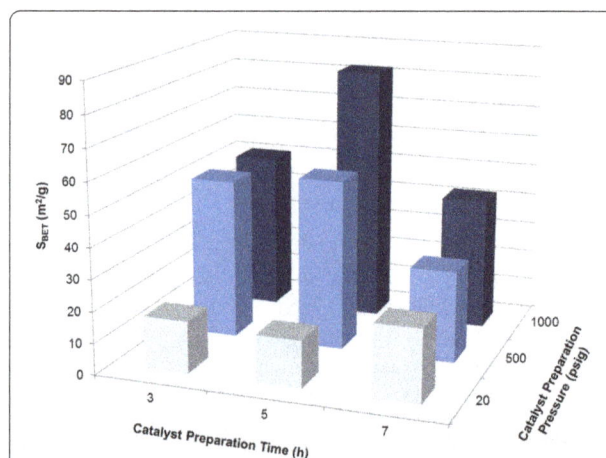

Figure 2 Change in specific surface area (S_{BET}) vs. decomposition time and H_2 pressure.

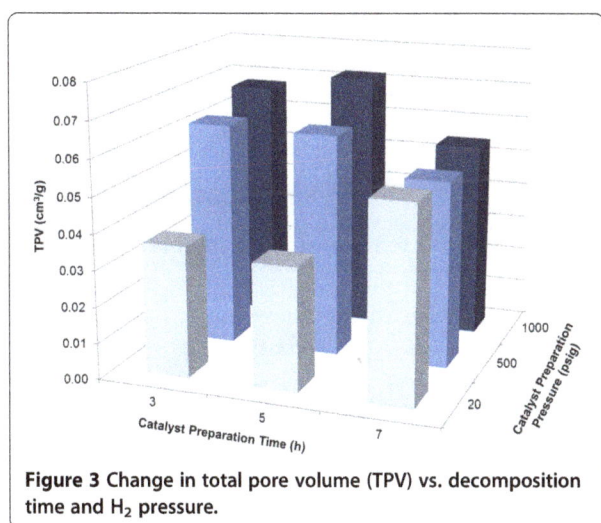

Figure 3 Change in total pore volume (TPV) vs. decomposition time and H₂ pressure.

change in pressure and with time; using the Debye-Scherrer equation applied to the broadening of the (002) diffraction peak (Table 1), it was found that with increasing decomposition time and pressure the influence on stacking height decreased. However, of note is that while for 3 and 5 h increasing decomposition pressure increased stacking height, for the longest time in this study (7 h), stacking height was found to *decrease* as decomposition pressure increased. The exact role of stacking height on the catalytic activity of MoS₂ is unclear with support both for and against its influence (Daage and Chianelli 1994; Afanasiev 2010).

FT-IR catalyst characterization

Five distinct peaks were observed in the FT-IR spectra of the samples in the region below ca. 700 cm^{-1}: 655, 594, 462, 385, and 378 cm^{-1}. All samples were found to contain the first three peaks but varied in the latter two,

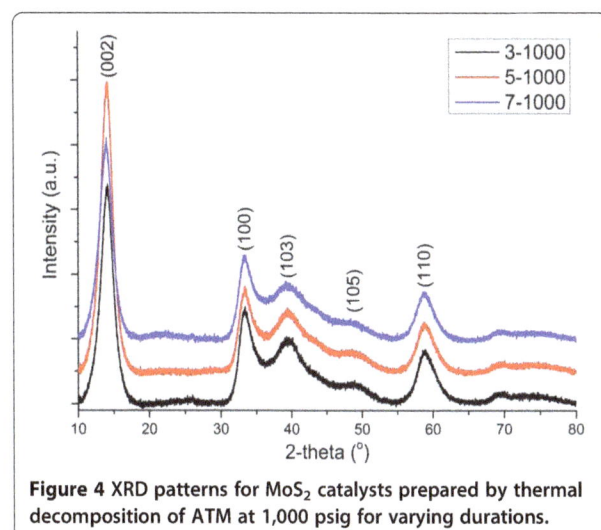

Figure 4 XRD patterns for MoS₂ catalysts prepared by thermal decomposition of ATM at 1,000 psig for varying durations.

containing 378 and/or 385 cm^{-1}. The FTIR spectra for MoS₂ catalysts prepared for 3-h decomposition time and 1,000 psig are shown in Figures 5 and 6, respectively (normalized against the peak at 378 cm^{-1} for ease of illustration). The peaks at 378 and 385 cm^{-1} have been assigned to Mo-S stretching vibrations along the basal plane (Berhault et al. 2002). With increasing heating time and pressure, the peak(s) at 378 and/or 385 cm^{-1} shifted towards a single peak at 378 cm^{-1}. The peak at 462 cm^{-1} is generally assigned to the Mo-S vibration perpendicular to the basal plane, i.e., the bridging Mo-S bond (Fedin et al. 1989). The presence of intermediate MoS₃ (with a peak at 385 cm^{-1}) is discounted due to the lack of corroborating peaks such as a peak at 525 cm^{-1} (Weber et al. 1995). The peaks at 655 and 594 cm^{-1} can be attributed to sulfur-containing peaks, with that at 655 cm^{-1} assigned to S-H vibrations (from Mo-SH) and that at 594 cm^{-1} attributed to S-S bonding strongly coupled to Mo-S (Müller et al. 1982).

Catalyst activity

HDS activity of each MoS₂ catalyst was tested, and the %DBT conversion of each catalyst is given in Table 2. HDS reaction conditions were set such that catalytic activity was kept below 20%, primarily to remove uncertainties associated with produced H₂S, which could limit the forward reaction and could increase the pressure in the batch reactor. A trend was observed of a general increase in HDS catalytic activity of MoS₂ prepared for longer decomposition times (i.e., across the row), with the exception of 7-*1,000*, as well as at higher H₂ pressure (i.e., down the column), excluding 7-*500* and 7-*1,000*. The amount of partial HYD is also given below (values in parentheses), and it can be seen that these percentages change depending upon the MoS₂ preparation conditions. As an example, the chromatogram of reaction product for *5-500* showed a reduction of DBT (retention time = 20.4 min) concentration of 12.0% and an increase in HYD (retention time = 20.2 min) product of 2.8%; thus, direct desulfurization (DDS) accounts for 9.2% of DBT removal.

Diffusion rates of gaseous products from thermal decomposition of solids are known to decrease with an increase in pressure (Oyumi and Brill 1987). In the case of ATM decomposing, gas is released from each step (see Equations 1 and 2) leading to an increase in pressure which could slow down diffusion of gaseous by-products. This is expected to have an impact on the resulting MoS₂ formed.

Analysis of results

A general increase in S_{BET} with an increase in H₂ pressure (Figure 2) was observed across all decomposition times, though to varying degrees. The influence of decomposition time on S_{BET} at low pressure was minimal, though as

Table 1 Crystalline order along the basal direction and apparent stacking heights in the c-axis direction

Pressure (psig)	20			500			1,000		
Time (h)	(110)	(002)	SA (m²/g)	(110)	(002)	SA (m²/g)	(110)	(002)	SA (m²/g)
3	51	23	350	61	28	290	63	30	270
5	54	25	320	63	30	270	61	31	270
7	64	32	260	65	31	260	62	29	280

Crystalline order along the basal direction (Å) and apparent stacking heights in the c-axis direction (Å) calculated using the Debye-Scherrer equation to the broadening of the (110) and (002) diffraction peaks, respectively, for MoS2 catalysts. Surface Area (SA) was calculated in m²/g using the formula mentioned in the work by Iwata et al (2001).

decomposition pressure increased, the influence of decomposition time became more pronounced. Based on the experimental parameters studied herein, it appears that 5 h was the optimal time and 1,000 psig the optimal pressure to produce a catalyst with the largest specific surface area. Increasing H_2 pressure was also found to produce larger pore volumes in the catalyst (Figure 3) leading to the conclusion that textural properties of the catalyst can be controlled by optimizing ATM decomposition time and pressure.

While increasing H_2 decomposition pressure increased S_{BET} within each decomposition time series, S_{BET} did not increase within each decomposition pressure series, particularly from 5 to 7 h. Intuitively, it is not unreasonable to expect an increase in pressure to result in a greater propensity for pore collapse (and subsequent decrease in surface area) which we see in 7-500 and 7-1,000, when compared against 5-500 and 5-1,000; however, the fact that pore collapse only happens at longer decomposition times again highlights the importance of the combined and sometimes conflicting roles of time and pressure and the necessity of varying ATM decomposition parameters to ensure greater control of the resulting MoS2. A similar trend was observed for TPV of MoS2 samples (Figure 3) in that the greatest increase in TPV was for the 5-h series and the lowest was for the 7-h series and likewise a

decrease in TPV for the high-pressure 7 h series compared to that for the 5-h series (e.g., compare 5-500 with 7-500 and 5-1,000 with 7-1,000).

The change in stacking height with a change in pressure is not a novel concept having been noted before on supported hydrotreating catalysts, with HDS process conditions determined as the main cause of destacking (De la Rosa et al. 2004). Hydrothermal synthesis of MoS2 in an autoclave was also found to result in destacking, and in that study, the presence of hydrocarbons was presented as a possible contributor (Peng et al. 2001) while, in a separate study, Chianelli et al. note that possible intercalation of H_2 at high pressures could result in MoS2 layers simply sliding apart over time (Chianelli et al. 2006). However, all of these analyses were conducted on catalysts under HDS conditions whereas, in this case, stacking is not measured as a function of reaction conditions but as a function of thermal decomposition parameters on the original ATM starting material.

For any crystalline solid (in this case poorly crystalline), it can be expected that with an increase in stacking there should be a corresponding increase in S_{BET}; however, the degree to which S_{BET} increases would not be by the same factor as the increase in stacking, simply on the basis that it is only the exposed edge surface which will add to S_{BET} whereas the basal planes are 'covered' by the extra stacks

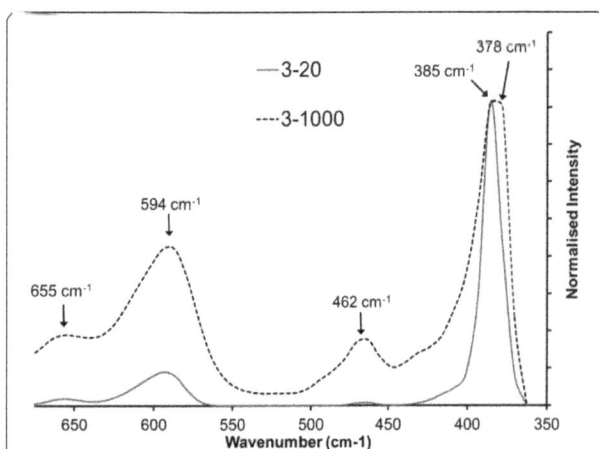

Figure 5 FT-IR spectra for specimens 3-20 and 3-1,000. FT-IR spectra for specimens 3-20 and 3-1,000 showing variation of Mo-S peak vibrations (378 and/or 385 cm⁻¹) and S-S peak (592 cm⁻¹); spectra normalized against peak at 378 cm⁻¹.

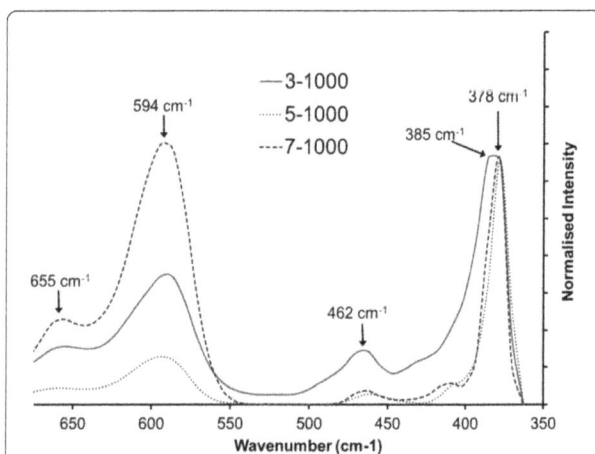

Figure 6 FT-IR spectra for 3-1,000, 5-1,000 and 7-1,000. FT-IR spectra for 3-1,000, 5-1,000, and 7-1,000 showing variation of Mo-S peak vibrations (378 and/or 385 cm⁻¹) and S-S peak (592 cm⁻¹); spectra normalized against peak at 378 cm⁻¹.

Table 2 Catalytic activity of MoS$_2$ samples

Pressure (psig)	20	500	1,000
Time (h)			
3	1.7 (0)	5.8 (1.4)	12.0 (1.7)
5	5.8 (0)	12.0 (2.8)	15.0 (2.0)
7	7.7 (0)	10.0 (1.2)	5.2 (1.3)

Catalytic activity of MoS$_2$ samples defined as % conversion of DBT in hexadecane at 573 K, 500 psig (H$_2$), for 3 h. Values in parentheses represent the % of total conversion which is attributable to hydrogenated DBT (HYD).

(this of course infers perfect alignment of stacks). The use of S_{BET}, however, assumes that there is no agglomeration. Iwata et al. have observed vastly different S_{BET} from the theoretical values of surface area obtained from utilizing data from XRD (Iwata et al. 2001); applying their formula, a similar pattern is evident in our samples, i.e., agglomeration is occurring (compare Figure 2 and SA values in Table 1). While S_{BET} *increases* with an increase in decomposition pressure, it can be seen from Table 1 that the XRD-determined surface area *decreases*, appearing to level off close to 270 m^2 g^{-1}. Thus, the pattern emerges within each time series such that the extent of agglomeration is decreasing with an increase in decomposition pressure. Agglomeration is assumed to be prevalent in the solid state, i.e., during N$_2$ sorption, though less so during activity measurements due to the presence of solvent and high temperatures.

Previously reported modelling studies of poorly crystalline MoS$_2$ have shown that interlayer rotation about the *a*-axis results in little change for the 110 peak but in a shift of the 002 peak towards lower angles (Liang et al. 1986). The same authors model interlayer rotation about the *c*-axis, with changes observed in the 100-103-105 region, with only a small effect on the 002 and 110 peaks. XRD patterns of our samples display slight variations in the angle of 002, as well changes in I_{103}:I_{002} and I_{105}:I_{002} indicating interlayer rotation about the *a*- and *c*-axes, respectively, though by how much exactly is unknown.

The presence of two distinct peaks for Mo-S bonds implies a variation in strength and/or length; based on FT-IR vibrational energies, we assign 385 cm^{-1} to the stronger (i.e., shorter) Mo-S bond, with the weaker (longer) Mo-S bond at 378 cm^{-1}. Mo-S vibrations are usually assigned to the region ca. 380 cm^{-1}, with no literature evidence on FT-IR of MoS$_2$ found distinguishing between these peaks. In a related study, however, laser Raman studies of alumina-supported MoS$_2$ by Payen et al. observed a shift in the Raman band from 380 to 385 cm^{-1} with an increase in Mo loading (Payen et al. 1987); the authors attributed their shift (and broadening) to the lateral growth of MoS$_2$ particles without making reference to whether this 'crystallite size' effect is an actual broadening of the basal plane or merely side-to-side stacking of MoS$_2$ crystals. In our samples, it can be seen

that the crystallite sizes do increase with an increase in decomposition pressure though the values do not correlate well with the above conclusion - our results show a general increase in basal plane size but the results for 7-20 in particular and all samples prepared at 500 psig in general show similar crystalline orders than the samples prepared at 1,000 psig; thus at present, it is inconclusive that the peak shift is due (at least primarily) to lateral growth.

Since FT-IR spectra are of the bulk material, it could be argued that there is an increase in the concentration of weaker (longer), more reactive Mo-S bonds produced with increasing decomposition pressure. While this finding is intuitively unappealing as one would reasonably expect a shortening of bond lengths with increase in pressure (Pietosa et al. 2008), a possible explanation is that pressure induces structural changes which in turn induce creation of new catalytically active sites. Though recent investigations of MoS$_2$ nanoclusters using direct space DFT calculations have found that an increase in S atom coordination of Mo atom results in increasing Mo-S bond lengths (McBride and Head 2009), no such investigations were carried out in this study. Work is ongoing with a view to quantifying the interlayer rotations observed using XRD and the creation of new catalytically active sites and the unique FT-IR shifts observed through the preparation of more ATM-derived MoS$_2$ using more discreet changes in decomposition pressures.

One theory for the proposed catalytic activity of MoS$_2$ is that the presence of a coordinatively unsaturated site (CUS), with nearby SH groups, is a requirement for HDS (Lipsch and Schuit 1969). This CUS is formed by removal of sulfur from a molybdenum atom and occurs in the presence of H$_2$ (Alonso et al. 1998). Logically, therefore, the weaker the Mo-S bond the greater the concentration of sulfur vacancies that can be produced resulting in a higher activity (Nørskov et al. 1992). One can expect an improved HDS activity of MoS$_2$ with an FT-IR peak at 378 cm^{-1} over MoS$_2$ with a stronger Mo-S bond at 385 cm^{-1}, when comparing similar activity amongst catalysts of comparable texture and with the same strength of Mo-S peak. This was observed in the present study as well, with the exception of specimen 7-*1,000*, which exhibited different textural properties from other specimens. From the conditions under consideration in this study, all catalysts prepared at high pressure exhibited the weaker Mo-S bond and the largest S_{BET} and the largest TPV were found in 5-*1,000*; thus, it was surmised to be the best catalyst prepared for HDS of DBT. While 5-*1,000* did in fact have the highest activity in real terms (Table 2), as well as a function of TPV, it did not as a function of S_{BET} (Figure 7A,B, respectively). However, we have already shown that agglomeration occurs during S_{BET} measurements, so a more accurate representation would be to

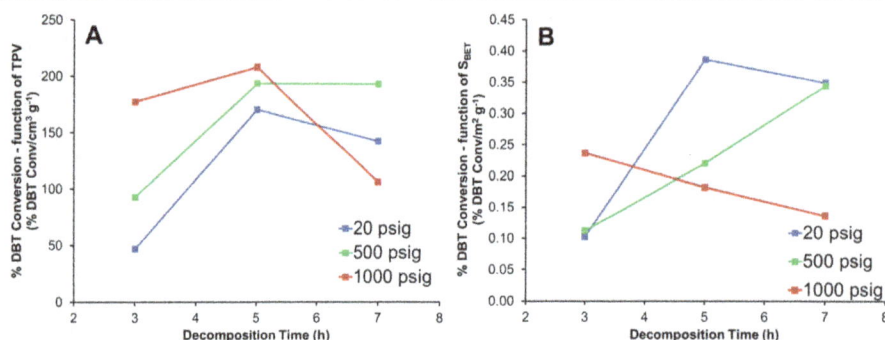

Figure 7 ATM-derived MoS2 activity as a function of TPV and S_{BET}. ATM-derived MoS2 activity as a function of total pore volume (TPV; shown in **(A)**) and BET-derived specific surface (S_{BET}; shown in **(B)**).

compare activity against the theoretically calculated surface area (from XRD). On this basis, 5-1,000 has the highest activity per unit area of MoS_2.

The increase in HYD:DDS ratio, as confirmed by chromatographic analysis, can be partially explained by a possible increase in the number of rim sites available due to interlayer rotation of the layers of MoS_2 in the stacks. Another possibility is that the reduced agglomeration from samples prepared at higher decomposition pressure simply exposes more rim sites to the DBT molecule. Of the samples which produce the hydrogenated DBT, 5-1,000 has one of the lowest HYD:DDS ratios (0.15) compared to say 3-500 (0.32). Thus, not only does 5-1,000 have a more active surface for HDS of DBT, but it also has a higher preference towards the DDS pathway compared to HYD which leads to the assumption that the exposure of rim sites for MoS_2 prepared from reductively decomposed ATM can be optimized by varying decomposition time and pressure.

Conclusions

We have shown herein the role played by both time and pressure for reductive thermal decomposition of ATM for the formation of MoS_2 and their subsequent impact on HDS activity. The influence of decomposition time serves to both enable an increase in surface area as well as an increased likelihood of sintering. Pressure increases slow down thermal decomposition by limiting gaseous by-product diffusion while at the same time facilitating the collapse of produced pores. Based on FT-IR vibrational energies, FT-IR spectral analysis shows that catalysts prepared at higher pressures have weaker Mo-S bonds ($378\ cm^{-1}$) than those prepared at lower pressure ($385\ cm^{-1}$). Evidence from XRD indicates both time and pressure induce interlayer rotation of stacks along both the a- and c-axes and that ATM decomposition pressure plays a role in determination of MoS_2 layer stacking. Using XRD-derived values for crystallite sizes, theoretical surface area values were determined; the

changes evident lead us to conclude that agglomeration is occurring. Optimal conditions were found producing a catalyst with weak Mo-S bonds, the largest (theoretical) surface area and largest pore volume which unsurprisingly resulted in the highest HDS activity of model dibenzothiophene. It was found that catalytic activity increased with a decrease in theoretical surface area, with 5-1,000 having the highest activity per unit area. Samples prepared at low pressures yielded no detectable HYD product, but this increased in samples prepared at higher decomposition pressure. An optimal system was found which gave the lowest HYD:DDS ratio, again 5-1,000. There is no doubt that there are other parameters which can impact both morphology and catalytic activity, such as ramp rates and variously substituted thiomolybdates; we have shown that the role of decomposition time and pressure for ATM-derived MoS_2 can in fact be a useful tool in optimizing catalyst synthesis with certain morphologies and activities.

Additional file

Additional file 1: XRD spectra from all synthesized MoS_2 catalysts.
Figure S1. XRD patterns for MoS_2 catalysts prepared by thermal decomposition of ATM for 3 h at varying pressures **Figure S2.** XRD patterns for MoS_2 catalysts prepared by thermal decomposition of ATM for 5 h at varying pressures. **Figure S3.** XRD patterns for MoS_2 catalysts prepared by thermal decomposition of ATM for 7 h at varying pressures.

Competing interests

The authors declare that they have no competing interests.

Authors' contributions

JW: catalyst synthesis and characterization and manuscript writing; IB: catalyst testing; GEL: FTIR characterization; NDS: catalyst testing; SS: experimental design and execution; AT: XRD characterization; SAH: original idea and data interpretation; RW: original idea and design of work; MSK: data interpretation and manuscript writing; SMA: overall supervision. All authors read and approved the final manuscript.

Acknowledgements

The authors would like to acknowledge financial support from the Abu Dhabi Oil Refining Company (TAKREER) and from the Department of Chemical Engineering at The Petroleum Institute, Abu Dhabi, United Arab Emirates.

Author details
[1]Department of Chemical Engineering, The Petroleum Institute, P.O. Box 2533, Abu Dhabi, United Arab Emirates. [2]Department of Chemistry, New York University Abu Dhabi, P.O. Box 129188, Abu Dhabi, UAE. [3]Department of Chemical and Biochemical Engineering, University Politehnica of Bucharest, 313 Spl. Independentei, sector 6, 060042, Bucharest, Romania. [4]Center for Organic Chemistry "C.D. Nenitzescu", 060023 Bucharest, Romania.

References

Afanasiev P (2008) Synthetic approaches to the molybdenum sulfide materials. Comptes Rendus Chimie 11(1–2):159–182, http://dx.doi.org/10.1016/j.crci.2007.04.009

Afanasiev P (2010) The influence of reducing and sulfiding conditions on the properties of unsupported MoS2-based catalysts. J Catal 269(2):269–280, http://dx.doi.org/10.1016/j.jcat.2009.11.004

Alekseevskii NE, Dobrovol'skii NM, Eckert D, Tsebro VI (1977) Investigation of critical currents of ternary molybdenum sulfides. J Low Temp Phys 29(5–6):565–572, doi:10.1007/bf00661547

Alonso G, Del Valle M, Cruz J, Petranovskii V, Licea-Claverie A, Fuentes S (1998) Preparation of MoS2 catalysts by in situ decomposition of tetraalkylammonium thiomolybdates. Catalysis Today 43(1–2):117–122, http://dx.doi.org/10.1016/S0920-5861(98)00140-0

Álvarez L, Berhault G, Alonso-Nuñez G (2008) Unsupported NiMo sulfide catalysts obtained from Nickel/Ammonium and Nickel/Tetraalkylammonium thiomolybdates: synthesis and application in the hydrodesulfurization of dibenzothiophene. Catal Lett 125(1–2):35–45, doi:10.1007/s10562-008-9541-2

Berhault G, Cota Araiza L, Duarte Moller A, Mehta A, Chianelli R (2002) Modifications of unpromoted and cobalt-promoted MoS2 during thermal treatment by dimethylsulfide. Catal Lett 78(1–4):81–90, doi:10.1023/a:1014910105975

Breysse M, Geantet C, Afanasiev P, Blanchard J, Vrinat M (2008) Recent studies on the preparation, activation and design of active phases and supports of hydrotreating catalysts. Catalysis Today 130(1):3–13, http://dx.doi.org/10.1016/j.cattod.2007.08.018

Brunet S, Mey D, Pérot G, Bouchy C, Diehl F (2005) On the hydrodesulfurization of FCC gasoline: a review. Appl Catal Gen 278(2):143–172, http://dx.doi.org/10.1016/j.apcata.2004.10.012

Camacho-Bragado GA, Elechiguerra JL, Olivas A, Fuentes S, Galvan D, Yacaman MJ (2005) Structure and catalytic properties of nanostructured molybdenum sulfides. J Catal 234(1):182–190, http://dx.doi.org/10.1016/j.jcat.2005.06.009

Chianelli RR, Siadati MH, De la Rosa MP, Berhault G, Wilcoxon JP, Bearden R, Abrams BL (2006) Catalytic properties of single layers of transition metal sulfide catalytic materials. Catalysis Rev 48(1):1–41, doi:10.1080/01614940500439776

Chianelli RR, Berhault G, Torres B (2009) Unsupported transition metal sulfide catalysts: 100 years of science and application. Catalysis Today 147(3–4):275–286, http://dx.doi.org/10.1016/j.cattod.2008.09.041

Criado J, González M, Málek J, Ortega A (1995) The effect of the CO2 pressure on the thermal decomposition kinetics of calcium carbonate. Thermochimica Acta 254(0):121–127, http://dx.doi.org/10.1016/0040-6031(94)01998-V

Daage M, Chianelli RR (1994) Structure-function relations in molybdenum sulfide catalysts: the "Rim-Edge" model. J Catal 149(2):414–427, http://dx.doi.org/10.1006/jcat.1994.1308

De la Rosa MP, Texier S, Berhault G, Camacho A, Yácaman MJ, Mehta A, Fuentes S, Montoya JA, Murrieta F, Chianelli RR (2004) Structural studies of catalytically stabilized model and industrial-supported hydrodesulfurization catalysts. J Catal 225(2):288–299, http://dx.doi.org/10.1016/j.jcat.2004.03.039

Devers E, Afanasiev P, Jouguet B, Vrinat M (2002) Hydrothermal syntheses and catalytic properties of dispersed molybdenum sulfides. Catal Lett 82(1–2):13–17, doi:10.1023/a:1020512320773

Egorova M, Prins R (2006) The role of Ni and Co promoters in the simultaneous HDS of dibenzothiophene and HDN of amines over Mo/γ-Al2O3 catalysts. J Catal 241(1):162–172, http://dx.doi.org/10.1016/j.jcat.2006.04.011

Fedin VP, Kolesov BA, Mironov YV, Fedorov VY (1989) Synthesis and vibrational (IR and Raman) spectroscopic study of triangular thio-complexes [Mo3S13]2– containing 92Mo, 100Mo and 34S isotopes. Polyhedron 8(20):2419–2423, http://dx.doi.org/10.1016/S0277-5387(89)80005-1

Iwata Y, Araki Y, Honna K, Miki Y, Sato K, Shimada H (2001) Hydrogenation active sites of unsupported molybdenum sulfide catalysts for hydroprocessing heavy oils. Catalysis Today 65(2–4):335–341, http://dx.doi.org/10.1016/S0920-5861(00)00554-X

Klimov OV, Pashigreva AV, Fedotov MA, Kochubey DI, Chesalov YA, Bukhtiyarova GA, Noskov AS (2010) Co–Mo catalysts for ultra-deep HDS of diesel fuels prepared via synthesis of bimetallic surface compounds. J Mol Catalysis A Chem 322(1–2):80–89, http://dx.doi.org/10.1016/j.molcata.2010.02.020

Liang KS, Chianelli RR, Chien FZ, Moss SC (1986) Structure of poorly crystalline MoS2 — a modeling study. J Non Cryst Solids 79(3):251–273, http://dx.doi.org/10.1016/0022-3093(86)90226-7

Lipsch JMJG, Schuit GCA (1969) The CoO MoO3 Al2O3 catalyst: III. Catalytic properties. J Catal 15(2):179–189, http://dx.doi.org/10.1016/0021-9517(69)90022-0

McBride KL, Head JD (2009) DFT investigation of MoS2 nanoclusters used as desulfurization catalysts. Int J Quantum Chem 109(15):3570–3582, doi:10.1002/qua.22328

Mdleleni MM, Hyeon T, Suslick KS (1998) Sonochemical synthesis of nanostructured molybdenum sulfide. J Am Chem Soc 120(24):6189–6190, doi:10.1021/ja9800333

Müller A, Jaegermann W, Enemark JH (1982) Disulfur complexes. Coord Chem Rev 46:245–280

Nørskov JK, Clausen BS, Topsøe H (1992) Understanding the trends in the hydrodesulfurization activity of the transition metal sulfides. Catal Lett 13(1–2):1–8, doi:10.1007/bf00770941

Oyumi Y, Brill TB (1987) Thermal decomposition of energetic materials 22. The contrasting effects of pressure on the high-rate thermolysis of 34 energetic compounds. Combustion Flame 68(2):209–216, http://dx.doi.org/10.1016/0010-2180(87)90058-7

Payen E, Grimblot J, Kasztelan S (1987) Study of oxidic and reduced alumina-supported molybdate and heptamolybdate species by in situ laser Raman spectroscopy. J Phys Chem 91(27):6642–6648, doi:10.1021/j100311a018

Peng Y, Meng Z, Zhong C, Lu J, Yu W, Yang Z, Qian Y (2001) Hydrothermal synthesis of MoS2 and its pressure-related crystallization. J Solid State Chem 159(1):170–173, http://dx.doi.org/10.1006/jssc.2001.9146

Piermarini GJ, Block S, Miller PJ (1987) Effects of pressure and temperature on the thermal decomposition rate and reaction mechanism of.beta.-octahydro-1,3,5,7-tetranitro-1,3,5,7-tetrazocine. J Phys Chem 91(14):3872–3878, doi:10.1021/j100298a028

Pietosa J, Dabrowski B, Wisniewski A, Puzniak R, Kiyanagi R, Maxwell T, Jorgensen JD (2008) Pressure effects on magnetic and structural properties of pure and substituted SrRuO3. Phys Rev B 77(10):104410

Polyakov M, van den Berg MWE, Hanft T, Poisot M, Bensch W, Muhler M, Grünert W (2008) Hydrocarbon reactions on MoS2 revisited, I: activation of MoS2 and interaction with hydrogen studied by transient kinetic experiments. J Catal 256(1):126–136, http://dx.doi.org/10.1016/j.jcat.2008.03.007

Sánchez V, Benavente E, Lavayen V, O'Dwyer C, Sotomayor Torres CM, González G, Santa Ana MA (2006) Pressure induced anisotropy of electrical conductivity in polycrystalline molybdenum disulfide. Appl Surf Sci 252(22):7941–7947, http://dx.doi.org/10.1016/j.apsusc.2005.10.011

Topsøe H, Clausen B, Massoth F (1996) Hydrotreating catalysis. In: Anderson J, Boudart M (eds) Catalysis, vol 11, Catalysis-science and technology. Springer, Berlin Heidelberg, pp 1–269, doi:10.1007/978-3-642-61040-0_1

Walton RI, Dent AJ, Hibble SJ (1998) In situ investigation of the thermal decomposition of ammonium tetrathiomolybdate using combined time-resolved X-ray absorption spectroscopy and X-ray diffraction. Chem Mater 10(11):3737–3745, doi:10.1021/cm980716h

Weber T, Muijsers JC, Niemantsverdriet JW (1995) Structure of amorphous MoS3. J Phys Chem 99(22):9194–9200, doi:10.1021/j100022a037

Zhang F, Vasudevan PT (1995) TPD and HYD studies of unpromoted and co-promoted molybdenum sulfide catalyst ex ammonium tetrathiomolybdate. J Catal 157(2):536–544, http://dx.doi.org/10.1006/jcat.1995.1317

16

NMR studies of a Glutaredoxin 2 from Clostridium oremlandii

Eun Hye Lee[1,2], Hae-Kap Cheong[1] and Hye-Yeon Kim[1*]

Abstract

Background: Grx2 is a glutaredoxin from gram positive bacterium *Clostridium oremlandii* (strain OhILAs), which is Cys-homolog of selenoprotein Grx1. Grx2 is a poor reductant of selenoprotein MsrA not like Grx1 while the reducing activity is reversed in two Grxs for Cys version of MsrA.

Methods: The wild-type Grx2 and the C15S mutant were overexpressed in *E.coli* and purified by affinity chromathography and gel filtration. The 3D NMR spectra was collected and assigned all the backbone chemical shifts including Cα, Cβ, CO, HN, and N of Grx2 and C15S mutant. The protein folding of two proteins were evaluated by circular dichroism.

Results: Here we report the protein purification and NMR spectroscopic study of recombinant Grx2 and the C15S mutant. The HSQC spectrum of two proteins show chemical shift difference for residues 8-19, 52-55,66. The circular dichroism result shows that recombinant proteins are well folded.

Conclusion: The conformation of two proteins resembles the oxidized form (wild-type Grx2) and the reduced form (the C15S mutant). The residues showing chemical shift difference will join the conformational change of Grx2 upon a disulfide formation.

Keywords: Grx2, MsrA, *Clostridium oremlandii*, Backbone assignment, NMR

Introduction

Glutaredoxins (Grxs) have been studied in decades and described as glutathionine-dependent reductases of the disulfide formed during its catalytic cycle (Holmgren et al. 2005). Grxs are able to restore the growth of *E.coli* in a mutant lacking thioredoxin (Trx) (Holmgren 1976). Trxs and Grxs share several functions but Grxs are more versatile in choice of substrate and reaction mechanisms (Holmgren 1989). Two groups of Grxs, dithiol and monothiol Grxs, are divided upon catalytic site and functional mechanism (Lillig et al. 2008). Dithiol Grxs contain the characteristic CPYC active site motif and monothiol Grxs lack the C-terminal active site cysteine in the CGFS motif. Both Grxs utilize glutathionine (GSH) as a substrate and share structural elements of binding GSH. GSH is a major biological compound and has a pivotal role in cellular redox homeostasis (Meister 1994). The ratio of GSH and the oxidized form of GSH,

glutathionine disulfide (GSSG), are major determinants of cellular redox state. Grxs could regulate the cellular processes related with the GSH-GSSG redox state. Many organisms contain a unique composition of Grxs. *E.coli* contains four Grxs, two classical dithiol Grxs (Grx1 and Grx3), one unusual dithiol Grx (Grx2), and one monothiol Grx (Grx4) (Vlamis-Gardikas & Holmgren 2002; Fernandes & Holmgren 2004). The structures of Grxs have been studied by X-ray crystallography and NMR spectroscopy. Grxs belong to the Trx fold family which consists of a four stranded β-sheet surrounded by three α-helices. In addition to the active site motif, two additional regions are present for binding of GSH; the residues preceding the *cis*-proline (consensus: TVP) and the residues following the GG-motif (consensus: GGxdD) (Lillig et al. 2008).

Clostridium oremlandii (strain OhILAs) is a selenoprotein-rich organism and contains selenoprotein MsrA and selenoprotein Grx1 (Kim et al. 2006). *C.oremlandii* has a Cys-homolog protein of selenoprotein Grx1 which is defined as glutaredoxin 2 (Grx2). MsrA catalyzes the

* Correspondence: hyeyeon@kbsi.re.kr
[1]Division of Magnetic Resonance Research, Korea Basic Science Institute, Ochang, Chungbuk, Korea
Full list of author information is available at the end of the article

reduction of oxidized methionine residue in cellular proteins. A cysteine residue at the active site of MsrA is oxidized after the catalysis and then recycled by reductases like Trx. Selenoprotein MsrA shows 20-fold higher catalytic activity than its Cys-containing form instead of selenocysteine (Sec). This organism uses Grx proteins, Grx1 or Grx2, for reduction of the oxidized MsrA instead of Trxs. Selenoprotein Grx1 is a strong reductant of selenoprotein MsrA while Grx2 shows poor reducing activity for selenoprotein MsrA (Boschi-Muller et al. 2000). Although Grx1 and Grx2 share sequence homology of 55%, the reducing activity for selenoprotein MsrA is extremely different. Interestingly, the reducing activity of Grxs is reversed between Cys vesion of Grx1 and wild-type Grx2 for Cys version of MsrA. Grx2 shows high reducing activity whereas Cys version Grx1 shows almost no activity in reduction of Cys version of MsrA (Kim et al. 2011). Previously, we reported the backbone assignment result of Cys version Grx1 (Lee et al. 2012). To investigate the structural characteristics of Grx2, we have performed the NMR spectroscopy of Grx2 and its C15S mutant. Grx2 consists of 85 amino acid residues including three cysteine residues in its sequence and contains a conserved CGPC motif of dithiol Grxs. Two cysteine residues are

defined as catalytic and resolving cysteines depending on the role during the cataylsis. Catalytic cysteine reduces the substrate and then the oxidized cysteine is recovered by the resolving cysteine. The resolving cysteine C15 is introduced to obtain the advantages in monitoring the molecular interaction between catalytic cysteines of Grx2 and MsrA. The wild-type and the C15S mutant of Grx2 are subjected to NMR experiments and circular dichroism. Here, we report purification and NMR backbone assignment of recombinant Grx2 proteins.

Methods

Cloning, expression and purification

Grx2 (residues 1–85) from genomic DNA of *Clostridium oremlandii* was cloned into the expression vector pET21b (Novagen). The recombinant plasmids were transformed to *E.coli* BL21(DE3) cells for protein overexpression. The wild-type Grx2 and the C15S mutant of Grx2 (the C15S mutant) were expressed with the C-terminal Histag (LEHHHHHH). The cells were grown in M9 minimal media containing 100 μg/ml ampicilin for $^{13}C/^{15}N$ double labeling at 37°C until OD_{600} reached 0.6. Then protein overexpression was induced by addition of 0.5 mM IPTG at 18°C for 20 h. The cells was harvested by centrifugation at 4,500 rpm for 20 min and resuspended in the ice-cold buffer A (20 mM Tris–HCl, pH 7.5, 300 mM NaCl, 4 mM $MgCl_2$). Harvested cells were disrupted by sonication and centrifuged at 13,000 rpm for 50 min at 4°C. The supernatant was loaded onto HisTrap column (GE Healthcare) equilibrated with buffer A and recombinant protein was eluted by gradient increasing of imidazole concentration. The protein was concentrated to ~2 ml and applied to HiLoad 16/60 Superdex-75 (GE healthcare) equilibrated with 20 mM HEPES, pH 7.0, 100 mM NaCl. The eluted protein was concentrated to 1 mM for NMR study.

NMR data acquisition and analysis

NMR experiments were performed at 25°C using 1 mM of $^{13}C,^{15}N$-labeled Grx2 and the C15S mutant samples in 20 mM HEPES, pH 7.0, 100 mM NaCl. 10% D_2O of total sample volume and 5 mM DTT were added to both samples before experiments. NMR data were collected by Bruker Avance 800-MHz NMR spectrometer (Korea Basic Science Institute, Korea) for three days. The backbone chemical shift were obtained by three-dimensional heteronuclear correlation experiments: HNCO, HN(CA)CO, HNCA, HN(CO)CA, HNCACB, CBCA(CO)NH (Wishart et al. 1995). NMR experiments of Grx2 including three spectra, HSQC, HNCACB and CBCA(CO)NH, were performed at same condition. All NMR data were processed and analyzed by TopSpin (Bruker BioSpin), NMRPipe (Delaglio et al. 1995) and then applied to AutoAssign server (Zimmerman et al. 1997) and further

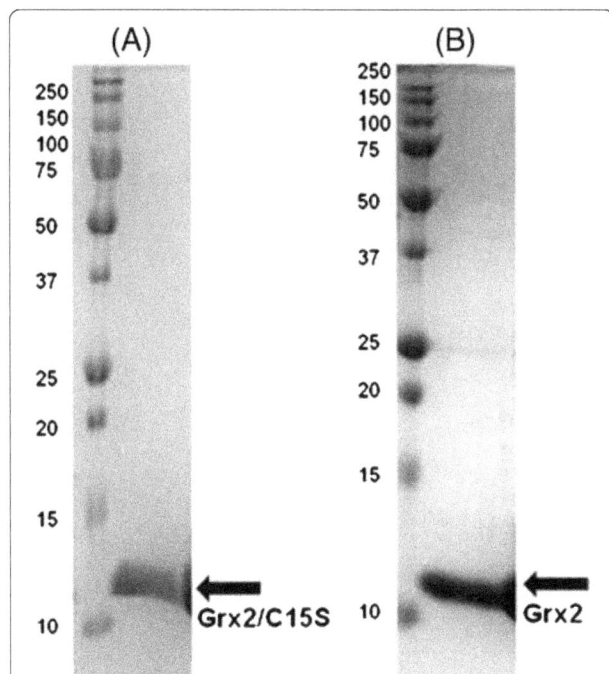

Figure 1 Protein purification. Samples from all purification steps were confirmed by the SDS-PAGE analysis. The expressed Grx2 proteins were purified using the HisTrap column and then applied to the Superdex 75 gel chromatography column. The purified C15S mutant (**A**) and wild-type Grx2 (**B**) proteins show >98% purity. The migration of the molecular mass markers is indicated on the left.

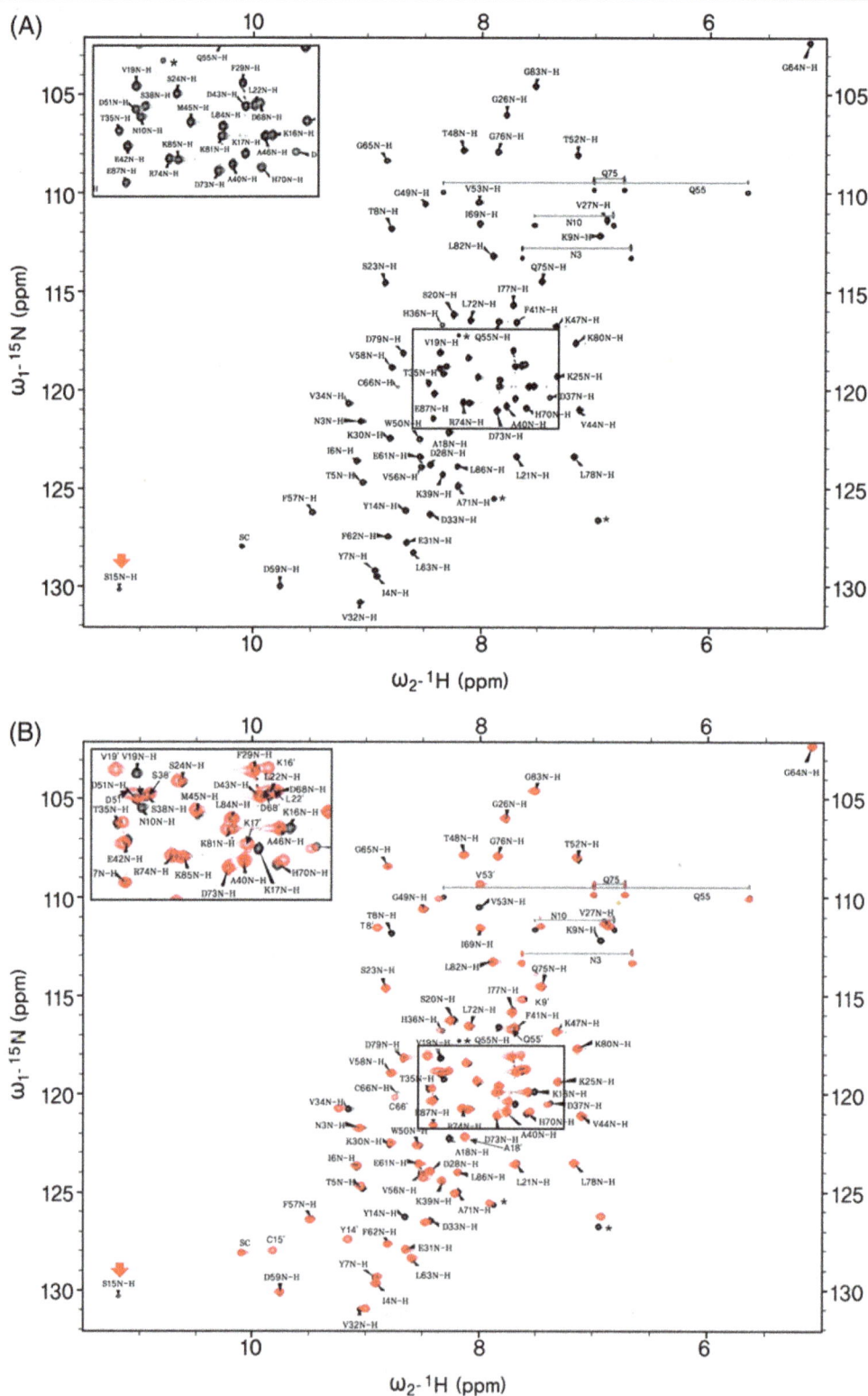

Figure 2 **¹H-¹⁵N HSQC spectra of the C15S mutant and wild-type Grx2.** (**A**) Assigned HSQC spectrum of the C15S mutant. (**B**) HSQC spectra overlay of the C15S mutant (black) and wild-type Grx2 (red). Several residues of wild-type Grx2 protein are represented with prime(') marks. All assigned residues are labeled and one crowded region is magnified (insets). The mutated residue C15S is indicated by red arrow. The assigned set of cross peaks from amide side-chains of Asn and Gln residues is indicated using a gray horizontal bar. The unassigned peaks are marked by '*' and the tryptophan side chain is marked by 'sc'.

Table 1 Assigned backbone chemical shifts (1HN, 15 N, 13CO, 13Cα and 13Cβ) of the C15S mutant

AA	HN	N	Cα	Cβ	CO	AA	HN	N	Cα	Cβ	CO
K2	-	-	53.11	31.01	172.9	A46	7.573	119.8	51.64	15.38	176.3
N3	9.051	121.6	50.24	36.27	171.9	K47	7.341	116.7	55.65	30.68	175.9
I4	8.905	129.5	58.24	36.53	172.6	T48	8.153	107.8	59.14	68.14	173.8
T5	9.033	124.7	58.69	68.94	169.6	G49	8.49	110.5	42.89	-	171.7
I6	9.087	123.6	55.28	39.13	169.5	W50	8.535	122.5	53.42	27.5	172.8
Y7	8.926	129.2	54.69	36.8	173.5	D51	8.356	118.9	49.69	38.2	173.4
T8	8.784	111.8	57.11	69.57	170.6	T52	7.153	108	57.08	68.83	170.9
K9	6.958	112.2	52.91	34.43	175.1	V53	8.021	110.5	55.83	30.89	170
N10	8.323	119.2	52.42	35.54	172.7	P54	-	-	59.2	33.52	173.8
P13	-	-	61.69	29.38	176.9	Q55	7.844	116.5	54.31	31	172
Y14	8.659	126.1	58.27	35.19	176.2	V56	8.518	123.9	59.31	30.42	170.6
S15	11.18	130.2	61.41	51.86	172.3	F57	9.482	126.2	53.6	40.89	172.5
K16	7.612	120.4	56.83	29.69	176.5	V58	8.779	118.8	58.27	30.67	173.3
K17	7.694	120.4	56.84	30.24	176.4	D59	9.754	130	54.44	36.77	173.1
A18	8.277	122.1	52.92	16.91	175.6	E60	-	-	54.66	26.15	172.9
V19	8.354	118.1	64.72	28.92	175.6	E61	8.533	123.4	53.16	28.25	172.4
S20	8.237	116.1	59.22	59.93	174.3	F62	8.81	127.5	52.56	36.32	172.9
L21	7.68	123.4	55.33	37.92	177.2	L63	8.59	128.3	51.63	40.3	172.3
L22	7.636	118.8	55.57	37.86	176.6	G64	5.136	102.3	41.28	41.28	169.3
S23	8.838	114.5	59.36	60.24	175.3	G65	8.823	108.3	40.98	41.03	171.3
S24	8.109	118.4	58.38	60.28	172.7	C66	8.721	119.9	60.96	35.07	-
K25	7.329	119.3	52.69	30.37	174.8	D67	-	-	55.04	36.66	176.3
G26	7.779	106	43.67	-	171.7	D68	7.602	118.7	54.92	38.57	176.4
V27	7.012	112	56.67	30.7	172.2	I69	8.009	111.5	62.98	35.16	175.1
D28	8.438	123.8	51.44	38.58	173.1	H70	7.594	120.9	59.86	25.44	175
F29	7.711	118	52.92	39.09	169.9	A71	8.196	124.9	52.91	14.83	178
K30	8.796	122.4	51.96	31.66	171.5	L72	8.091	116.4	54.66	39.86	177.1
E31	8.648	127.8	51.43	28.48	173	D73	7.863	121	54.4	39.05	177
V32	9.056	130.8	58.79	29.63	171.2	R74	8.153	120.6	56.52	27.33	175.8
D33	8.44	126.3	50.56	38.56	176	Q75	7.462	114.5	53.4	27.95	173.6
V34	9.159	120.7	58.59	28.05	173.5	G76	7.854	107.9	42.97	-	172.2
T35	8.458	119.7	64.95	66.01	172.4	I77	7.713	115.7	58.9	36.87	174
H36	8.335	116.7	52.67	28.19	172.2	L78	7.18	123.4	55.31	37.16	175.1
D37	7.393	120.4	49.88	37.87	172.1	D79	8.68	118.1	55.5	37.08	175.5
S38	8.297	118.8	58.21	60.13	174.5	K80	7.165	117.6	56.33	29.42	177.8
K39	8.33	124.3	56.29	28.85	176	K81	7.843	119.8	55.12	29.3	175.3
A40	7.775	120.8	51.76	15.74	178.1	L82	7.896	113.1	52.22	39.01	173.2
F41	7.683	116.6	56.17	36.15	174.1	G83	7.521	104.5	42.96	-	171.8
E42	8.404	120.2	57.2	26.4	176.8	L84	7.835	119.5	52.36	39.76	173.9
D43	7.692	118.8	54.38	37.61	175.6	K85	8.096	120.6	52.74	30.37	173
V44	7.135	121	63.45	28.52	174.6	L86	8.2	123.9	52.29	39.69	174.5
M45	8.028	119.4	56.38	30.65	177	E87	8.413	121.4	53.69	27.68	173.3

Table 2 Assigned backbone chemical shifts (1HN, 15 N, 13Cα and 13Cβ) of Grx2

AA	HN	N	Cα	Cβ	AA	HN	N	Cα	Cβ
K2	-	-	53.23	31.02	A46	7.585	119.8	51.66	15.39
N3	9.061	121.6	50.28	36.4	K47	7.343	116.7	55.71	30.68
I4	8.912	129.5	58.31	36.49	T48	8.155	107.8	59.24	68.11
T5	9.047	124.5	63.84	-	G49	8.507	110.5	42.94	-
I6	9.084	123.5	55.37	39.11	W50	8.558	122.5	53.47	27.49
Y7	8.903	129.2	54.97	36.88	D51	8.375	118.7	49.65	38.21
T8	8.907	111.5	56.84	69.69	T52	7.168	108	57.09	68.89
K9	7.542	114.8	52.83	34.3	V53	8.015	109.4	55.83	30.74
N10	8.344	118.8	52.17	35.64	P54	-	-	59.17	33.67
P13	-	-	61.83	29.48	Q55	7.721	116.6	54.55	30.74
Y14	9.096	127.1	58.64	34.98	V56	8.494	124.1	59.31	30.37
C15	9.988	128.1	62.55	25.84	F57	9.494	126.2	53.62	40.9
K16	7.625	118.2	56.97	29.52	V58	8.79	118.8	58.31	30.64
K17	7.752	120.3	56.91	30.23	D59	9.758	129.9	54.55	36.8
A18	8.143	122.1	53	16.86	E60	-	-	54.74	26.25
V19	8.465	118	64.75	28.91	E61	8.54	123.4	53.27	28.24
S20	8.269	116.1	60	59.79	F62	8.814	127.5	52.62	36.31
L21	7.687	123.4	55.41	37.91	L63	8.601	128.1	51.66	40.33
L22	7.6	118.7	55.69	37.85	G64	5.129	102.3	41.37	-
S23	8.838	114.6	59.33	60.05	G65	8.818	108.4	41.08	-
S24	8.136	118.3	58.39	60.29	C66	8.751	120	61.06	24.51
K25	7.326	119.3	52.77	30.38	D67	-	-	55.07	36.64
G26	7.786	106	43.72	-	D68	7.63	118.6	54.99	38.61
V27	6.905	111.3	56.66	30.72	I69	8.015	111.5	62.95	35.16
D28	8.442	123.8	51.56	38.57	H70	7.563	120.8	59.94	25.43
F29	7.726	118	52.98	39.14	A71	8.227	124.9	53.03	14.85
K30	8.791	122.4	51.98	31.75	L72	8.113	116.4	54.73	39.76
E31	8.652	127.8	51.55	28.36	D73	7.856	121	54.46	39.09
V32	9.006	130.8	58.84	29.09	R74	8.169	120.6	56.53	27.34
D33	8.479	126.3	50.68	38.67	Q75	7.475	114.4	53.47	27.94
V34	9.243	120.6	58.56	28.09	G76	7.856	107.9	43.01	-
T35	8.424	119.6	64.91	65.99	I77	7.719	115.8	58.92	36.85
H36	8.36	116.7	52.76	28	L78	7.188	123.4	55.39	37.1
D37	7.419	120.4	49.91	37.86	D79	8.676	118.1	55.6	37.11
S38	8.28	118.7	58.31	60.15	K80	7.157	117.6	56.29	29.4
K39	8.338	124.3	56.3	28.85	K81	7.865	119.8	55.23	29.29
A40	7.771	120.8	51.83	15.75	L82	7.9	113.2	52.3	38.96
F41	7.7	116.5	56.24	36.16	G83	7.53	104.6	43.01	-
E42	8.425	120.2	57.29	26.38	L84	7.841	119.5	52.41	39.72
D43	7.678	118.8	54.45	37.61	K85	8.116	120.7	52.85	30.36
V44	7.118	121	63.5	28.54	L86	8.2	123.9	52.35	39.69
M45	8.04	119.2	56.4	30.71	E87	8.412	121.5	53.73	27.68

backbone assignment was performed by Sparky (Goddard & Kneller 2004) software packages.

CD analysis

CD spectra (190–250 nm) were measured at 25°C on a Jasco J-715 apparatus, using a 1.0 mm path length quartz cell. Recombinant proteins were diluted 20 times with water at a protein concentration of 50 μM. The buffer contained 1 mM HEPES, pH 7.0, 5 mM NaCl. The averaged blank spectra were subtracted.

Results and discussion

Sample preparation

The C-terminal Histag fused Grx2 and the C15S mutant proteins were overexpressed in *E.coli* BL21(DE3). The recombinant proteins were purified by nickel affinity chromatography (HisTrap column) and then applied to size-exclusion column (HiLoad 16/60 Superdex-75 column). The purified protein contained the C-terminal histag which was not removed by further treatment. Through gel filtration, Grx2 protein was eluted at a protein size of 10 kD and it means that Grx2 present as a monomer in solution. The eluted protein showed >98% purity at SDS-PAGE and concentrated to 1 mM for NMR measurements. The final purified proteins are shown in Figure 1.

Backbone assignment

The HSQC spectrum of the C15S mutant shows doublet peaks generated by intermolecular disulfide bond in oxidative condition. The doublet peaks disappear after addtion of DTT to the sample at concentration of 5 mM. We have assigned 92% of the expected backbone ^{1}H-^{15}N correlations (77 out of 83; Grx2 contains 2 proline residues) and 96% of all ^{13}CO, ^{13}Cα and ^{13}Cβ (239 out of 249; Figure 2). The six residues, M1, K2, Y11, C12, E60 and D67, are not visible in HSQC spectrum. The two residues of C-terminal histag (86LEHHH-HHH93) were assigned the backbone chemical shifts (Figure 2A). In HSQC spectrum, three ^{1}H-^{15}N correlations are unassigned which lost their conectivity between assigned residues. The assigned chemical shifts (Cα, Cβ, CO, HN, and N) of the C15S mutant were summarized in Table 1. NH$_2$ group of Asn and Gln side-chains generally produce two split HSQC cross peaks that were identified in the measured HSQC spectrum. All possible 4 set of amide side-chains peaks were identified in the HSQC spectrum. Residues N3, N10, Q55 and Q75 made two split HSQC cross peaks which are indicated by gray line between two peaks. There is one tryptophan residue in Grx2 protein and the side chain NH resonance of W50 residue was assigned in HSQC spectrum. The missing residues in HSQC spectrum are expected to be partially solvent-exposed or have possible conformational

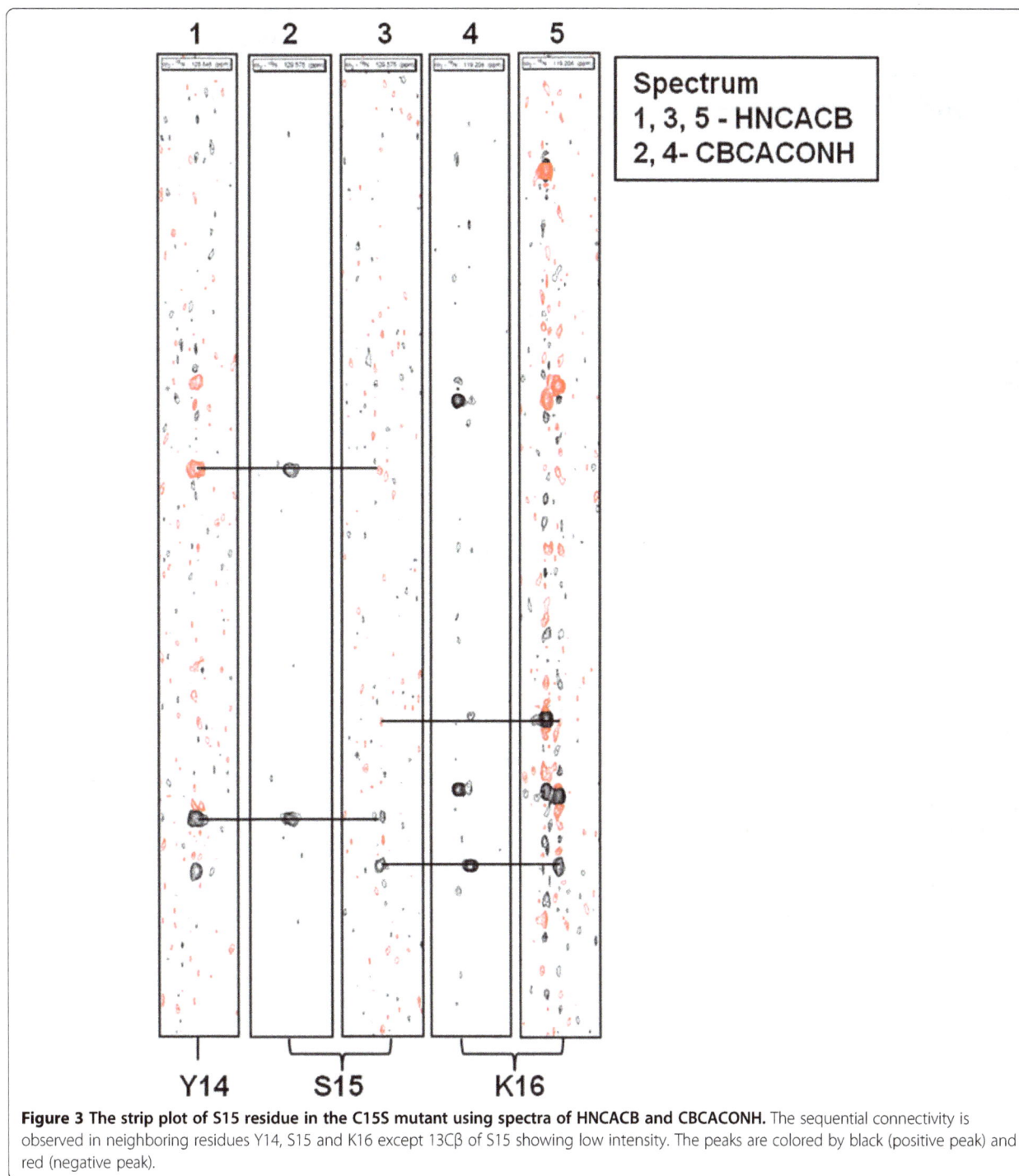

Figure 3 The strip plot of S15 residue in the C15S mutant using spectra of HNCACB and CBCACONH. The sequential connectivity is observed in neighboring residues Y14, S15 and K16 except 13Cβ of S15 showing low intensity. The peaks are colored by black (positive peak) and red (negative peak).

exchange within NMR time scale. The unassigned three peaks may originated from the remained hexahistidine tag. The ^{1}H-^{15}N correlations of Grx2 are assigned on HSQC spectrum based on the C15S mutant assignments and HSQC spectra of two proteins are superposed (Figure 2B). Some ambigouos peaks are assigned by additional experiments of HNCACB, CBCA(CO)NH using ^{13}C,^{15}N-labeled Grx2. The assigned chemical shifts

(Cα, Cβ, HN, and N) of Grx2 were summarized in Table 2. The ^{1}H-^{15}N correlations of Grx2 are assigned execept two correlations which are remained in unassigned in the C15S mutant spectrum. In HSQC spectrum of Grx2, ^{1}H-^{15}N correlations of 77 residues are shown and they are common residues in the C15S mutant. Most residues are represented at the identical position of HSQC spectrum while some residues show large chemical shift

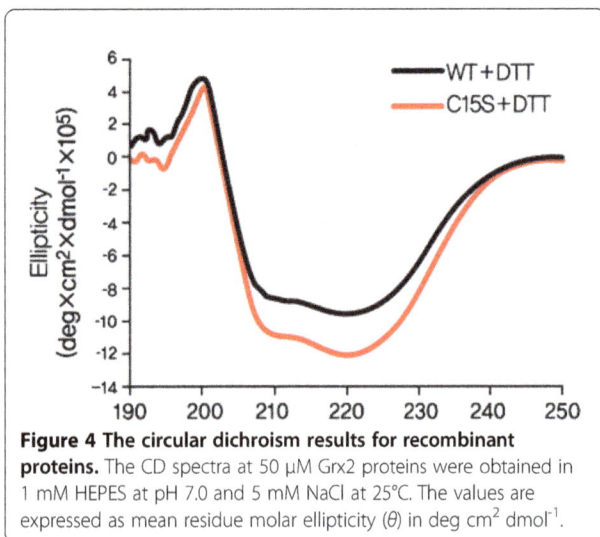

Figure 4 The circular dichroism results for recombinant proteins. The CD spectra at 50 μM Grx2 proteins were obtained in 1 mM HEPES at pH 7.0 and 5 mM NaCl at 25°C. The values are expressed as mean residue molar ellipticity (θ) in deg cm^2 dmol^{-1}.

change between wild-type Grx2 and the C15S mutant. The chemical shift of S15 residue has extremely high ^{1}H chemical shift of 11.1 ppm than 9.8 ppm of C15 residue. The 11.1 ppm can be observed in serine residue which has 1H chemical shift range of 3.76 ppm 12.33 ppm according to Biological Magnetic Resonance data Bank. The magnitude of the chemical shift depends upon the type of nucleus and the details of the electron motion in the nearby atoms and molecules (Hobbie 1998). The >1 ppm chemical shift difference may caused by extensive alteration of circumstance near proton in amino group of S15 residue. The strip plot of S15 residue with adjacent residues are represented in Figure 3. The residues K9, Y14 and C15 have chemical shift difference over 0.5 ppm and T8, K16, A18, V19, V53, Q55 and C66 residues have over 0.1 ppm. These residues could be grouped to three regions, residues 8–19 including C15 residue, residues 52TVPQ55, and residue C66. The substitution of resolving cysteine to serine may induce the conformational change near active site that is related to oxidation state of Grx2. However, there is a possibility that the chemical shift difference is occurred by the simple change of chemical environments near C15 or S15 residue without no structural change. In addition, two Grx2 proteins have well-folded structure which are validated by circular dichroism (Figure 4).

Conclusions

The substitution of resolving cysteine to serine occured conformational change and these residues may be related to oxidation state of Grx2. Two proteins show different HSQC spectrum even in the reduced condition made by DTT addition. The addition of 5 mM DTT was not enough to break the intramolecular disulfide bond but the intermolecular disulfide bond. The resoliong C15 residue makes intramolecular disulfide bond with

catalytic C12 residue in wild-type Grx2. Wild-type Grx2 keeps two cysteine residues which can form a disulfide bond while the C15S mutant keeps one cysteine residue and is not able to form it. The conformation of two proteins resembles the oxidized form (wild-type Grx2) and the reduced form (the C15S mutant). The residues showing chemical shift difference will join the conformational change of Grx2 upon a disulfide formation. These results will be useful to the structural study of oxidized and reduced Grx2 and the interaction study with MsrA

Competing interests

The authors declare that they have no competing interests.

Authors' contributions

EHL carried out the smaple preparation, NMR studies and circular dichroism analysis. EHL, HKJ. and H-YK. drafted the manuscript. All authors read and approved the final manuscript.

Acknowledgements

This work was supported by the NMR research program of Korea Basic Science Institute to H.-Y.K. We thank Kim Hwa-Young (Yeungnam University) for providing the Grx2 constructs.

Author details

[1]Division of Magnetic Resonance Research, Korea Basic Science Institute, Ochang, Chungbuk, Korea. [2]Division of Biotechnology, College of Life Sciences and Biotechnology, Korea University, Seoul, Korea.

References

Boschi-Muller S, Azza S, Sanglier-Cianferani S, Talfournier F, Van Dorsselear A, Branlant G (2000) A sulfenic acid enzyme intermediate is involved in the catalytic mechanism of peptide methionine sulfoxide reductase from Escherichia coli. J Biol Chem 275:35908–35913

Delaglio F, Grzesiek S, Vuister GW, Zhu G, Pfeifer J, Bax A (1995) NMRPipe: a multidimensional spectral processing system based on UNIX pipes. J Biomol NMR 6:277–293

Fernandes AP, Holmgren A (2004) Glutaredoxins: glutathione-dependent redox enzymes with functions far beyond a simple thioredoxin backup system. Antioxid Redox Signal 6:63–74

Goddard ID, Kneller DG (2004) SPARKY 3. University of California, San Francisco

Hobbie RK (1998) Intermediate Physics for Medicine and Biology. 2nd Ed. Wiley

Holmgren A (1976) Hydrogen donor system for Escherichia coli ribonucleoside-diphosphate reductase dependent upon glutathione. Proc Natl Acad Sci U S A 73:2275–2279

Holmgren A (1989) Thioredoxin and glutaredoxin systems. J Biol Chem 264:13963–13966

Holmgren A, Johansson C, Berndt C, Lonn ME, Hudemann C, Lillig CH (2005) Thiol redox control via thioredoxin and glutaredoxin systems. Biochem Soc Trans 33:1375–1377

Kim HY, Fomenko DE, Yoon YE, Gladyshev VN (2006) Catalytic advantages provided by selenocysteine in methionine-S-sulfoxide reductases. Biochemistry 45:13697–13704

Kim MJ, Lee BC, Jeong J, Lee KJ, Hwang KY, Gladyshev VN, Kim HY (2011) Tandem use of selenocysteine: adaptation of a selenoprotein glutaredoxin for reduction of selenoprotein methionine sulfoxide reductase. Mol Microbiol 79:1194–1203

Lee EH, Kim EH, Kin HY, Hwang KY, Kim HY (2012) NMR spectroscopic study of a Glutaredoxin1 from Clostridium oremlandii. JAST 3:154–159

Lillig CH, Berndt C, Holmgren A (2008) Glutaredoxin systems. Biochim Biophys Acta 1780:1304–1317

Meister A (1994) Glutathione-ascorbic acid antioxidant system in animals. J Biol Chem 269:9397–9400

Vlamis-Gardikas A, Holmgren A (2002) Thioredoxin and glutaredoxin isoforms. Methods Enzymol 347:286–296

Wishart DS, Bigam CG, Yao J, Abildgaard F, Dyson HJ, Oldfield E, Markley JL, Sykes BD (1995) 1H, 13C and 15N Chemical Shift Referencing in Biomolecular NMR. J Biomol NMR 6:135–140

Zimmerman DE, Kulikowski CA, Feng W, Tashiro M, Chien C-Y, Ríos CB, Moy FJ, Powers R, Montelione GT (1997) Artificial intelligence methods for automated analysis of protein resonance assignments. J Mol Biol 269:592–610

17

Sm-Nd isotopic analysis of mixed standard solutions by multi-collector inductively coupled plasma mass spectrometry: evaluations on isobaric interference correction of Nd isotopic composition and external calibration of Sm/Nd ratio

Jong-Sik Ryu, Min Seok Choi, Youn-Joong Jeong and Chang-sik Cheong[*]

Abstract

Background: The Sm-Nd isotope system has long been used to provide information on the age and geochemical evolution of terrestrial rocks and extraterrestrial objects. Traditional thermal ionization mass spectrometry requires a refined chemical separation of Sm and Nd. Here, we present multi-collector inductively coupled plasma mass spectrometry (MC-ICP-MS) Sm-Nd isotopic results for a series of mixed standard solutions with different Sm/Nd ratios to test the validity of isobaric interference corrections of Nd isotopic composition and external calibration of Sm/Nd inter-elemental ratio.

Findings: Reliable $^{143}Nd/^{144}Nd$ and $^{145}Nd/^{144}Nd$ ratios of the mixed solutions were obtained by using the exponential law and selected Sm isotopic compositions. The Sm/Nd ratios of the mixed solutions corrected by the standard bracketing method were consistent with the gravimetric values mostly within 1% difference.

Conclusions: This study provides a simple and high-throughput technique that can simultaneously measure Nd isotopic composition and Sm/Nd ratio without chemical separation between Sm and Nd.

Keywords: Sm-Nd, MC-ICP-MS, Isobaric interference, Isotopic composition, Inter-elemental ratio

Introduction

Sm and Nd are rare earth elements presenting in only small amounts in most rock-forming minerals. Sm and Nd each have seven naturally occurring isotopes (^{144}Sm, ^{147}Sm, ^{148}Sm, ^{149}Sm, ^{150}Sm, ^{152}Sm, ^{154}Sm; ^{142}Nd, ^{143}Nd, ^{144}Nd, ^{145}Nd, ^{146}Nd, ^{148}Nd, ^{150}Nd). One isotope of Sm (^{147}Sm) decays by α-emission to one isotope of Nd (^{143}Nd) with a half-life of 106 Ga (Lugmair & Marti 1978; Begemann et al. 2001). The Sm-Nd decay system has been efficiently used for determining the timing of major events occurred during the chemical evolution of planets and probing into the earth's interior (DePaolo

1988). The application of this system demands highly accurate Sm-Nd isotope data because its half-life is very long and natural variations in Sm/Nd inter-elemental ratio are typically quite limited.

Although the traditional thermal ionization mass spectrometry (TIMS) is still regarded as the benchmark technique for Sm-Nd isotopic measurement (Chu et al. 2009; Harvey & Baxter 2009; Ali & Srinivasan 2011), more recent multi collector-inductively coupled plasma-mass spectrometry (MC-ICP-MS) has also become a routine technique with high sample throughput and comparable precision to TIMS (Walder et al. 1993; Vance & Thirlwall 2002; Yang et al. 2010; Yang et al. 2011). The classic Sm-Nd isotope analysis requires a separation of two elements from the sample matrix by refined chemical

* Correspondence: ccs@kbsi.re.kr
Division of Earth and Environmental Sciences, Korea Basic Science Institute, Chungbuk 363-883, South Korea

procedures. Recently, however, it was reported that the ^{143}Nd/^{144}Nd ratio of geological samples could be measured accurately by MC-ICP-MS without Sm and Nd separation (Yang et al. 2010). This study further evaluates the validity of Nd isotopic and Sm/Nd elemental ratio measurements for a series of Sm + Nd mixed standard solutions by MC-ICP-MS technique, and revisited various sets of reported Sm isotopic composition.

Instrumentation

The Sm-Nd isotopic analysis of this study was conducted by using a Neptune MC-ICP-MS installed at the Korea Basic Science Institute (KBSI) in Ochang. This double focusing high-resolution ICP-MS is equipped with eight movable Faraday collectors and one fixed axial channel where the ion beam intensities can be measured with either a Faraday collector or an ion counting electron multiplier. The Faraday collectors were statically set to simultaneously detect the required isotopes: ^{140}Ce (L4), ^{142}Nd (L3), ^{143}Sm (L2), ^{144}(Sm + Nd) (L1), ^{145}Nd (axial), ^{146}Nd (H1), ^{147}Sm (H2), ^{148}(Sm + Nd) (H3), and ^{149}Sm (H4). The sensitivity on ^{145}Nd was typically around 5 V/Nd ppm ($10^{11}\Omega$ resistors) in a low-resolution mode. Details of the other operational parameters are summarized in Table 1.

Measurement of Nd standard solutions

The basic performance of KBSI Neptune was tested by using the JNdi standard solution with Nd concentration of 100 µg/L. The mass bias was exponentially normalized to ^{146}Nd/^{144}Nd = 0.7219. One measurement consists of 9 blocks of 10 cycles with an integration time of 4.194 s. The average ^{143}Nd/^{144}Nd ratio was 0.512100 ± 0.000004 (n = 10, 2σ S.E.), in reasonable agreement with the recommended value (0.512115 ± 0.000007) (Tanaka et al. 2000).

Table 1 Instrumental setting and operational parameters

RF forward power	1200 W
RF reflected power	< 2 W
Cooling gas	15 L/min
Auxiliary gas	0.75 - 0.80 L/min
Sample gas	0.985 - 0.990 L/min
Extraction	−2 kV
Focus	−0.654 kV
Acceleration voltage	10 kV
Interface cones	Nickel
Spray chamber	Quartz dual cyclonic
Nebulizer	ESI PFA MicroFlow
Sample uptake rate	100 µL/min
Instrumental resolution	ca. 400
Mass analyzer pressure	2.9×10^{-9} mbar

The in-house Nd standard solution of 100 µg/L was prepared from the AccuTrace™ Nd Reference Standard (lot no. B9035110, plasma emission standard). It yielded an average ^{143}Nd/^{144}Nd ratio of 0.512204 ± 0.000005 (n = 9, 2σ S.E.) with the same analytical design as above (9 blocks of 10 cycles with an integration time of 4.194 s). Two diluted in-house Nd solutions of 50 and 10 µg/L also yielded comparable results of ^{143}Nd/^{144}Nd = 0.512212 ± 0.000006 (n = 5, 2σ S.E.) and 0.512207 ± 0.000004 (n = 5, 2σ S.E.), respectively.

Isobaric interference correction

The contribution of ^{144}Sm imposed on the ^{144}Nd peak should be carefully corrected for accurate determination of ^{143}Nd/^{144}Nd ratio. The first step of correction in this study was to calculate the Sm mass bias factor, β(Sm), for which the exponential law (Russel et al. 1978) was applied as the following.

$$\beta(Sm) = \ln \left[\left(^{147}Sm/^{149}Sm\right)_{true} / \left(^{147}Sm/^{149}Sm\right)_{measured} \right]$$
$$\div \ln \left(M_{147}/M_{149}\right), \quad (1)$$

where M denotes the mass of the isotope.

The exponential law also yields an equation for $(^{144}Sm/^{149}Sm)_{measured}$:

$$\left(^{144}Sm/^{149}Sm\right)_{measured} = \left(^{144}Sm/^{149}Sm\right)_{true}$$
$$\times \left(M_{149}/M_{144}\right)^{\beta(Sm)} \quad (2)$$

The ^{144}Sm intensity was calculated as multiplying Eq (2) by measured ^{149}Sm intensity. Then, ^{144}Nd intensity

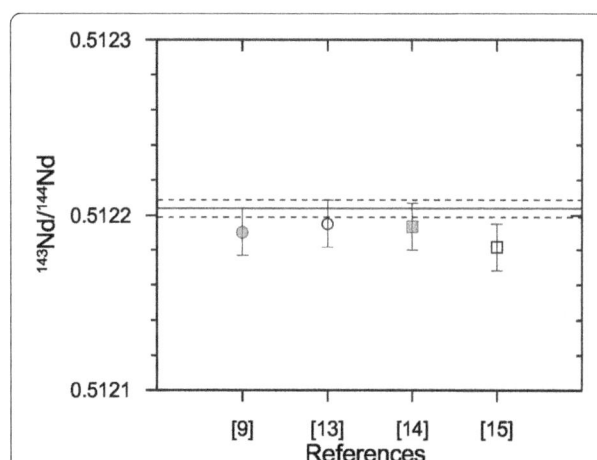

Figure 1 The ^{143}Nd/^{144}Nd ratios of a Sm-doped Nd standard solution with 100 µg/L Nd and Sm/Nd of 0.2041. The isobaric interference was corrected using reported Sm isotopic compositions ([9] Yang et al. 2010; [13] Wasserburg et al. 1981; [14] McFarlane & McCulloch 2007; [15] Berglund & Wieser 2011). Solid and dashed lines respectively represent an average measured ^{143}Nd/^{144}Nd ratio and 2σ S.D. of the unspiked Nd standard solution.

Table 2 Nd isotope ratios of the Sm-doped Nd standard solutions with the Sm/Nd ratio of 0.2

	Gravimetric Sm/Nd	^{143}Nd/^{144}Nd	2σ S.E.	^{145}Nd/^{144}Nd	2σ S.E.	n
100 µg/L Nd	0.2041	0.512195	0.000011	0.348415	0.000005	140
200 µg/L Nd	0.2022	0.512195	0.000022	0.348419	0.000010	20
50 µg/L Nd	0.2036	0.512208	0.000038	0.348420	0.000031	20

was calculated by subtracting the ^{144}Sm intensity from the intensity on mass 144 using the equation.

$$^{144}Nd_{measured} = {}^{144}(Sm + Nd)_{measured}$$
$$- \left[{}^{149}Sm_{measured} \times \left({}^{144}Sm/{}^{149}Sm \right)_{true} \right.$$
$$\left. \times (M_{149}/M_{144})^{\beta(Sm)} \right] \quad (3)$$

Finally, the ^{144}Sm-corrected ^{143}Nd/^{144}Nd ratio was exponentially normalized to ^{146}Nd/^{144}Nd = 0.7219.

The Sm isotope ratios (^{147}Sm/^{149}Sm and ^{144}Sm/^{149}Sm) have not been uniformly reported. The following sets of reported Sm isotopic composition were evaluated in this study.

$$^{147}Sm/{}^{149}Sm = 1.0868 \text{ (Yang et al. 2010)},$$
$$1.0851 \text{ (Wasserburg et al. 1981)},$$
$$1.06119 \text{ (MCFarlane McCulloch 2007)},$$
$$1.0847 \text{ (Berglund Wieser 2011)}$$
$$(4)$$

$$^{144}Sm/{}^{149}Sm = 0.22332 \text{ (Yang et al. 2010)},$$
$$0.22249 \text{ (Wasserburg et al. 1981)},$$
$$0.2103 \text{ (McFarlane McCulloch 2007)},$$
$$0.22214 \text{ (Berglund Wieser 2011)},$$
$$(5)$$

To evaluate these Sm isotopic compositions, the in-house Nd standard solution of 100 µg/L was doped with AccuTrace^{TM} Sm Reference Standard (lot no. B8085072, plasma emission standard), in which the concentration ratio of Sm to Nd was 0.2041. As depicted in Figure 1, analytical results (7 measurements, 1 block of 20 cycles with an integration time of 4.194 s) of this solution were different according to the employed Sm isotopic compositions (Yang et al. 2010; Wasserburg et al. 1981; McFarlane & McCulloch 2007; Berglund & Wieser 2011). Sm isotopic compositions reported in (Yang et al. 2010; Wasserburg et al. 1981; McFarlane & McCulloch 2007) yielded the ^{143}Nd/^{144}Nd ratios comparable with the unspiked value, which were 0.512190 ± 0.000014 (2σ S.E.), 0.512195 ± 0.000014 (2σ S.E.), and 0.512194 ± 0.000014 (2σ S.E.), respectively.

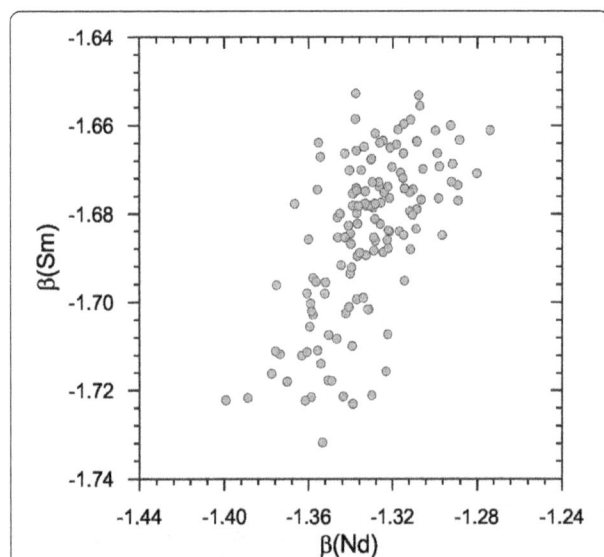

Figure 2 The correlation between the Sm and Nd mass bias factors (β(Sm) and β(Nd)) measured for Sm-doped Nd standard solutions with the Sm/Nd ratio of 0.2041.

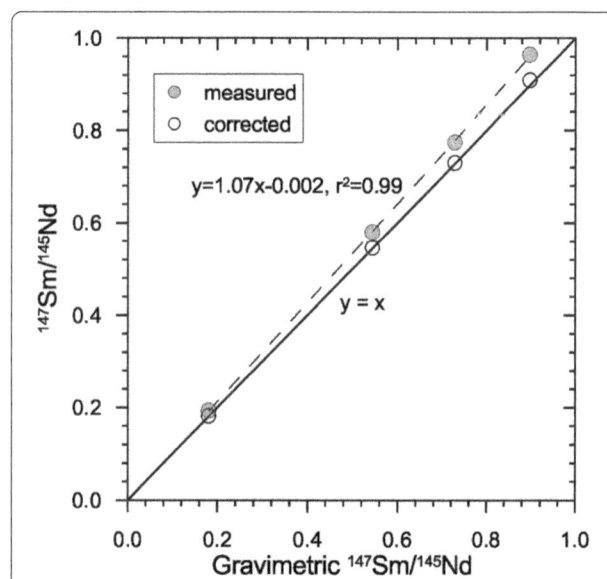

Figure 3 Comparisons of the measured and corrected ^{147}Sm/^{145}Nd ratios with gravimetric values.

Table 3 Sm-Nd isotopic data of the Sm-doped Nd standard solutions of 100 µg/L Nd

$^{143}Nd/^{144}Nd$	2σ S.E.	n	$^{147}Sm/^{145}Nd$			Nd (µg/L)	
			Gravimetric	Measured	Corrected	Gravimetric	Calculated
0.512185	0.000022	20	0.1805	0.1934	0.1818	100	101
0.512191	0.000026	20	0.5441	0.5796	0.5457	100	103
0.512214	0.000028	20	0.7275	0.7744	0.7302	100	103
0.512223	0.000026	20	0.8978	0.9641	0.9091	101	103

Sm isotopic compositions were iteratively solved to minimize the residual sum of squares between corrected $^{143}Nd/^{144}Nd$ ratio of Sm-doped Nd standard solution and the unspiked value using the Excel Solver. The result suggests that the ratios of ^{147}Sm to ^{149}Sm and ^{144}Sm to ^{149}Sm would be 1.0844 and 0.22233, respectively. Because these values are the closest to the recommended values in (Wasserburg et al. 1981), we hereafter use 1.0851 and 0.22249 as the $(^{147}Sm/^{149}Sm)_{true}$ and $(^{144}Sm/^{149}Sm)_{true}$ ratios for correcting mass fractionation of Sm and calculating its isobaric contribution to ^{144}Nd.

The $^{143}Nd/^{144}Nd$ ratios of the Sm-doped Nd standard solutions with similar Sm/Nd ratio of around 0.20 but different Nd concentrations (200 and 50 µg/L) were 0.512195 ± 0.000022 and 0.512208 ± 0.000038, respectively, corroborating the validity of this correction design (Table 2). Furthermore, the corrected $^{145}Nd/^{144}Nd$ ratios of the mixed solutions were well consistent with a constant value of 0.348417 obtained by TIMS (Wasserburg et al. 1981). The correlation between β(Sm) and β(Nd) values indicates that the two factors are not identical and are roughly positively correlated with each other (β(Sm) = 0.516 × β(Nd)-0.997) (Figure 2).

We further analyzed a series of Sm-doped Nd standard solutions of 100 µg/L Nd with different Sm/Nd ratios (Sm/Nd = ca. 0.1, 0.3, 0.4, and 0.5) to test the validity of correction scheme described above. The results show that the correction protocol is reasonable (Table 3). However, there is a systematic increasing trend in the corrected $^{143}Nd/^{144}Nd$ ratio with increasing Sm/Nd ratios, implying that the mass bias may not be perfectly corrected by the exponential law for high-Sm/Nd (> 0.5) samples.

Calibration of Sm/Nd ratio

The instrumental mass bias on isotope measurements could be corrected by using either double-spike or standard bracketing methods. The latter method consists in interpolating the mass bias of an unknown sample between the biases inferred from two standard runs, one preceding and one following the sample analysis (Albarede & Beard 2004).

In order to correct the inter-elemental mass bias on the measurement, this study considered the Sm-doped

Nd standard solution with the Sm/Nd of 0.2 as the bracketing standard and various mixed solutions with different Sm/Nd values (Sm/Nd = ca. 0.1, 0.3, 0.4, and 0.5) as unknown samples. During the measurements, the average correlation factor in the instrumental mass bias inferred from the standard runs was 0.943 ± 0.002 (n = 7, 2σ S.E.), which yielded consistent Sm/Nd ratios with gravimetric Sm/Nd values mostly within 1% difference (Table 3; Figure 3). This result indicates that the mass bias in the measurement of the Sm/Nd ratio can be reasonably corrected by the standard bracketing method.

The Nd concentrations of the mixed solutions were calculated based on the intensity of the bracketing standard of 100-101 µg/L. Calculated Nd concentrations were consistent with gravimetric values within 3% difference (Table 3).

Conclusions

We evaluated the capability of a Neptune MC-ICP-MS to obtain accurate Nd isotopic composition and Sm/Nd elemental ratio using a series of Sm + Nd mixed standard solutions with different Sm/Nd ratios. The isobaric interference correction using the exponential law and selected Sm isotopic composition yielded accurate $^{143}Nd/^{144}Nd$ and $^{145}Nd/^{144}Nd$ ratios for the mixed solutions, although there is a systematic increasing trend in the corrected $^{143}Nd/^{144}Nd$ ratios with increasing Sm/Nd ratios. The Sm/Nd ratios of the Sm-doped Nd standard solutions could be reliably calibrated by the standard bracketing method mostly within 1% difference from the gravimetric values. These results indicate that accurate Nd isotopic composition and Sm/Nd ratio can be simultaneously measured by a simple and high-throughput technique without chemical separation of Sm and Nd.

Competing interests
The authors declare that they have no competing interests.

Authors' contributions
CSC, JSR and YJJ designed the study. JSR and MSC made the sample solutions and carried out isotope measurements. CSC and JSR drafted the manuscript. All authors read and approved the final manuscript.

Acknowledgements
This study was supported by the KBSI grants (G33200 and C33710).

References

Albarede F, Beard B (2004) Analytical methods for Non-traditional isotopes. Rev Mineral Geochem 55:113–152

Ali A, Srinivasan G (2011) Precise thermal ionization mass spectrometric measurements of $^{142}Nd/^{144}Nd$ and $^{143}Nd/^{144}Nd$ isotopic ratios of Nd separated from geological standards by chromatographic methods. Int J Mass Spectrom 299:27–34

Begemann F, Ludwig KR, Lugmair GW, Min K, Nyquist LE, Patchett PJ, Renne PR, Shin C-Y, Villa IM, Walker RJ (2001) Call for an improved set of decay constants for geochronological use. Geochim Cosmochim Acta 65:111–121

Berglund M, Wieser ME (2011) Isotopic compositions of the elements 2009 (IUPAC Technical Report). Pure Appl Chem 83:397–410

Chu Z, Chen F, Yang Y, Guo J (2009) Precise determination of Sm, Nd concentrations and Nd isotopic compositions at the nanogram level in geological samples by thermal ionization mass spectrometry. J Anal At Spectrom 24:1534–1544

DePaolo DJ (1988) Neodymium isotope geochemistry. Springer-Verlag, Berlin, Heidelberg

Harvey J, Baxter EF (2009) An improved method for TIMS high precision neodymium isotope analysis of very small aliquots (1–10 ng). Chem Geol 258:251–257

Lugmair GW, Marti K (1978) Lunar initial $^{143}Nd/^{144}Nd$: Differential evolution of the lunar crust and mantle. Earth Planet Sci Lett 39:349–357

McFarlane CRM, McCulloch MT (2007) Coupling of in-situ Sm-Nd systematics and U-Pb dating of monazite and allanite with applications to crustal evolution studies. Chem Geol 245:45–60

Russel WA, Papanastassiou DA, Tombrello TA (1978) Ca isotope fractionation on the earth and other solar system materials. Geochim Cosmochim Acta 42:1075–1090

Tanaka T, Togashi S, Kamioka H, Amakawa H, Kagami H, Hamamoto T, Yuhara M, Orihashi Y, Yoneda S, Shimizu H, Kunimaru T, Takahashi K, Yanagi T, Nakano T, Fujimaki H, Shinjo R, Asahara Y, Tanimizu M, Dragusanu C (2000) JNdi-1: a new neodymium isotopic reference in consistency with LaJolla neodymium. Chem Geol 168:279–281

Vance D, Thirlwall M (2002) An assessment of mass discrimination in MC-ICPMS using Nd isotopes. Chem Geol 185:227–240

Walder A, Platzner I, Freedman PA (1993) Isotope ratio measurement of lead, neodymium and neodymium-samarium mixtures, hafnium and hafnium-lutetium mixtures with a double focusing multiple collector inductively coupled plasma mass spectrometer. J Anal At Spectrom 8:19–23

Wasserburg GJ, Jacobsen SB, DePaolo DJ, McCulloch MT, Wen T (1981) Precise determination of Sm/Nd ratios, Sm and Nd isotopic abundances in standard solutions. Geochim Cosmochim Acta 45:2311–2323

Yang Y, Wu F, Xie L, Zhang Y (2010) High-precision measurements of the $^{143}Nd/^{144}Nd$ isotope ratio in certified reference materials without Nd and Sm separation by multiple collector inductively coupled plasma mass spectrometry. Anal Lett 43:142–150

Yang Y-H, Chu Z-Y, Wu F-Y, Xie L-W, Yang J-H (2011) Precise and accurate determination of Sm, Nd concentrations and Nd isotopic compositions in geological samples by MC-ICP-MS. J Anal At Spectrom 26:1237–1244

18

ICH guideline practice: application of novel RP-HPLC-DAD method for determination of olopatadine hydrochloride in pharmaceutical products

Pawan K Basniwal[1,2*] and Deepti Jain[1]

Abstract

Background: A novel reverse-phase high-performance liquid chromatography (RP-HPLC)-DAD method was developed, validated and applied to quantify olopatadine hydrochloride in pharmaceutical products.

Methods: The RP-HPLC analyses were carried out using a mixture of 0.1% formic acid and methanol (35:65) as a mobile phase on ZORBAX Eclipse Plus C18 (250 mm × 4.6 mm, 5 μm), with a flow rate of 1.0 mL/min and UV detection at 300 nm. The developed method was validated as per the International Conference on Harmonisation of Technical Requirements for Registration of Pharmaceutical for Human Use guidelines for linearity, range, accuracy, precision, robustness, limit of detection, limit of quantitation and specificity.

Results: The validated method was applied to quantify the drug content in raw material, tablets and eye drops which was found to be 99.36% to 101.02%, 98.99% to 100.56% and 99.09% to 100.91%, respectively.

Conclusion: The method was found to be efficient, precise, accurate, specific and economic and useful for the routine analysis of olopatadine hydrochloride in pharmaceutical industries.

Keywords: Olopatadine hydrochloride; RP-HPLC; Pharmaceutical products

Background

Olopatadine (OLO) is a new histamine H1 receptor-selective antagonist, chemically, 11-((Z)-3-(dimethyl-amino) propylidene)-6,11-dihydro-dibenz[b,e]oxepin-2-acetic acid (Ohshima et al. 1992) (Figure 1), used to treat allergic conjunctivitis (itching eyes) (Scoper et al. 2007; Kajita et al. 2002; McGill 2004; Takahashi et al. 2008; Ohishi et al. 1995). Very few assay methods were reported for the analysis of olopatadine, *viz.* radioimmunoassay method for humans (Tsunoo et al. 1995).

However, it had several problems, such as cross-reactivity of metabolites and low precision, and so it was considered that plasma concentrations of olopatadine measured by RIA needed to be confirmed by an alternative method.

High-performance liquid chromatography (HPLC) with tandem mass spectrometry has been applied for the determination of a number of compounds in biological fluids (Zhu et al. 2011). Other assay methods for olopatadine and its metabolites in human plasma by HPLC with electrospray ionisation tandem mass spectrometry were reported (Fujimaki et al. 2006; Fujita et al. 1999). Varghese et al. (2011) have used 0.1% orthophosphoric acid (pH 4.5) with triethylamine/acetonitrile (75:25) for the determination of olopatadine hydrochloride. Triethylamine should be avoided as its addition to the mobile phase requires longer column equilibration times, which is not advisable for the routine use of the developed method. It occasionally introduces additional problems such as erratic baselines and poor peak shape and complicates the preparation of the mobile phase (Synder et al. 1997). A complicated buffer is a component of the mobile phase for the HPLC method, which includes monobasic potassium phosphate (6.8 g), 1-pentane sulphonic acid sodium

* Correspondence: pawanbasniwal@gmail.com
[1]School of Pharmaceutical Sciences, Rajiv Gandhi Technological University, Bhopal, Madhya Pradesh 462 033, India
[2]LBS College of Pharmacy, Jaipur, Rajasthan 302 004, India

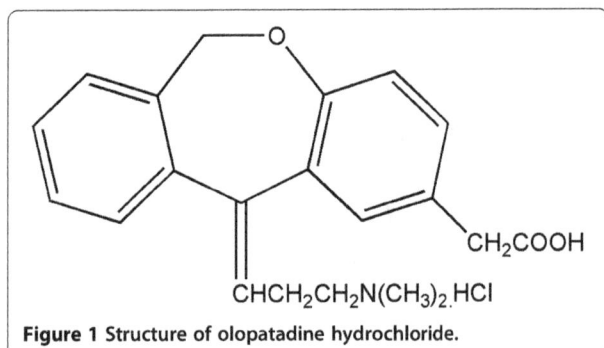

Figure 1 Structure of olopatadine hydrochloride.

salt monohydrate (1.28 g) and triethylamine (3 mL), and the pH is adjusted to 3.0 with orthophosphoric acid (Rele and Warkar 2011). Thus, both the above methods cannot be useful for routine analysis as tedious mobile phase composition and problem arise from triethylamine.

Hitherto, the objective of the present research work was to develop a simple, precise, accurate and fast reverse-phase high-performance liquid chromatography (RP-HPLC) assay method for the analysis of olopatadine hydrochloride in different pharmaceutical products including raw material, tablets and eye drops, and to compare the assay results by statistical analysis, which may be useful for routine analysis.

Methods
Instrumentation and chromatograph
The HPLC chromatograph used was Agilent Infinity 1260 series (Agilent Technologies, Inc., Santa Clara, CA, USA) equipped with 1260 binary pump VL (400 bar), 1260 manual injector (600 bar), Rheodyne 7725i seven-port sample injection valve with 20-μL fixed loop, ZORBAX Eclipse Plus C18 (250 mm × 4.6 mm, 5 μm), 1260 DAD VL, 20-Hz detector, standard flow cell (10 mm, 13 μL, 120 bar), OpenLab CDS EZChrom Ed. Workstation and syringe (50.0 μL, FN, LC tip). All weighing for analysis was performed on Shimadzu electronic analytical balance AX-200 (Kyoto, Japan). Water used for analysis was prepared by triple distillation assembly. All dilutions, mobile phase and other solutions that were used for the analysis were filtered through a 0.2-μm nylon filter (Ultipor®N66 Nylon 6,6 membrane, Pall Sciences, Pall India Pvt. Ltd., Mumbai, India).

Chemicals and reagent
The working standard used was OLO which was supplied by Ranbaxy Laboratories Limited (Gurgaon, Harayana, India) as a gift sample. Formic acid and methanol were procured from Merck Specialties Private Limited (Mumbai, India). The mobile phase was prepared from the combination of formic acid (0.1%) and methanol.

Chromatography
Accurately weighed 50 mg of OLO was dissolved in 50% aqueous methanol to prepare stock I (1,000 μg/mL) in a

50-mL volumetric flask. Stock II (100 μg/mL) was prepared from stock I, which was used to prepare further dilutions containing 1, 5, 10, 15 and 20 μg/mL. All dilutions were filtered through the 0.2-μm nylon filter (Ultipor®N66 Nylon 6,6 membrane, Pall Sciences) and chromatographed by a set of conditions on Agilent Infinity 1260 series. The mixture of 0.1% formic acid and methanol (35:65) was used as the mobile phase for the elution of the drug on Zorbax Eclipse Plus C18 column (250 mm × 4.6 mm, 5 μm) at 1.0 mL/min flow rate. OLO was successfully eluted at 3.77 min with a run time of 7 min, and detection was performed using a photodiode array detector (PDA) at 300 nm.

Method validation
According to the International Conference on Harmonisation of Technical Requirements for Registration of Pharmaceutical for Human Use (ICH) guidelines (ICH 2000a, b), the developed method was validated to assure the reliability of the results of analysis for the different parameters, *viz.* linearity, range, accuracy, precision, robustness, limit of quantization (LOQ), limit of detection (LOD) and specificity. Linearity was determined by serial dilutions (1 to 20 μg/mL) of the OLO in 50% aqueous methanol in triplicate. The range of OLO was validated between 5 and 15 μg/mL with triplicates of dilutions. The recovery method was used to determine the accuracy of the developed method by spiking the standard solution to the pre-analysed samples (5, 10 and 15 μg/mL), which was repeated six times. Repeatability and intermediate precision were studied to assure the precision of the method. Six replicates of the standard dilution (5 μg/mL) were chromatographed subsequently to assure repeatability, which were further chromatographed after 5 h to assure the stability of the drug in the solvent system. The standard dilutions were analysed by different analysts in subsequent days to study intermediate precision in the linearity range. A change in temperature (20°C, 25°C and 30°C) and acidic content of the aqueous part of the mobile phase (5% change in 0.1% aqueous formic acid) was observed. Different serial dilutions of OLO (0.1 to 1,000 ng/mL) were chromatographed to calculate the signal-to-noise ratio to determine LOD and LOQ. Alkaline-degraded OLO samples were chromatographed to ascertain the specificity of the developed method for OLO.

Analysis of pharmaceutical products
Raw material
As per the 'Chromatography' subsection, the samples of raw material have been prepared and analysed in the set of condition of analysis, which was repeated in six batches. The response to chromatographic analysis was used to calculate the concentration with the help of a regression equation.

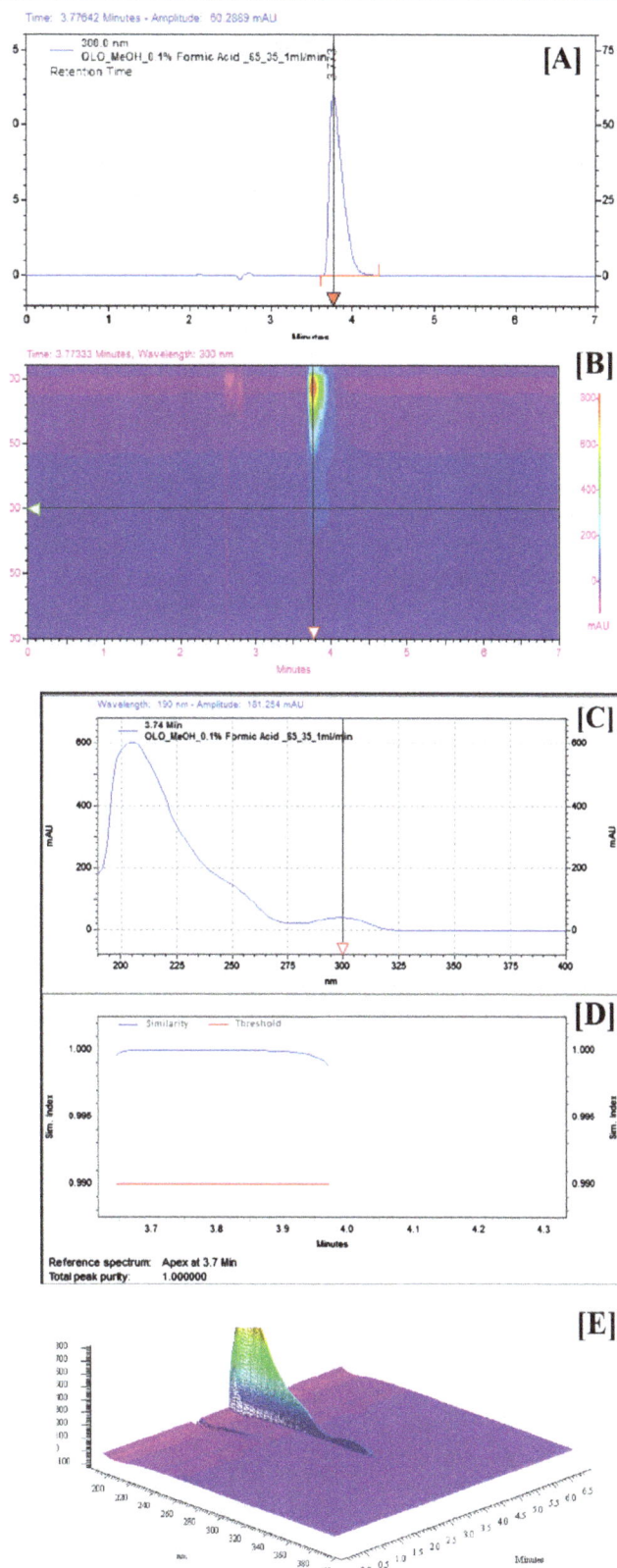

Figure 2 Representative chromatogram (A), counterplot (B), Gaussian spectra (C), peak purity curve (D) and three-dimensional view (E) of OLO.

Tablets

Powdered tablets were weighed equivalently to 50 mg of OLO and sonicated to dissolve the drug content in methanol to extract the complete drug content from the tablet powder. The sonicated solution was filtered through Whatman filter no. 41 to remove the un-dissolved excipients of the tablet dosage form, and different serial dilutions were prepared by subsequent dilution with 50% aqueous methanol. All dilutions were filtered through the 0.2 µm nylon filter and chromatographed. The drug content was determined from the regression equation.

Eye drops

An accurately measured volume of ophthalmic solution (Olodin, FDC Limited, Aurangabad, India), equivalent to about 10 mg of OLO, was transferred to a 100 mL 163 volumetric flask and diluted with diluent to the volume. The solution was mixed and sonicated for 10 min. An appropriate dilution was prepared from the stock solution and filtered (stock P, 100 µg/mL). Aliquots of stock P were diluted to get sample concentrations (5, 10 and 15 µg/mL) in the range of linearity for the developed method and filtered through the 0.2 µm nylon filter. All these dilutions were chromatographed, and the area under the curve (AUC) of the peak of OLO was placed in the regression equation to get the concentration of the samples.

Results and discussion

Optimization of chromatography

The aim of this research work was to develop a novel RP-HPLC method for the determination of OLO in different matrices by eliminating the triethylamine component in the mobile phase, which improves the peak shape associated with other number of troubles to the column. Keeping the view of the results with triethylamine use in the mobile phase, the physical properties of OLO were used to improve the chromatographic parameters. On the basis of the solubility of OLO, different combinations of the mobile phase were tried to elute on C18 column. Broadening and splitting of the peak have been seen with the mixture of methanol and water (50:50) and the mixture of acetonitrile and water (50:50). The pK_a value (4.29) has been taken into account to design the mobile phase composition as OLO has a carboxylic group. So 0.1% formic acid was added to the aqueous phase of the mixture of acetonitrile and water (50:50), but the same broadening of peak with a little bit splitting of peak was observed. Tailing was found with the mixture of methanol and water (50:50) along with the acidic content of the aqueous phase which was improved by increasing the concentration of methanol content in the mobile phase. A very sharp peak shape was found with 70% content of methanol in the mobile phase, but it was merging with the diluent peak when a higher value was present at 60%. Thus, chromatographic

conditions were concluded to be better than the reported methods.

The mixture of 0.1% formic acid and methanol (35:65) was selected to elute OLO on C18 column with 1 mL/min flow rate, where it was eluted at 3.77 min with acceptable peak shape and tailing factor (Figure 2A). A counterplot of the chromatogram was able to show the exact position of the elution point where time and wavelength cross each other (Figure 2B). The detection wavelength was 300 nm, which was the λmax of OLO (Figure 2C).

The peak purity of OLO in the chromatogram was 1 unit which was supported by the peak purity curve (Figure 2D). A three-dimensional view of the chromatogram was the proof for no interference to the peak of OLO (Figure 2E).

System suitability parameters

Acceptable system suitability results for a chromatographic run establish that the method is performing adequately and can be used to generate reportable data. It includes the number of theoretical plates, tailing factor, retention time and peak purity of the analyte. The number of theoretical plates for the C18 column was 8,578 ($n = 6$) with an acceptable relative standard deviation (%RSD) value of 1.09, which indicates that the column performance was excellent. OLO should have tailing in the chromatogram on C18 column if the mobile phase is without diethylamine or triethylamine as it has a tertiary amino functional group. The formic acid content of the aqueous phase of the mobile phase was solved to have an acceptable limit of tailing factor (1.31) with a %RSD of 0.49. The retention time for OLO was 3.77 min in the 7 min run time of analysis. The peak purity of the OLO was always 1 at 3.77 min (Table 1).

Method validation

A linear relationship was found between the OLO concentrations and the response to chromatographic analysis which was demonstrated by high regression coefficients ($r^2 = 0.999$) for the concentration of 1 to 20 µg/mL and the mean regression equation was found as AUC = 79,991X – 64,340. The working range for the drug was selected to be 5 to 15 µg/mL. Accuracy was investigated by the recovery of standard addition to pre-analysed samples which was near 100% with acceptable %RSD. Intra-day variation (repeatability) and intermediate

Table 1 System suitability parameters for OLO in 0.1% formic acid and methanol (35:65) on C18 column

Parameters	Value ($n = 6$)	SD	%RSD
Number of theoretical plates	8,578	42.63	1.09
Tailing factor	1.31	0.94	0.49
RT (min)	3.77	0.046	0.021
Peak purity	1	0	0

SD standard deviation, *RSD* relative standard deviation, *RT* retention time.

Table 2 Validation parameters for olopatadine hydrochloride

Parameters	Values[a] ± SD, ± %RSD
Linearity	1 to 20 µg/mL
Regression equation	AUC = 79,991X − 64,340
Correlation coefficient	r^2 = 0.999 ± 0.001, ±0.100
Range	5 to 15 µg/mL ± 1.08, ±0.51
Accuracy	100.11 ± 1.065, ±0.784
Precision	
Repeatability	99.94 ± 0.742, ±0.482
Intermediate precision	
Inter-day	100.08 ± 0.825, ±0.091
Analyst to analyst	99.89 ± 0.929, ±0.027
Robustness	
Temperature (20°C, 25°C and 30°C)	99.91 ± 0.816, ±0.089
Formic acid concentration (±5%)	100.06 ± 0.794, ±0.296
LOQ	5 ng/mL ± 1.098, ±0.566
LOD	0.5 ng/mL ± 1.691, ±0.295
Specificity	Ascertained by analysing standard drug and degraded sample of equivalent concentration

[a]Mean of six replicates. *SD* standard deviation, *RSD* relative standard deviation, *AUC* area under the curve, *LOQ* limit of quantification, *LOD* limit of detection.

precision (days and analyst variation) were evaluated by analysing quality control samples containing low, medium and high concentrations of OLO.

For intra-day variation, sets of the six replicates of the three concentrations were analysed on the same day; for intermediate precision, the six replicates were analysed on three different days by three different analysts. All results of precision were between 99.89% and 100.08% within the acceptable limits of %RSD values, and there was no significant difference in the results of the analysis when drug samples were analysed after 5 h. The developed method is robust when it was unaffected by small changes in operating conditions of the analysis. The experimental conditions were deliberately altered

at three different levels, and chromatographic response was evaluated.

Changes in temperature of analysis time and formic acid percent of the aqueous part of the mobile phase were studied as robustness factors, and one factor at a time was changed to study the effect on the result of the method. The results of robustness vary between 99.91% and 100.06% with less than 1 unit of the %RSD value (Table 2). The LOD and LOQ were determined by considering the signal-to-noise ratio of 3 and 10, respectively. The developed method was highly sensitive to OLO as LOD and LOQ values were found to be 0.5 and 5 ng/mL, respectively. The method was specific to the drug as PDA analyses proved that the peak purity for the drug peak in a mixture of stressed samples was 1 unit. The purity threshold curve hereby indicated that the drug peak was free from any co-eluting peak (Figure 2E).

Analysis of products

The validated chromatographic method was applied to determine OLO in raw material, tablets and eye drops, where six batches were prepared for each quality control sample (5, 10, and 15 µg/mL) for all pharmaceutical products.

OLO was determined in raw material within the range of 99.36% to 101.02% with a standard deviation of 0.556. In the tablet dosage form, the drug content was found to be within the range of 98.99% to 100.56% with a standard deviation of 0.404. In a similar fashion, the OLO content in the eye drop was estimated to be in the range of 99.09% to 100.91% with a standard deviation of 0.498 (Table 3). Thus, all the pharmaceutical products have been analysed within the acceptable limits.

Conclusion

Hence, the simple, fast, precise, accurate and novel reverse-phase liquid chromatographic method was developed and validated according to ICH guidelines. The

Table 3 Analysis of olopatadine hydrochloride in pharmaceutical products

Batch	Concentration of quality control samples (%)								
	Raw material (µg/mL)			Tablet (µg/mL)			Eye drop (µg/mL)		
	5	10	15	5	10	15	5	10	15
A	100.23	100.92	99.83	99.93	99.99	100.19	100.83	99.48	100.03
B	101.02	99.28	100.12	98.99	99.63	99.92	100.41	100.69	100.28
C	99.36	100.04	99.94	100.29	100.59	100.46	99.98	100.83	99.56
D	98.94	100.91	100.46	100.06	100.48	100.56	99.74	99.93	99.09
E	100.32	99.76	99.83	99.89	99.67	99.89	100.46	100.91	100.06
F	100.19	99.89	100.11	100.56	100.16	100.15	100.29	100.02	100.04
Mean	100.01	100.13	100.05	99.95	100.09	100.20	100.29	100.31	99.84
SD		0.556			0.404			0.498	

SD standard deviation.

validated method was successfully applied to determine the OLO content in pharmaceutical products including raw material, tablets and eye drops with acceptable limits. As previous reported methods may not be applied for routine analysis due to the use of the triethylamine component in the mobile phase, this novel RP-HPLC method might be applied for assays, dissolution studies, bio-equivalence studies as well as routine analysis of OLO in pharmaceutical industries.

Competing interests
Both authors declare that they have no competing interests.

Authors' contributions
Both authors equally contributed in experimental design, framing, writing, proofing and approval of the manuscript. Experimental work was done by PKB.

Acknowledgements
One of the authors, Pawan Kumar Basniwal, is earnestly indebted to the Science and Engineering Research Board (SERB), DST, New Delhi, for the financial support for this research work under Fast Track Scheme for Young Scientists. The authors are highly thankful to the Head of the School of Pharmaceutical Sciences, RGPV, Bhopal, and the Principal of the LBS College of Pharmacy, Jaipur, for providing the experimental facilities for this research work.

References
Fujimaki K, Lee XP, Kumazawa T, Sato J, Sato K (2006) Determination of some anti-allergic drugs in human plasma by direct-injection high-performance liquid chromatography-tandem mass spectrometry. Forensic Toxicol 24:8–16

Fujita K, Magara H, Kobayashi H (1999) Determination of olopatadine, a new anti-allergic agent, and its metabolites in human plasma by high-performance liquid chromatography with electrospray ionization tandem mass spectrometry. J Chromatogr B 731:345–352, S0378-4347(99)00236-4

ICH (2000a) Q2A: text on validation of analytical procedures. International Conference on Harmonisation of Technical Requirements for Registration of Pharmaceutical for Human Use, Geneva

ICH (2000b) Q2B: validation of analytical procedure: methodology. International Conference on Harmonisation of Technical Requirements for Registration of Pharmaceutical for Human Use, Geneva

Kajita J, Inano K, Fuse E, Kuwahara T, Kobayashi H (2002) Effects of olopatadine, a new anti-allergic agent, on human liver microsomal cytochrome p450 activities. Drug Metabo Disposit 30:1504–1511

McGill JI (2004) A review of the use of olopatadine in allergic conjunctivitis. Int Ophthalmology 25(3):171–179

Ohishi T, Magara H, Yasuzawa T, Kabayashi H, Yamaguchi K, Kobayashi S (1995) Disposition of KW-4679 (4): metabolism of KW-4679 in rats and dogs. Xenobiol Metab Dispos 10:689–706

Ohshima E, Sato H, Obase H, Uchimura T, Kuwabara T, Kobayashi S (1992) Synthesis of a dibenz [b, e]oxepin-bovine serum albumin conjugate for radioimmunoassay of KW-4679 ((Z)-11-[3-(dimethylamino)propylidene]-6, 11-dihydrodibenz[b, e]oxepin-2-acetic acid hydrochloride). Chem Pharm Bull 40:2552–2554

Rele RV, Warkar CB (2011) Application of high performance liquid chromatographic technique for olopatadine hydrochloride and its impurity in ophthalmic solution. Int J Chem Sci 9(2):601–614

Scoper SV, Berdy GJ, Lichtenstein SJ, Rubin JM, Bloomenstein M, Prouty RE, Vogelson CT, Edwards MR, Waycaster C, Pasquine T, Gross RD, Robertson SM (2007) Perception and quality of life associated with the use of olopatadine 0.2% (Pataday™) in patients with active allergic conjunctivitis. Adv Ther 24:1221–1232

Synder LR, Kirkland JJ, Glajch JL (1997) Practical HPLC method development, 2nd edn. Wiley, New York, p 430

Takahashi H, Zhang Y, Morita E (2008) Evaluation of the anti-histamine effects of olopatadine, cetirizine and fexofenadine during a 24 h period: a double-blind, randomized, crossover, placebo-controlled comparison in skin responses induced by histamine iontophoresis. Arch Dermatol Res 300:291–295

Tsunoo M, Momomura S, Masuo M, Iizuka H (1995) Phase I clinical study on KW-4679, an anti-allergic drug: safety and pharmacokinetics in the single and repeated administration study to healthy subjects. Kiso To Rinsho 29:4129–4147

Varghese SJ, Kumar AM, Ravi TK (2011) Stability-indicating high-performance column liquid chromatography and high-performance thin-layer chromatography methods for the determination of olopatadine hydrochloride in tablet dosage form. J AOAC Int 94(6):1815–1820

Zhu P, Wen Y, Fan XP, Zhou ZL, Fan RX, Chen JM, Huang KL, Zhu XL, Chen YF, Zhuang J (2011) A rapid and sensitive liquid chromatography–tandem mass spectrometry method for determination of olopatadine concentration in human plasma. J Ana Toxicol 35:113–118

19

Kinetic spectrophotometric determination of an important pharmaceutical compound, pregabalin

Raafia Najam[1†], Gh Mohd Shah[1†] and S Muzaffar Ali Andrabi[2*†]

Abstract

Background: Pregabalin (PGB), an anticonvulsant, was studied throughout this work using spectrophotometric method.

Methods: The spectrophotometric method is based on the condensation reaction of PGB with p-dimethylaminobenzaldehyde (pDMAB) in acid medium. The condensation product showed λ_{max} at 420 nm.

Results: The different parameters affecting the stability of the condensation product were carefully studied and optimized. The calibration plots were constructed over the concentration range of 40 to 120 µg ml^{-1}.

Conclusions: A simple, reliable, sensitive and accurate spectrophotometric method has been developed for the determination of an anticonvulsant drug, PGB. The proposed method was successfully applied to the analysis of the drug in dosage form. The high sensitivity of the proposed method allows determination of PGB in bulk and in pharmaceutical preparations.

Keywords: PGB; pDMAB; Spectrophotometric determination; Capsules

Background

Pregabalin (PGB), (S)-3-(aminomethyl)-5-methyl hexanoic acid is an antiepileptic and structurally related to the inhibitory neurotransmitter aminobutyric acid (GABA). It is a white crystalline solid with molecular formula $C_8H_{17}NO_2$, molecular mass of 159.23 g/mol and melting point from 190°C to 192°C. It was approved in the year 2007 for adjunctive treatment of partial seizures in adults (Tassone et al. 2007; Hamandi and Sander 2006; Barona et al. 2008) in United States and Europe, and for the treatment of neuropathic pain from post-therapeutic neuralgia and diabetic neuropathy.

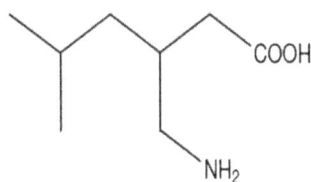

PREGABALIN

* Correspondence: muzaffar2000@gmail.com
†Equal contributors
²University Science Instrumentation Centre, University of Kashmir, Srinagar, Jammu and Kashmir 190006, India
Full list of author information is available at the end of the article

The wide use of this drug has prompted many researches to develop sensitive and accurate analytical methods for its determination, especially for routine quality control in the analysis of pharmaceutical products. Several methods have been developed for the determination of the drug in pure and pharmaceutical preparations which are mostly based on chromatographic, spectrofluorimetric and spectrophotometric methods listed elsewhere (Bali and Gaur 2011). A detailed literature survey shows that few spectrophotometric methods have been developed for the determination of PGB in bulk and pharmaceutical preparation. A sensitive and selective spectrophotometric method, based on the reaction of the drug with 7-chloro-4-nitrobenzofuran, has been developed for the determination of PGB by Onal and Sagirli (2009). The relation between the absorbance of the reaction product at 460 nm and the concentration is rectilinear over the range 0.5 to 7.0 µg/ml. Gujral et al. (2009) developed a simple and sensitive method for the determination of PGB in bulk and pharmaceutical formulations. The method is based on the reaction of the drug with a mixture of potassium iodate and potassium iodide. The method is linear over the range 0.5 to 3.5 µg/ml. Onal (2009) developed three methods for the determination of PGB in pharmaceutical preparations. Two methods are based on the charge transfer complexation of the drug with

2,3-dichloro-5,6-dicyano-1,4-benzoquinone (DDQ) and 7,7, 8,8-tetracyanoquinodimethane (TCNQ), and the third method was based on the reaction of ninhydrin with the primary amine group on the drug molecule. While the first two methods were linear over the concentration ranges of 2.0 to 30 and 1.5 to 10 μg/ml, respectively, the third method was linear over a much wider concentration range of 40 to 180 μg/ml. Two simple spectrophotometric methods for the quantitative estimation of PGB in bulk and pharmaceutical formulations were developed by Sowjanya et al. (2011). The first method is based on the condensation of PGB with 1,2-naphthaquinone-4-sulfonic acid sodium in alkaline medium, and the second method is based on the oxidation of 2,4-dinitrophenyhydrazine and the coupling of the oxidation product with the drug to give intensely coloured chromogen. The first method is linear over the concentration range of 5 to 45 μg/ml, and the second method is linear over the range of 50 to 450 μg/ml. Reddy (2013) developed a spectrophotometric method for determination of PGB in bulk and pharmaceutical dosage form. The method is based on the reaction of PGB with DDQ to form red colour charge-transfer complex. Beer's law is obeyed in the concentration range of 50 to 250 μg/ml for the method. UV-visible spectroscopy is the technique of choice for the accurate and cost-effective determination of pharmaceutical compounds especially in third world countries. Consequently, there is scope for the development of simple and accurate spectrophotometric methods for the determination of pregabalin in bulk and pharmaceutical formulations.

In this study, p-dimethylaminobenzaldehyde (pDMAB) has been used as a chromogenic agent for the determination of pregabalin. pDMAB possesses some peculiar structural features which account for its applicability in a wide range of reactions and processes. Its condensation reactions have been utilized for the spectrophotometric determination of many drugs (Adegoke and Umoh 2009; Adegoke and Nwoke 2008). An attempt has been made to develop a simple, accurate, rapid and economical method for determination of pregabalin in pure and pharmaceutical formulations. The method is based on the reaction of pregabalin with pDMAB in acidic medium. The method involves a one-step reaction, does not involve any extraction or heating steps and does not require any costly chemicals and equipment. The reaction is monitored spectrophotometrically, and the change in absorbance with time is measured at 420 nm.

Methods

Instrumentation

A Systronics UV-visible spectrophotometer (model 118, Gujarat, India) with 1-cm matched quartz cells was used for the absorbance measurements. Shimadzu electronic balance (Kyoto, Japan) was used for weighing the samples.

Materials

All the chemicals and materials were of analytical grade and were purchased from Qualigens Fine Chemicals Pvt. Ltd. (Mumbai, India), and Deccan Fine Chemicals India Limited (Hyderabad, India). All the solutions were

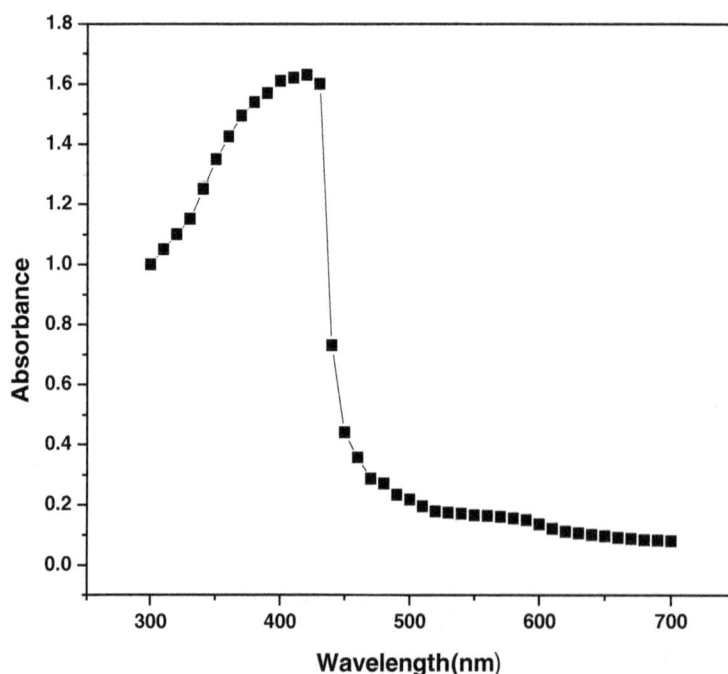

Figure 1 UV-visible spectrum of the product of PGB and pDMAB (λ_{max} 420 nm).

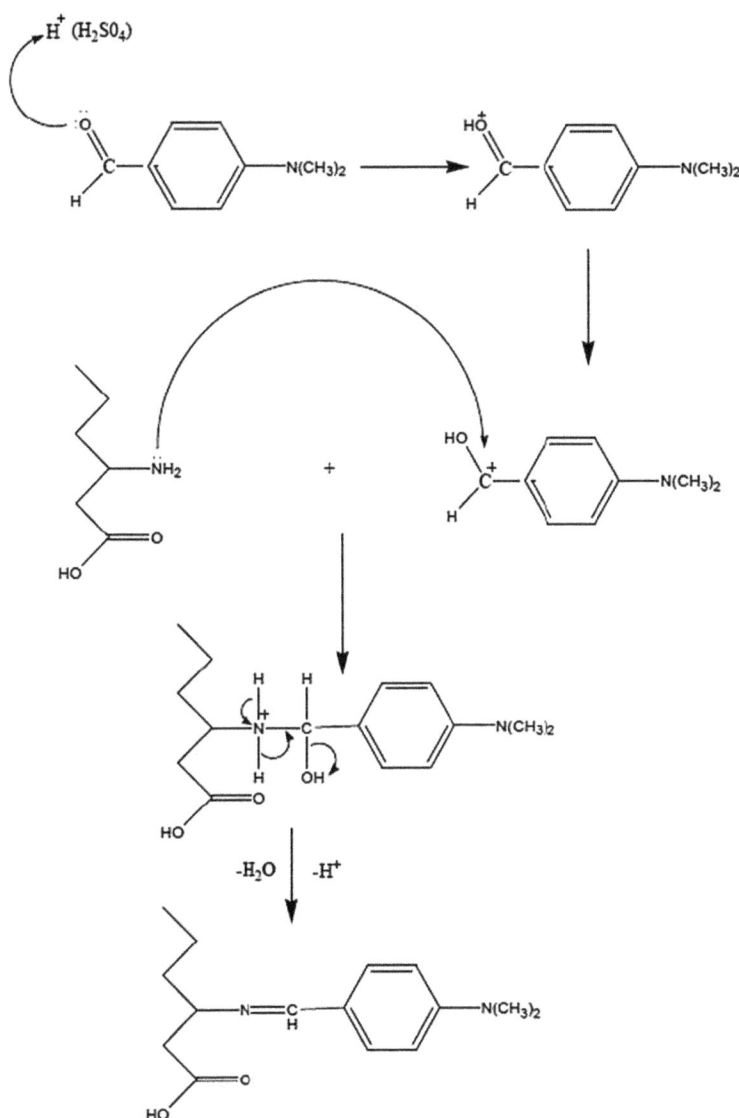

Scheme 1 Probable mechanism of the reaction between *p*DMAB and PGB in acid medium.

freshly prepared. PGB, AR grade, was purchased from Himedia Laboratories (Mumbai, India), and PGB 75 capsules (label amount 75 mg PGB/capsule) of various pharmaceutical manufactures were purchased from the market.

Preparation of the standard solutions

Stock solution of PGB (1,000 μg/ml) was prepared by dissolving 100 mg of drug in 10 ml of 0.5 M H_2SO_4 and diluting up to the mark by ethanol in a 100-ml calibrated flask. The stock solution was further diluted appropriately to get working concentrations. *p*DMAB (0.3% *w/v*) was made by dissolving 0.3 g in 100 ml of 0.5 M H_2SO_4.

General procedure
Construction of calibration curve

To a set of 10-ml volumetric flasks, appropriate aliquots of the standard working solution were transferred to obtain concentrations in the range 40 to 120 μg ml^{-1} of PGB. Aliquots of standard solution of pregabalin were mixed with 2 ml of 0.3% *p*DMAB, and the contents were diluted up to 10 ml with ethanol and time was noted. The reaction mixture was rapidly transferred into a cuvette, and absorbance at 420 nm was recorded after every 5 min against the reagent blank prepared simultaneously in the same manner without the analyte. First, absorbance was taken exactly 5 min after mixing PGB and *p*DMAB solutions. The procedure was repeated for different concentrations of the drug solution, with a constant concentration of *p*DMAB

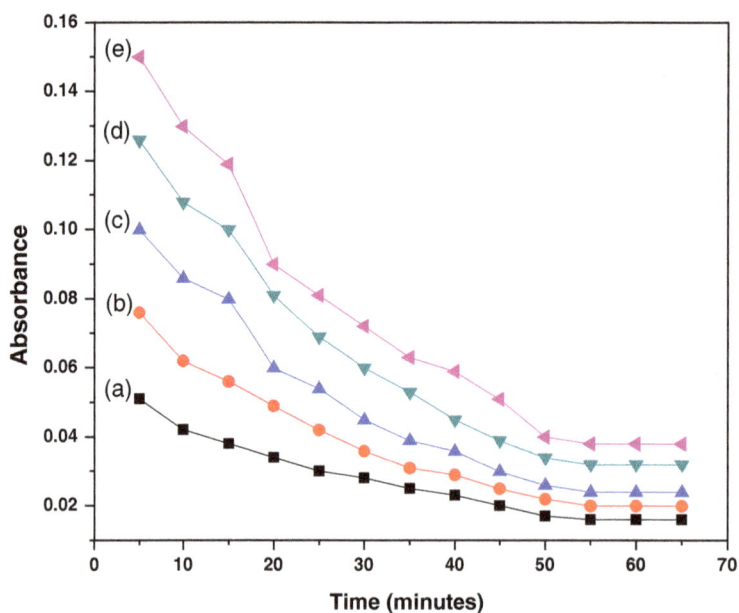

Figure 2 Variation of absorbance of drug-reagent mixture with time. **(a)** 40 µg/ml, **(b)** 60 µg/ml, **(c)** 80 µg/ml, **(d)** 100 µg/ml, and **(e)** 120 µg/ml.

solution. All the experiments are carried out at room temperature. The regression equations of calibration graphs were calculated using the method of least squares.

Assay of capsules

An accurately weighed portion of powder from tablets purchased from open market equivalent to 100 mg of PGB was put in a 100-ml volumetric flask containing 10 ml of H_2SO_4 and was diluted up to the mark using ethanol. It was shaken thoroughly for about 5 to 10 min, filtered through a Whatman paper to remove insoluble matter and used to prepare 1,000 µg/ml using ethanol for dilution. An aliquot of this solution was diluted with ethanol to obtain a required concentration (40 to 120 µg/ml). Then, to a solution of particular concentration, 2 ml of 0.3% pDMAB was added and gently shaken. The contents were diluted

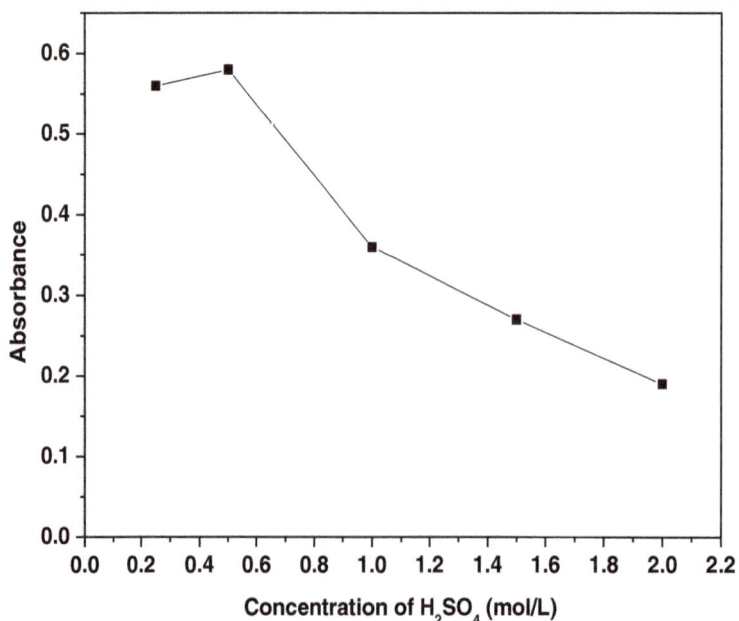

Figure 3 Effect of acid concentration on absorbance of drug-reagent mixture.

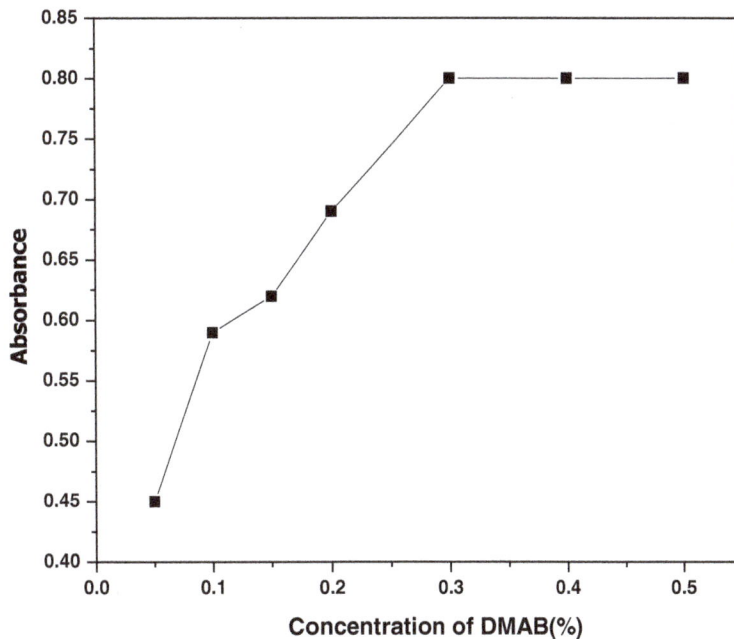

Figure 4 Effect of concentration of *p*DMAB on absorbance of drug-reagent mixture.

up to 10 ml with ethanol. The nominal content of the capsules was determined using the corresponding regression equations or the calibration graphs.

Results and discussions

In an effort to develop a spectrophotometric method for quantification of pregabalin, its reaction with *p*DMAB in an acid medium for the generation of a chromophoric product was studied. PGB reacts instantly with *p*DMAB in an acid medium to give a light yellow colour (λ_{max} at 420 nm). PGB shows a λ_{max} at 180 nm and does not absorb in the visible region at all, while *p*DMAB shows λ_{max} at 280 nm. The UV-visible spectrum of the product of the reaction between PGB and *p*DMAB is given in Figure 1. The probable mechanism of the reaction between *p*DMAB and PGB in acid medium is given in Scheme 1.

The condensation reaction requires the presence of an acid for the protonation of the carbonyl oxygen and thereby leaving the carbonyl carbon fully positively charged. The PGB then donates a lone pair of electrons to the carbon. Internal rearrangement thereafter results in the formation

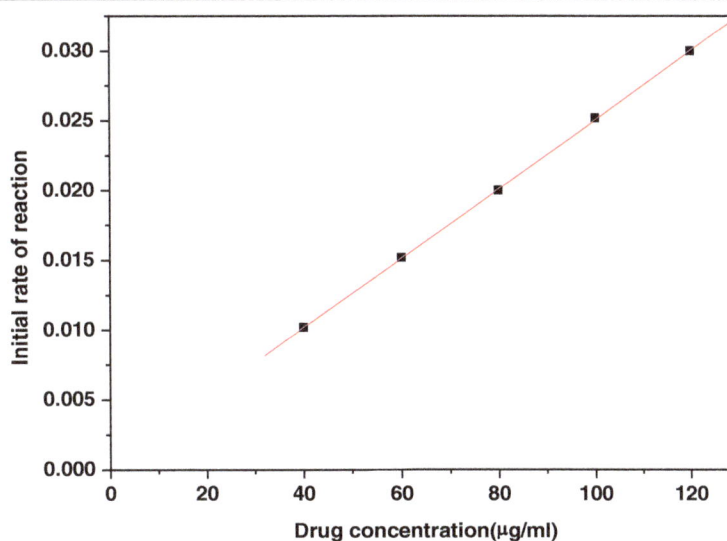

Figure 5 Calibration plot of the initial rate of reaction versus drug concentration.

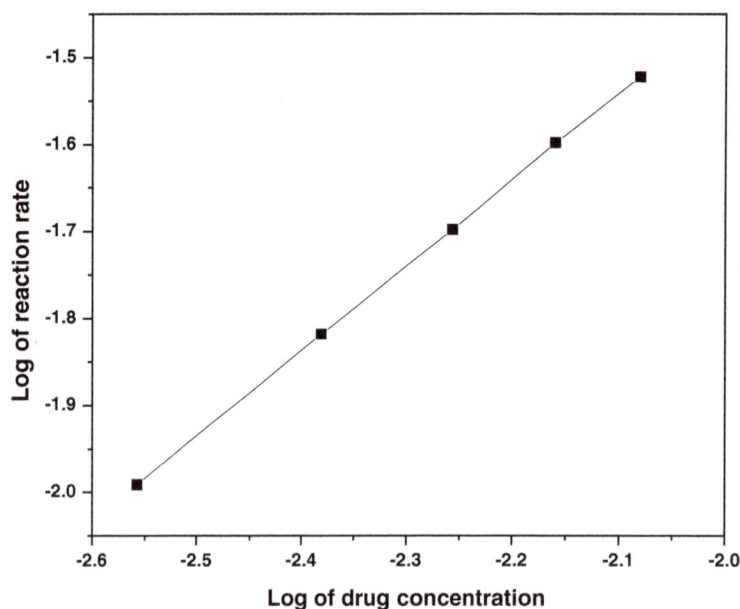

Figure 6 Plot of log of reaction rate versus log of drug concentration (mol/l).

of condensation product, giving water and H^+ as by-product. The intensity of colour decreases with time (Figure 2) and provides a basis for kinetic study. The decrease in the intensity of yellow colour and hence absorbance is perhaps due to partial decomposition of the reaction product into the reagents on standing. This was confirmed by measuring the λ_{max} of the reaction mixture at different time intervals, *viz.*, 5, 15, 30, 65 min, after mixing the reagents. The λ_{max} has been found to remain unchanged at 420 nm. The rate of reaction was monitored spectrophotometrically at 420 nm at room temperature with various concentrations of the drug, while *p*DMAB was kept in excess and constant.

Optimization of reaction conditions
Effect of acid concentration
The stability of the condensation product was checked with HCl, HNO_3, oxalic acid and H_2SO_4. The best results were obtained when H_2SO_4 was used. After selecting H_2SO_4, the stability was checked with its varying concentrations. Lower acid concentrations gave low absorbance values, while absorbance declined with increasing acid concentrations beyond 0.5 M H_2SO_4. The best results were obtained with 0.5 M H_2SO_4 (Figure 3). For the sake of ease, the experiments were carried out with $\approx$ 500-μg/ml drug concentration.

Effect of pDMAB concentration
It was found that the reaction is dependent on the *p*DMAB concentration. The absorbance of the reaction solution increases as the reagent concentration increases, and the

highest absorption intensity is attained at 0.3% (*w/v*) reagent concentration. A higher reagent concentration up to 1% has no effect on the absorption values. Further experiments were carried out using 0.3% (*w/v*) of the reagent. The results obtained are shown in Figure 4. The experiments were carried out with $\approx$ 600-μg/ml drug concentration.

Reaction rate method
A plot of the initial rate of reaction versus concentration of the drug (Figure 5) gives a straight line and serves as a

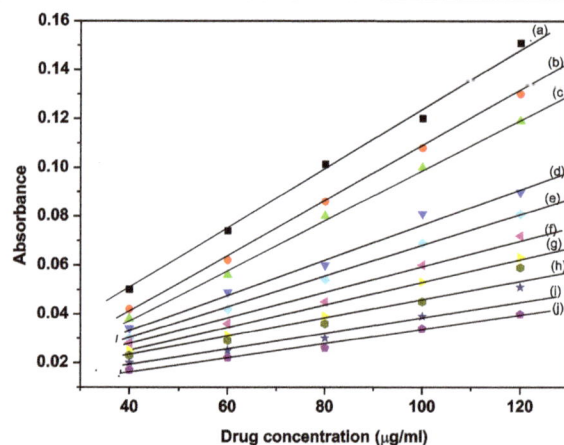

Figure 7 Calibration plots of absorbance versus drug concentration at fixed time. **(a)** 5 min, **(b)** 10 min, **(c)** 15 min, **(d)** 20 min, **(e)** 25 min, **(f)** 30 min, **(g)** 35 min, **(h)** 40 min, **(i)** 45 min, and **(j)** 50 min.

Table 1 Regression equations for the reaction rate and fixed time methods for the determination of pregabalin

Method	Regression equation	r^2
Reaction rate method	Rate $= 2.8 \times 10^{-4} + 2.48 \times 10^{-4} \times$ drug concentration	0.999
Fixed time method, time (min)		
5	$A = 0.00106 + 0.00123 \times$ drug concentration	0.999
10	$A = -0.0032 + 0.00111 \times$ drug concentration	0.999
15	$A = -0.0038 + 0.00103 \times$ drug concentration	0.999
20	$A = 0.0052 + 7.2 \times 10^{-4} \times$ drug concentration	0.993
25	$A = 0.0036 + 6.4 \times 10^{-4} \times$ drug concentration	0.999
30	$A = 0.0034 + 5.6 \times 10^{-4} \times$ drug concentration	0.992
35	$A = 0.003 + 4.9 \times 10^{-4} \times$ drug concentration	0.989
40	$A = 0.0032 + 4.4 \times 10^{-4} \times$ drug concentration	0.984
45	$A = 0.0026 + 3.8 \times 10^{-4} \times$ drug concentration	0.979
50	$A = 0.0046 + 2.9 \times 10^{-4} \times$ drug concentration	0.993

A Absorbance.
The drug concentration is represented in µg/ml.

calibration curve. The rate of the reaction was calculated from the variable time method (Presez-Bendito and Silva 1988; Martin and Bustamante 1993) of measurement as $\Delta A / \Delta t$, where A is the absorbance, and t is the time in seconds. In the present study, $\Delta A / \Delta t$ was obtained by dividing the absorbance measured 300 s (5 minutes) after mixing the drug and the reagent solutions by 300 s, assuming that the absorbance of the coloured product at $t = 0$ is zero. The regression equation for the reaction rate-versus-concentration (µg/ml) graph is

Table 2 Evaluation of accuracy and precision by the proposed method: determination of PGB in pharmaceutical preparations

Method	Amount taken (µg/ml)	Amount[a] found (µg/ml)	%Recovery	SD	RSD (%)
Reaction rate method	40	39.32	98.3	1.071	2.7
	60	59.08	98.46	1.318	2.2
	80	80.58	100.7	1.714	2.1
	100	96.04	96.04	2.210	2.3
	120	120.64	100.53	0.724	0.6
Fixed time method, time (min)					
5	40	39.92	99.8	1.081	2.5
	60	59.83	99.7	1.325	2.2
	80	81.51	101.89	1.756	2.1
	100	97.09	97.09	2.22	2.2
	120	121.89	101.5	0.72	0.5
10	40	40.10	100.25	1.085	2.6
	60	58.28	97.13	0.492	0.8
	80	80.20	100.25	1.750	2.1
	100	99.87	99.87	1.356	1.3
	120	120.6	100.5	0.734	0.6
15	40	40.90	102.25	0.50	1.2
	60	57.72	96.21	1.004	1.7
	80	82.32	102.9	2.129	2.5
	100	101.25	101.25	1.337	1.3
	120	119.70	99.75	0.811	0.6

[a]An average of six determinations.

$$\text{Rate} = 2.8 \times 10^{-4} + 2.48 \times 10^{-4}\,\text{drug conc.}(\mu g/ml),$$
$$r^2 = 0.999.$$

A plot of log of reaction rate versus log of drug concentration gives a straight line (Figure 6) which shows that the reaction rate of the drug obeys the following equation:

$$\text{Rate} = K'[\text{drug}]^n, \qquad (1)$$

where K' is the rate constant, n is the order of the reaction and the drug concentration is in mol/L.

Taking logarithms of Equation (1),

$$\text{Log rate} = \log K' + n \log[\text{drug}]$$
$$\text{Log}\,\Delta A/\Delta t = \log K' + n \log[\text{drug}]$$
$$\text{Log}\,\Delta A/\Delta t = -3.5664 + 0.98 \log[\text{drug}],$$
$$r^2 = 0.999.$$

Thus, $K' = 0.00027$, and the reaction is first order ($n = 0.98$) with respect to drug concentration.

Fixed time method

Change in absorbance with time was followed for different concentrations of the drug. At a fixed time, which was accurately determined, the absorbance was measured. Calibration graphs of absorbance versus initial concentrations of the drug at fixed times of 5, 10, 15, 20,..., 50 min were drawn (Figure 7). The correlation coefficients of the curves were calculated. The regression equations for the calibration graphs corresponding to different fixed times are given in Table 1.

Validation of the proposed methods

Two different methods were tried to construct the calibration curves for the determination of the drug from the rate data, reaction rate method and fixed time method. The regression equations were calculated for every calibration curve. It is evident that in both methods, there is an excellent correlation between the analytical parameter and the concentration of the drug. The high correlation coefficients (r^2) obtained for most of the calibration curves indicate high linearity in the range 40 to 120 μg/ml, and hence, these are suitable methods for the assay of the drug. The above methods were performed in the concentration range of 40 to 120 μg/ml. At higher concentrations, Beer's law is not obtained.

Precision and accuracy

The precision, accuracy and the applicability of the proposed methods were evaluated by measuring five independent samples of pregabalin in pharmaceutical preparations (tablet form) at 40, 60, 80, 100 and 120-μg/ml drug concentrations. Six replicate measurements were made for each concentration. The precision and accuracy were evaluated in terms of the standard deviation and percent recovery. The results are given in Table 2. The calculated relative standard deviations are around 2% for most of the concentrations studied (except for 40 μg/ml where it reaches up to 2.7%), indicating excellent precision of the proposed methods. The percent recovery has been between 96.04% and 102.9%, indicating a close agreement between the measured and true values. Hence, the proposed methods will be effective for the determination of pregabalin in pharmaceutical formulations. The condensation reaction between the drug and the reagent involves the primary aliphatic amine group. The absence of primary aliphatic amine group in the common excipients of the drug namely lactose monohydrate, talc, gelatin, maize starch and glucose eliminates any chances of interferences in the determination of the drug because of their inability to react with the reagent. The excellent RSD and %recovery values obtained with samples of pharmaceutical formulations confirm that there is no potential interference of these excipients on the proposed methods.

Conclusion

The proposed methods are simple which preclude any use of harmful and costly solvents and reagents. &b_k'p-Dimethylaminobenzaldehyde is a suitable reagent for the spectrophotometric determination of pregabalin. It is not only cheap and safe but also is available in any analytical laboratory with excellent shelf life. The procedure of the proposed methods is simple and time saving. No tedious procedures, extractions, heating and long standing times etc. are involved. The proposed method is sensitive, accurate and reproducible; requires simple apparatus for its performance; and consequently is suitable for routine quality control of the drug.

Competing interests

The authors declare that they have no competing interests.

Authors' contributions

All authors read and approved the final manuscript.

Author details

[1]PG Department of Chemistry, University of Kashmir, Srinagar, Jammu and Kashmir 190006, India. [2]University Science Instrumentation Centre, University of Kashmir, Srinagar, Jammu and Kashmir 190006, India.

References

Adegoke OA, Nwoke CE (2008) Spectrophotometric determination of hydralazine using p- dimethylaminobenzaldehyde. J Iranian Chem Soc 5:316

Adegoke OA, Umoh OE (2009) A new approach to the spectrophotometric determination of metronidazole and tinidazole using p-dimethylaminobenzaldehyde. Acta Pharm 59:407–419

Bali A, Gaur P (2011) A novel method for spectrophotometric determination of pregabalin in pure form and in capsules. Chem Central J 5:59

Barona R, Brunnmüllerb U, Brasserb M, Mayc M, Bindera A (2008) Efficacy and safety of pregabalin in patients with diabetic peripheral neuropathy or postherpetic neuralgia, Open-label, non-comparative, flexible-dose studies. Eur J Pain 12:850

Gujral RS, Manirul Haque SK, Kumar S (2009) A novel method for the determination of pregabalin in bulk pharmaceutical formulations and human urine samples. Afr J Pharm Pharmacol 3:327–334

Hamandi K, Sander JW (2006) Pregabalin: a new antiepileptic drug for refractory epilepsy. Seizure Eur J Epilep 15:73

Martin A, Bustamante P (1993) Physical Pharmacy P: Physical Chemical Principles in the Pharmaceutical Sciences, 4th edition. Lea and Febiger, Philadelphia PA, p 287

Onal A (2009) Development and Validation of Selective Spectrophotometric methods for the determination of Pregabalin in pharmaceutical preparation. Chin J Chem 27:781–786

Onal A, Sagirli O (2009) Spectrophotometric and spectrofluorimetric methods for the determination of pregabalin in bulk and pharmaceutical preparation. Mol Bimol Spectros 72:68–71

Presez-Bendito D, Silva M (1988) Kinetic Methods in Analytical Chemistry. John Wiley and Sons, New York, pp 44–45. Ch.11

Reddy AJP (2013) New spectrophotometric determination of pregabalin bulk and Pharmaceutical dosage form. J Drug Discov and Therap 1:56–58

Sowjanya K, Thejaswini JC, Gurupadayya BM, Indu Priya M (2011) Spectrophotometric determination of Pregabalin using 1, 2-Napthaquinone-4-sulfonic acid Sodium and 2, 4 dinitrophenyl hydrazine in pharmaceuticaldosage form. Der Pharmacia Lettre 3:47–56

Tassone DM, Boyce E, Guyer J, Nuzum D (2007) Pregabalin: a novel gamma-aminobutyric acid analogue in the treatment of neuropathic pain, partial-onset seizures, and anxiety disorders. Clin Ther 29:26

20

ICH guideline practice: application of validated RP-HPLC-DAD method for determination of tapentadol hydrochloride in dosage form

Deepti Jain[1] and Pawan K Basniwal[1,2]*

Abstract

Background: Tapentadol is a novel centrally acting analgesic. There is no method for the determination of drug content in dosage form without any interference of any excipients and without using the diethylamine content in the mobile phase with UV detection.

Methods: A simple, precise, and accurate new reverse-phase high-performance liquid chromatography (RP-HPLC) method was developed and validated as per International Conference on Harmonisation of Technical Requirements for Registration of Pharmaceuticals for Human Use guidelines to determine tapentadol hydrochloride in tablet dosage form. It was successfully eluted at 5.34 min by mixture of 0.1% formic acid in water and acetonitrile (75:25) on C18 column (250 mm × 4.6 mm, 5 μm) at the flow of 1 ml/min.

Results: Drug content was determined in between 99.79% and 100.33% with standard deviation of 0.217 without using dimethylamine with UV detection.

Conclusions: The validated RP-HPLC method may be successfully applied for assay, dissolution studies, bioequivalence studies, as well as routine analysis in pharmaceutical industries.

Keywords: RP-HPLC; Tapentadol hydrochloride; Tablet

Background

Tapentadol (TAP), chemically 3-[(1R,2R)-3-(dimethyl-amino)-1-ethyl-2-methylpropyl]phenol (Figure 1), is a novel centrally acting analgesic with a dual mode of action: μ-opioid receptor agonism and noradrenaline reuptake inhibition. This combination of dual action effect not only provides effective analgesia in a broad range of acute and chronic pain conditions but also provides an 'opioid-sparing' effect, i.e., to lower the dose of TAP required to produce a given level of analgesia. TAP also exerted analgesic effects in patients undergoing moderate-to-acute, inflammatory, and chronic neuropathic pain (Schneider et al. 2010; Vadivelu et al. 2011; Wade and Spruill 2009). However, in veterinary practice, its use is still uncertain and controversial (Giorgi 2012a). Recently, a comprehensive review on tapentadol counting the

recent trends in synthesis, related substances, analytical methods, pharmacodynamics, and pharmacokinetics has been published (Jain and Basniwal 2013).

Only few studies were conducted to determine TAP, *viz.* in urine (Coulter et al. 2010), in urine and oral fluid (Bourland et al. 2010) by liquid chromatography-mass spectrometry (LC-MS), and in canine plasma by high-performance liquid chromatography (HPLC) with spectrofluorimetric detection (Giorgi et al. 2012b) and pharmacokinetic studies in dogs (Giorgi et al. 2012c). UV detection was performed in most pharmaceutical industries, while spectrofluorimetric detector is not widely applicable. Longer saturation time is needed when amino derivative (diethylamine or triethylamine) modifier is used as a component of mobile, which is not recommended for routine analysis of drug content in the pharmaceutical industry. It also causes bonus troubles during analysis such as erratic baselines and poor peak shape (Synder et al. 1997). In this context, very complex mobile phases were used for the separation of

* Correspondence: pawanbasniwal@gmail.com
[1]School of Pharmaceutical Sciences, Rajiv Gandhi Technological University, Bhopal, Madhya Pradesh 462033, India
[2]LBS College of Pharmacy, Jaipur, Rajasthan 302004, India

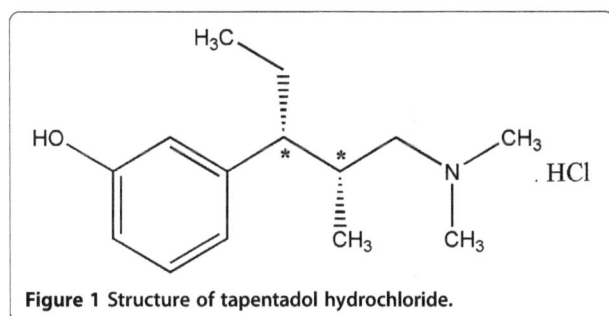

Figure 1 Structure of tapentadol hydrochloride.

TAP such as phosphate buffer and triethylamine (Marathe et al. 2013), potassium dihydrogen orthophosphate and potassium hydroxide (Kathirvel et al. 2013), and phosphate buffer with glacial acetic acid and triethylamine (Sherikar and Mehta 2012). As we have experienced, the working range for HPLC methods is near 10 μg/ml, while the mentioned phases have very high working ranges at 75 to 300 μg/ml (Kathirvel et al. 2013) and 5 to 100 μg/ml (Sherikar and Mehta 2012).

Thus, there is still a gap in research work; there is no method for the determination of TAP in dosage form, which claims that there is no interference of any excipients in determination without using complex mobile phase and with higher sensitivity. The new reverse-phase HPLC (RP-HPLC) method was developed and validated as per International Conference on Harmonisation of Technical Requirements for Registration of Pharmaceuticals for Human Use (ICH) guidelines without using diethylamine content in the mobile phase with DAD detection, which is simple, rapid, precise, and accurate for the determination of TAP in tablet dosage form.

Methods

Instrumentation and chromatograph

The HPLC chromatograph used was Agilent Infinity 1260 series (Agilent Technologies, Santa Clara, CA, USA) equipped with a 1260 binary pump VL (400 bar), 1260 manual injector (600 bar), Rheodyne 7725i seven-port sample injection valve with a 20-μl fixed loop, ZORBAX Eclipse Plus C18 (250 mm × 4.6 mm, 5 μm), 1260 DAD VL, 20-Hz detector, a standard flow cell (10 mm, 13 μl, and 120 bar; OpenLab CDS EZChrom Ed. Workstation), and 50-μl syringe (FN, LC tip). All weighing for analysis was performed on a Shimadzu electronic analytical balance AX-200 (Kyoto, Japan). Water used for analysis was prepared by triple distillation assembly. All dilutions, mobile phase and other solutions, used for the analysis were filtered through a 0.2-μm nylon filter (Ultipor®N66 Nylon 6,6 membrane, Pall Sciences, Pall India Pvt. Ltd. Mumbai, India).

Chemicals and reagent

The working standard used was TAP which was supplied by Ranbaxy Laboratories Limited, Gurgaon, Harayana, as a gift sample. Tablets of TAP (TRANSDOL 50, Lupin Ltd, Mumbai, India) were procured from the local market. Triple distilled water was prepared from distillation assembly. Formic acid and acetonitrile were procured from Merck Specialties Private Limited Mumbai, India. The mobile phase was prepared from the combination of formic acid (0.1%) and acetonitrile.

Sample preparation

Accurately weighed 50 mg of TAP was dissolved in triple distilled water to prepare stock I (1,000 μg/ml) in 50-ml volumetric flask. Stock II (100 μg/ml) was prepared from stock I, which was used to prepare further dilutions containing 0.2, 0.4, 0.8, 1.2, 1.6, and 2 μg/ml. All dilutions were filtered through 0.2-μm nylon filter (Ultipor®N66 Nylon 6,6 membranes, Pall Sciences).

Chromatography

The filtered dilutions were chromatographed by the set of conditions on Agilent Infinity 1260 series. The mixture of 0.1% formic acid and acetonitrile (75:25) was used as mobile phase for the elution of the drug on ZORBAX Eclipse Plus C18 column (250 mm × 4.6 mm, 5 μm) at 1 ml/min of flow rate. TAP was successfully eluted at 5.8 min with a run time of 7 min, and detection was performed by photodiode array detector (PDA) at 272 nm.

Method validation

According to the ICH guidelines (ICH Q2A 1994; ICH Q2B 1996), the developed method was validated to assure the reliability of the results of analysis for different parameters viz. linearity, range, accuracy, precision, robustness, ruggedness, limit of quantization (LOQ), limit of detection (LOD), and specificity. Linearity was determined by serial dilutions (0.2 to 2 μg/ml) of the TAP in distilled water in triplicates. The range of TAP was validated between 0.8 and 1.6 μg/ml with triplicates of dilutions. Accuracy was determined by recovery method by spiking the standard solution to the pre-analyzed samples. This procedure was repeated six times. Precision of the method was studied under the head of repeatability and intermediate precision. The six replicates of 0.8 μg/ml were chromatographed subsequently to assure the repeatability. Intermediate precision was determined by day-to-day analysis variation and analyst-to-analyst variation in the linearity range. Robustness of the method was studied with variation in temperature (20°C, 25°C, and 30°C) and content of formic acid (0.1%) in aqueous phase variation by a 5% change. Serial dilutions of TAP from 1 to 1,000 ng/ml were chromatographed, which was repeated three times to determine LOD and LOQ. Specificity was ascertained by

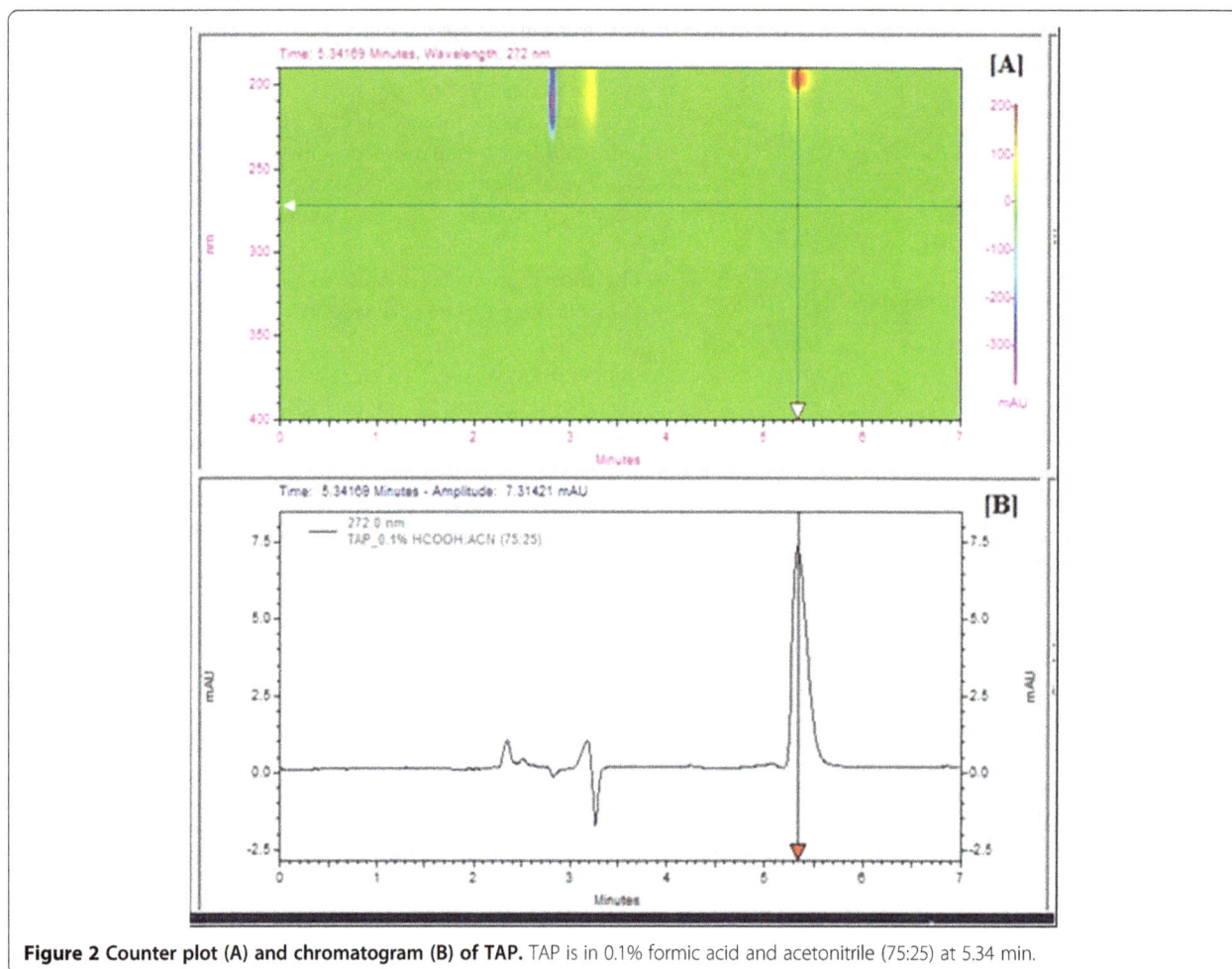

Figure 2 Counter plot (A) and chromatogram (B) of TAP. TAP is in 0.1% formic acid and acetonitrile (75:25) at 5.34 min.

degrading the drug sample in alkaline medium. Sample solution stability was demonstrated by analyzing six replicates of 0.8 μg/ml TAP standard samples at different time intervals (0, 12, 24, 36, and 48 h) with freshly prepared mobile phase on each time.

Analysis of dosage form

Powdered tablets were weighed equivalent to 50 mg of TAP and sonicated to dissolve drug content in triple distilled water. The sonicated solution was filtered through Whatman filter (no. 41), and different serial dilutions were

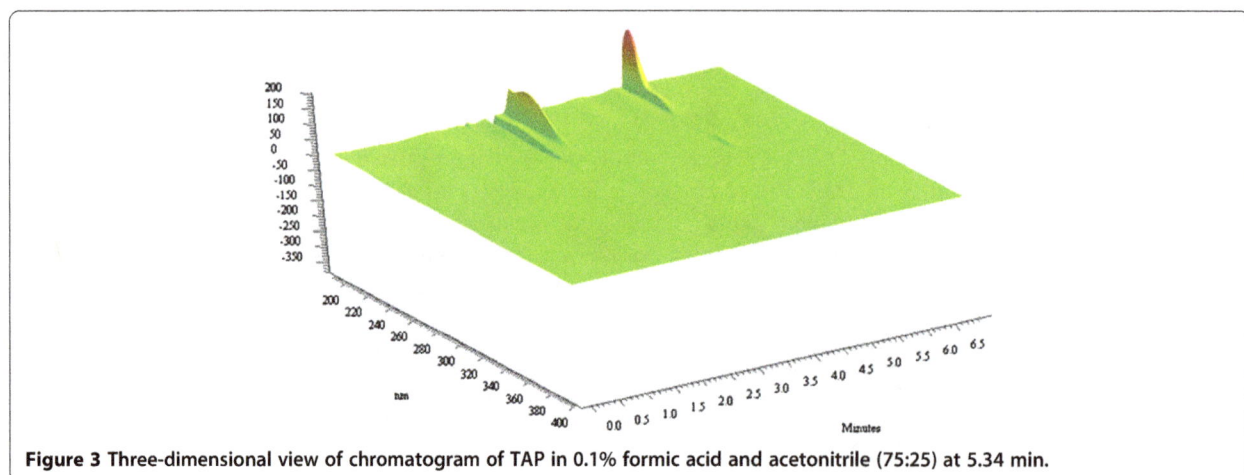

Figure 3 Three-dimensional view of chromatogram of TAP in 0.1% formic acid and acetonitrile (75:25) at 5.34 min.

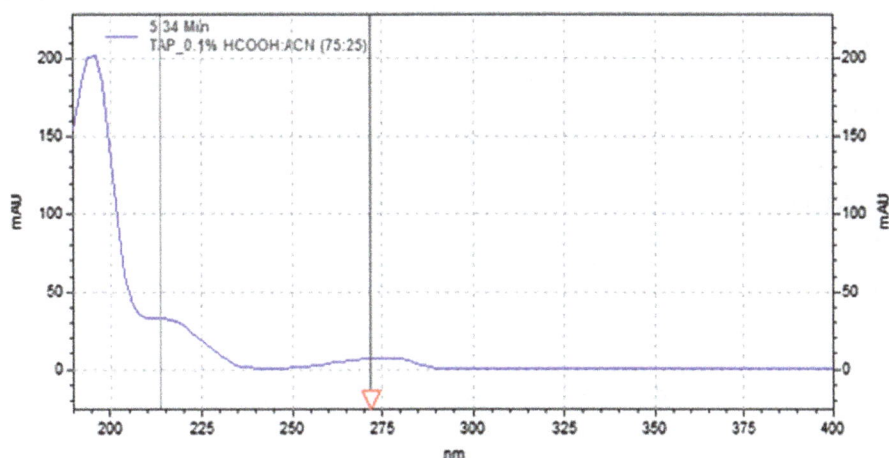

Figure 4 Spectrum of TAP at 5.34 min in 0.1% formic acid and acetonitrile (75:25).

prepared by subsequent dilution with triple distilled water. The dilutions were chromatographed, and percentages of drug content in tablets were determined by extrapolating the AUC values on regression line.

Results and discussion
Optimization of chromatography

The RP-HPLC method was optimized with the objective of developing a simple, precise, accurate, and fast assay method for TAP. On the basis of chemistry and solubility of TAP, the initial mixture of water and acetonitrile (50:50) was made to elute TAP on C18 column (250 mm × 4.6 mm, 5 μm) at the flow of 1 ml/min. The splitting of peak was observed, which indicates that the drug ionizes in the present mobile phase and the peak was highly broadened. Now, the pKa values (9.34 and 10.45) of the TAP have been taken into consideration to design the mobile phase (Synder et al. 1997), so the acidic pH should be favored to elute the drug in a single peak with an acceptable peak shape because in acidic pH, it should be present in nonionic form. Formic acid (0.1%) in water and acetonitrile (50:50) was run to elute TAP. The drug was eluted with a diluent peak which was splitting in nature. When aqueous content was decreased, more splitting was observed with diluent peaks, i.e., acidic content in the mobile phase should be increased. Thus, aqueous phase (acidic content) was increased to 70%; the single peak without splitting was observed which was near the diluent peak with acceptable peak shape but with tailing. Finally, TAP was better resolved from the diluent peak without splitting with acceptable peak shape (no tailing and fronting) in 0.1% formic acid in water and acetonitrile (75:25). Thus, we have excluded the use of amino derivative (diethylamine or triethylamine) as modifier of the mobile phase.

It was clearly shown in Figure 2A,B that the diluent peak comes in between 2.5 and 3.5 min and is well resolved from the TAP peak (5.34 min). Three-dimensional view (Figure 3) of the chromatogram also confirmed that there was no peak around the TAP elution time. The above mobile phase composition enabled the peak shape and

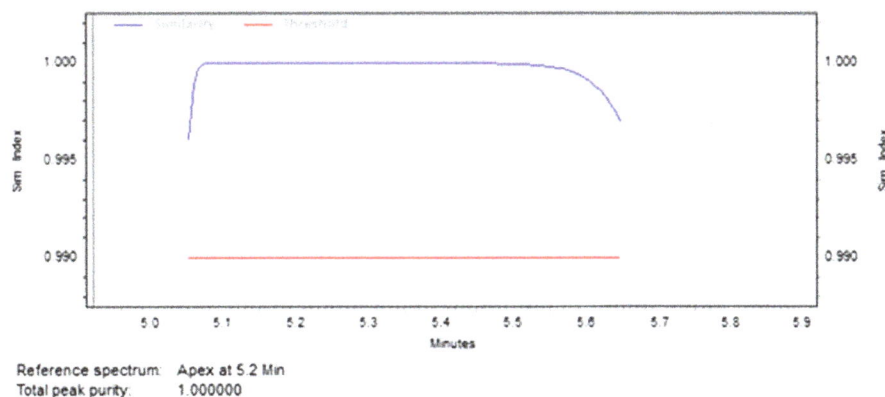

Figure 5 Peak purity curve of TAP at 5.34 min in 0.1% formic acid and acetonitrile (75:25).

elution of the drug, and in this separation, the UV detector has good spectra of the drug. The detection wavelength was confirmed at 272 nm by the spectrum of TAP at an elution time of 5.34 min (Figure 4), while previously reported methods have different detection, *viz.* spectrofluorimetric and LC-MS methods, which were costly than UV detection. The peak purity curve at the elution time of the TAP (Figure 5) indicated that there was no interference with the peak of TAP as the peak purity of the TAP was one unit.

System suitability parameters

System suitability parameters were analyzed to check the system performance consistency. For system suitability parameters, six replicates of high quality control sample of TAP was injected, and column performances like tailing factor, retention time, and number of theoretical plates were observed (Table 1); values of percentage of relative standard deviation (%RSD) for these parameters were found within the acceptance criteria of system performance. Higher theoretical plates (21,930) with a lower %RSD value indicate good separation of TAP on the C18 column in described chromatographic conditions. Tailing factors for most peaks should fall between 0.9 and 1.4, with a value of 1.0 indicating a perfectly symmetrical peak. Tailing factor for TAP was in between the range; thus, the TAP's peak was in symmetrical shape. The capacity factor was 16.44 ± 0.222, i.e., TAP has sufficient opportunity to interact with the stationary phase resulting in differential migrations. The co-elution of impurities or degradants is generally investigated by examining the peak purity using a PDA detector. Here, the peak purity at 5.34 min was 1.0; there was no interference with elution of TAP at retention time, or nothing was co-eluting along with TAP at 5.34 min. Thus, all system suitability parameters were within the acceptance criteria.

Linearity and range

Linearity was evaluated by analyzing different concentrations of the standard solutions of the TAP. Response was a linear function of concentration over the range of 0.2 to 2 µg/ml which was used as the working range of the method. Peak area and concentration were subjected to

Table 2 Validation parameters of RP-HPLC method for TAP

Parameters	Values[a] ± SD, ± %RSD
Linearity	0.2 to 2 µg/ml
Regression equation	AUC = 18,374.93x −62.59
Correlation coefficient	r^2 = 0.9998 ± 0.001, ± 0.100
Response ratio	2,377.778 ± 1.510, ± 0.063
Range	0.8 to 1.6 µg/ml ± 1.23, ± 0.02
Accuracy	100.05 ± 0.841, ± 0.841
Precision	
Repeatability	100.07 ± 0.319, ± 0.319
Intermediate precision	
Inter-day	99.89 ± 0.205, ± 0.205
Analyst to analyst	99.74 ± 0.125, ± 0.125
Robustness	
Temperature (20°C, 25°C, 30°C)	100.21 ± 0.75, ± 0.748
Formic acid concentration (±5%)	100.12 ± 0.54, ± 0.539
LOQ	8 ng/ml ± 0.93, ± 0.063
LOD	1 ng/ml ± 0.78, ± 0.067
Specificity	Ascertained by analyzing standard drug and samples of equivalent concentration
Stability in sample solution	
Response ratio	184.16 ± 1.83, ± 0.057

LOD limit of detection, *LOQ* limit of quantization. [a]Mean of six replicates.

linear least-squares regression analysis to calculate the calibration equation and correlation coefficient (Table 2). The linearity of the calibration plots was confirmed by the high value of correlation coefficients (r^2 = 0.9998 ± 0.001), and %RSD for the correlation coefficients was less than 2.

Accuracy

The accuracy of the method was ascertained by recovery method. When the method was used for extraction and subsequent analysis of the drug in the dosage form after

Table 1 System suitability parameters for TAP

Parameters	Value for TAP[a]	SD	%RSD
Number of theoretical plates	21,930	61.64	0.281
Tailing factor	1.12	0.051	0.956
Capacity factor	16.44	0.222	1.352
RT (min)	5.34	0.037	0.698
Peak purity	1.00	0.000	0.000

RT retention time, *SD* standard deviation, *%RSD* percentage of relative standard deviation. [a]Mean of six values.

Table 3 Result of assay of TAP dosage form

Batch	Concentration of tablet samples (µg/ml)	Concentration found (µg/ml)	Percentage found
I	0.8	99.75	99.75
II	0.8	100.125	100.125
III	0.8	99.625	99.625
IV	0.8	99.875	99.875
V	0.8	100.125	100.125
VI	0.8	100.25	100.25
Mean		99.96	99.96
SD		0.246	0.246
%RSD		0.2459	0.2459

spiking with 50%, 100%, and 150% of the drug, the recovery was 100.05% (99.7% to 100.9%).

Precision
The repeatability of sample injection and measurement of peak area were expressed as %RSD (Table 2). Repeatability and intermediate precision at three different concentrations (0.4, 0.6, and 0.8 µg/ml) for both within-day and day-to-day analysis were always <2%. These low values of the %RSD showed that the repeatability and intermediate precision of the method were within the acceptable value.

Robustness
There was no significant change in the result of developed method, after the introduction of small deliberate changes in temperature (±5°C) and formic acid content in aqueous phase of the mobile phase (±5%). The standard deviation of peak areas was calculated for each set of conditions and was found to be <2% (Table 2). The low values of %RSD indicate that the method is robust.

LOQ and LOD
The developed method was highly sensitive to detect and determine the TAP content. The LOD for signal-to-noise ratio of 3:1 was 1 ng/ml (RSD ± 0.067%), and the LOQ for signal-to-noise ratio of 10:1 was 8 ng/ml (RSD ± 0.063%) (Table 2).

Specificity
A different set of condition for elution of the TAP was changed as discussed in previous sections, *viz.* formic acid content and temperature; then in spite of these changes, no additional peak was found, although a very small change was observed in retention times and peak shapes. The specificity of the method was ascertained by analyzing drug standard solution and samples of equivalent concentration (0.8 µg/ml). The identity of the peak in the sample was confirmed by comparison of the retention time and UV spectrum of the peak from the sample with those of the peak from the standard. Peak purity for the drug was assessed by comparing the UV spectra acquired at the peak start, peak apex, and peak end. The specificity of the method was also ascertained by analyzing the alkaline degraded samples; when degraded sample was chromatographed, the concentration of the TAP was reduced and other peaks were observed at different retention time.

Sample solution stability
The response ratio of all samples was averaged as 184.16 (Table 2). The standard deviation and percentage of relative standard deviation were found to be less than 2: 1.83 and 0.057, respectively.

Analysis of dosage form
TAP is freely water soluble, so drug content from tablet powder was extracted by triple distilled water. Sonication of drug powder with triple distilled water has better extraction compared to the shaking of solution. TAP content was determined between 99.79% and 100.33% with a standard deviation of 0.217. Error of standard deviation was far less than the unit which was favorable in consistency with the result of the method.

Conclusions
Hence, the new liquid chromatographic method in reverse phase was developed and validated; (Table 3) it was simple, fast, precise, and accurate without having to use diethylamine in the mobile phase and with UV detection. The method was successfully applied to determine the TAP content in tablet dosage form within acceptable limits and may be applied for assay, dissolution studies, bio-equivalence studies, as well as routine analysis in pharmaceutical industries.

Competing interests
The authors declare that they have no competing interests.

Authors' contributions
Experimental work was done by PKB. Both authors equally contributed in experimental design, framing, writing, proofing and approval of the manuscript.

Acknowledgement
One of the authors, Pawan Kumar Basniwal, earnestly indebted to Department of Science and Technology (DST), Government of India, New Delhi, for the financial support for this research work under Fast Track Scheme for Young Scientists. Authors are highly thankful to Head, School of Pharmaceutical Sciences, RGPV, Bhopal and Principal, LBS College of Pharmacy, Jaipur for providing the experimental facilities for this research work.

References
Bourland JA, Collins AA, Chester SA, Ramachandran S, Backer RC (2010) Determination of tapentadol (Nucynta®) and N-desmethyltapentadol in authentic urine specimens by ultra-performance liquid chromatography-tandem mass spectrometry. J Anal Toxicol 34:450–457
Coulter C, Taruc M, Tuyay J, Moore C (2010) Determination of tapentadol and its metabolite N-desmethyltapentadol in urine and oral fluid using liquid chromatography with tandem mass spectral detection. J Anal Toxicol 34:458–463
Giorgi M (2012) Tramadol vs tapentadol: a new horizon in pain treatment? American J Animal Veterinary Sci 7(1):7–11
Giorgi M, Meizler A, Mills PC (2012a) Pharmacokinetics of the novel atypical opioid tapentadol following oral and intravenous administration in dogs. Vet J 194:309–313
Giorgi M, Meizler A, Mills PC (2012b) Quantification of tapentadol in canine plasma by HPLC with spectrofluorimetric detection: development and validation of a new methodology. J Pharm Biomed Ana 67–68:148–153
ICH Q2A (1994) Harmonised tripartite guideline: text on validation of analytical procedures, Proceedings of the international conference on harmonization, Geneva
ICH Q2B (1996) Harmonised tripartite guideline: validation of analytical procedures: methodology, Proceedings of the international conference on harmonization, Geneva
Jain D, Basniwal PK (2013) Tapentadol, a novel analgesic: review of recent trends in synthesis, related substances, analytical methods, pharmacodynamics and

pharmacokinetics. Bulletin Facult Pharmacy Cairo Univ. doi:10.1016/j.
bfopcu.2013.04.003

Kathirvel S, Satyanarayana SV, Devalarao G (2013) Application of a validated stability-
indicating LC method for the simultaneous estimation of tapentadol and its
process-related impurities in bulk and its dosage form. J Chem 2013:927814

Marathe GM, Patil PO, Patil DA, Patil GB, Bari SB (2013) Stability indicating
RP-HPLC method for the determination of tapentadol in bulk and in
pharmaceutical dosage form. Int J ChemTech Res 5(1):34–41

Schneider J, Jahnel U, Linz K (2010) Neutral effects of the novel analgesic
tapentadol on cardiac repolarization due to mixed ion channel inhibitory
activities. Drug Dev Res 71:197–208

Sherikar OD, Mehta PJ (2012) Development and validation of RP- HPLC,
UV-spectrometric and spectrophotometric method for estimation of
tapentadol hydrochloride in bulk and in laboratory sample of tablet dosage
form. J Chem Pharm Res 4(9):4134–4140

Synder LR, Kirkland JJ, Glajch JL (1997) Practical HPLC method development,
2nd edn. John Wiley & Sons, New York

Vadivelu N, Timchenko A, Huang Y, Sinatra R (2011) Tapentadol extended-release
for treatment of chronic pain: a review. J Pain Res 4:211–218

Wade WE, Spruill WJ (2009) Tapentadol hydrochloride: a centrally acting oral
analgesic. Clin Ther 31(12):2804–2818

21

Application of a modified graphene nanosheet paste electrode for voltammetric determination of methyldopa in urine and pharmaceutical formulation

Hadi Beitollahi[1*], Somayeh Tajik[2], Malek Hossein Asadi[3] and Pourya Biparva[4]

Abstract

Background: Electrochemical sensors and biosensors for pharmaceutical, food, agricultural and environmental analyses have been growing rapidly due to electrochemical behavior of drugs and biomolecules and partly due to advances in electrochemical measuring systems. In the present work, we describe the preparation of a new electrode composed of graphen (G) modified with 2,7-bis(ferrocenyl ethyl) fluoren-9-one (2,7-BFGPE) and investigate its performance for the electrocatalytic determination of methyldopa in aqueous solutions.

Methods: Experimental section was carried out using cyclic voltammetry, square wave voltammetry and chronoamperometry.

Results: Under the optimized conditions (pH 7.0), the square wave voltammetric peak current of methyldopa increased linearly with methyldopa concentration in the ranges of 9.0×10^{-8} to 5.0×10^{-4} M. The detection limit was 5.0×10^{-8} M methyldopa. The diffusion coefficient ($D = 9.35 \times 10^{-6}$ cm2/s) and electron transfer coefficient ($\alpha = 0.52$) for methyldopa oxidation were also determined.

Conclusions: The method shows the development of a sensor for selective and sensitive determination of methyldopa. This sensor was successfully applied to determine the methyldopa in some real samples.

Keywords: Methyldopa; Graphene nanosheets; Modified electrode; Voltammetry; Electrochemical sensor

Background

Methyldopa is an antihypertensive agent that is used in the treatment of high blood pressure or hypertension, especially when it is complicated with renal disease. Its antihypertensive properties are primarily due to its action on the central nervous system. Methyldopa inhibits the enzyme DOPA decarboxylase, which converts L-DOPA into dopamine, and is a precursor for norepinephrine and subsequently epinephrine. It is converted to α-methyl norepinephrine in adrenergic nerve terminals, and its antihypertensive action appears to be due to its stimulation of central adrenal receptors, which reduces sympathetic tone and produces a fall in blood pressure. The therapeutic concentration of methyldopa in human plasma is usually in the range of 0.1 to 0.5 mg L^{-1}, and its average terminal elimination half-life is 2 h (Kwan et al. 1976; Myhre et al. 1982). Clearly, detection and quantification of methyldopa is an important feature in pharmaceutical and clinical procedures (Rezaei et al. 2013; Gholivand and Amiri 2013). Several analytical procedures have been reported for the analysis of methyldopa in bulk form, pharmaceutical form, or biological fluids. These include titrimetry, chromatography, kinetic methods, spectrophotometry, and H NMR. However, these methods have disadvantages, including high costs, long analysis times, the requirement of complex and tedious sample pretreatments, and, in some cases, a low sensitivity and selectivity, that make them unsuitable for a routine analysis. On the other hand, electrochemical methods have attracted great interest because of

* Correspondence: h.beitollahi@yahoo.com
[1]Environment Department, Institute of Science and High Technology and Environmental Sciences, Graduate University of Advanced Technology, P.O. Box 76315-117, Kerman, Iran
Full list of author information is available at the end of the article

their simplicity, rapidness, and high sensitivity in detecting methyldopa and various other analytes without requiring tedious pretreatments (Athanasiou-Malaki and Koupparis 1984; Tajik et al. 2013a; Shahrokhian and Rastgar 2011; Molaakbari et al. 2014; Moccelini et al. 2011).

The use of carbon paste as an electrode was initially reported in 1958 by Adams. In afterward researches, a wide variety of modifiers including enzymes, polymers, and nanomaterials have been used with these versatile electrodes. Carbon paste electrodes (CPEs) are widely applicable in both electrochemical studies and electroanalysis, thanks to their advantages such as very low background current (compared to solid graphite or noble metal electrodes), facility to prepare, low cost, large potential window, simple surface renewal process, and easiness of miniaturization. Besides the advantageous properties and characteristics listed previously, the feasibility of incorporating different substances during paste preparation (which results in the so-called modified carbon paste electrode) allows the fabrication of electrodes with desired composition and, hence, with predetermined properties (Tajik et al. 2013b; Khoobi et al. 2013; Mokhtari et al. 2012; Díaz et al. 2013; Gholivand and Mohammadi-Behzad 2014; Mazloum-Ardakani et al. 2010; Thomas et al. 2013a; Raoof et al. 2007; Dönmez et al. 2014; Raoof et al. 2006a).

Electrochemical methods using chemically modified electrodes (CMEs) have been widely used as sensitive and selective analytical methods for the detection of trace amounts of biologically important compounds. One of the most important properties of CMEs is their ability to catalyze the electrode process via the significant decrease of overpotential with respect to the unmodified electrode. With respect to the relatively selective interaction of the electron mediator with the target analyte in a coordinated fashion, these electrodes are capable of considerably enhancing the selectivity of electroanalytical methods (Beitollahi et al. 2011a; Luo et al. 2013; Taleat et al. 2008; Huo et al. 2013; Thomas et al. 2013b; Raoof et al. 2006b; Oliveira et al. 2013; Beitollahi et al. 2011b; Thomas et al. 2013c; Mohammadi et al. 2013; Sanghavi et al. 2013; Beitollahi et al. 2014; Li et al. 2012; Ghoreishi et al. 2012; Yildiz et al. 2014).

As a new kind of two-dimensional carbon material, graphene has attracted increasing attention due to its unique properties including high surface area, excellent electrical conductivity, quick electron mobility at room temperature, high mechanical strength, and ease for functionalization (Joon et al. 2014). Graphene-based electrochemical sensors have been proved to possess excellent electrocatalytic ability and good performances (Ping et al. 2014; Ma et al. 2014; Silva et al. 2014; Zhu et al. 2013; Sun et al. 2012; Xi et al. 2013).

In the present work, we describe the preparation of a new electrode composed of graphene (G) modified with 2,7-bis(ferrocenyl ethyl)fluoren-9-one (2,7-BFGPE) and investigate its performance for the electrocatalytic determination of methyldopa in aqueous solutions.

Methods

Apparatus and chemicals

The electrochemical measurements were performed with an Autolab potentiostat/galvanostat (PGSTAT-302 N, Eco Chemie, Utrecht, The Netherlands). The experimental conditions were controlled with General Purpose Electrochemical System (GPES) software. A conventional three-electrode cell was used at $25°C \pm 1°C$. An Ag/AgCl/KCl (3.0 M) electrode, a platinum wire, and 2,7-BFGPE were used as the reference, auxiliary, and working electrodes, respectively. A Metrohm 691 pH/Ion Meter (Utrecht, The Netherlands) was used for pH measurements.

All solutions were freshly prepared with double-distilled water. Methyldopa and all other reagents were of analytical grade from Merck (Darmstadt, Germany). Graphite powder and paraffin oil (DC 350, density = 0.88 g cm^{-3}) as the binding agent (both from Merck) were used for preparing the pastes. The buffer solutions were prepared from orthophosphoric acid and its salts in the pH range of 2.0 to 11.0. 2,7-BF was synthesized in our laboratory as reported previously (Raoof et al. 2006a).

Synthesis of graphene nanosheets

Graphene nanosheets were synthesized from natural graphite flakes based on the modified Hummers and Offeman's method (Hummers and Offeman 1958). In a typical synthesis process, 1.0 g of pristine graphite flakes was immersed in 50 mL of formic acid and then sonicated for 2 h at room temperature. The resulting graphite plates were washed with acetone and then dried in an oven at 95°C for 12 h. Then, 100 mL H$_2$SO$_4$ (95%) was added into a 500-mL flask and cooled by immersion in an ice bath followed by stirring. About 1.0 g of treated graphite powder and 0.5 g NaNO$_3$ were added under vigorous stirring to avoid agglomeration. After the graphite powder was well dispersed, 3 g KMnO$_4$ was added gradually under stirring and cooling so that the temperature of the mixture was maintained below 10°C. The mixture was stirred for 2 h and diluted with deionized double-distilled water (in an ice bath). After that, 25 mL 15% H$_2$O$_2$ was slowly added to the mixture until the colour of the mixture changed to brilliant yellow, indicating fully oxidized graphite. The as-obtained graphite oxide slurry was re-dispersed in deionized double-distilled water and then exfoliated to generate graphene oxide nanosheets by sonication for 2 h. Then, the solution was filtered and washed with diluted HCl solution to remove metal ions. Finally, the product was washed with deionized double-distilled water until the solution became acid free and dried under vacuum at 50°C. A typical transmission

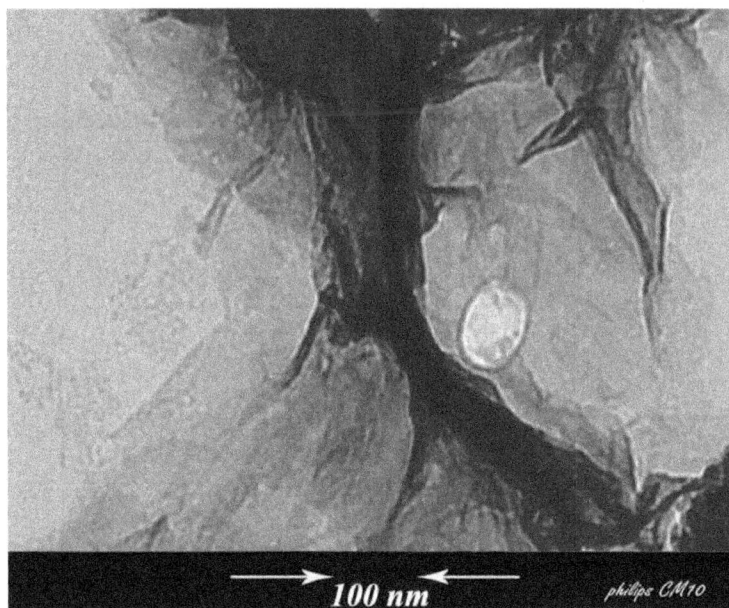

Figure 1 TEM image of the synthesized graphene nanosheets.

electron microscopy (TEM) image of the synthesized graphene nanosheets is shown in Figure 1.

Preparation of the electrode

2,7-BFGPEs were prepared by hand-mixing 0.01 g of 2,7-BF with 0.89 g graphite powder and 0.1 g G with a mortar and pestle. Then, approximately 0.7 mL of paraffin was added to the above mixture and mixed for 20 min until a uniformly wetted paste was obtained. The paste was then packed into the end of a glass tube (ca. 3.4 mm i.d. and 10 cm long). A copper wire inserted into the carbon paste provided the electrical contact. When necessary, a new surface was obtained by pushing an excess of the paste out of the tube and polishing with a weighing paper.

For comparison, 2,7-BF-modified CPE (2,7-BFCPE) without G, G paste electrode (GPE) without 2,7-BF, and unmodified CPE in the absence of both 2,7-BF and G were also prepared in the same way.

Results and discussion

Electrochemical behavior of 2,7-BFGPE

2,7-BFGPE was constructed and its electrochemical properties were studied in a 0.1 M phosphate-buffered saline (PBS; pH 7.0) by cyclic voltammetry (CV). The experimental results show well-defined and reproducible anodic and cathodic peaks related to the 2,7-bis(ferrocenyl ethyl)fluoren-9-one/2,7-bis(ferricenium ethyl)fluoren-9-one redox system, with E_{pa}, E_{pc}, and $E°'$ of 320, 260, and 290 mV vs. Ag/AgCl/KCl (3.0 M) respectively. The observed peak separation potential ($\Delta E_p = E_{pa} - E_{pc}$) of 60 mV was greater than the value of 59/n mV expected for a reversible system (Bard and Faulkner 2001), suggesting that the redox couple

of 2,7-BF in 2,7-BFGPE has a quasi-reversible behavior in aqueous medium.

In addition, the long-term stability of 2,7-BFGPE was tested over a 3-week period. When CVs were recorded after the modified electrode was stored in atmosphere at room temperature, the peak potential for methyldopa oxidation

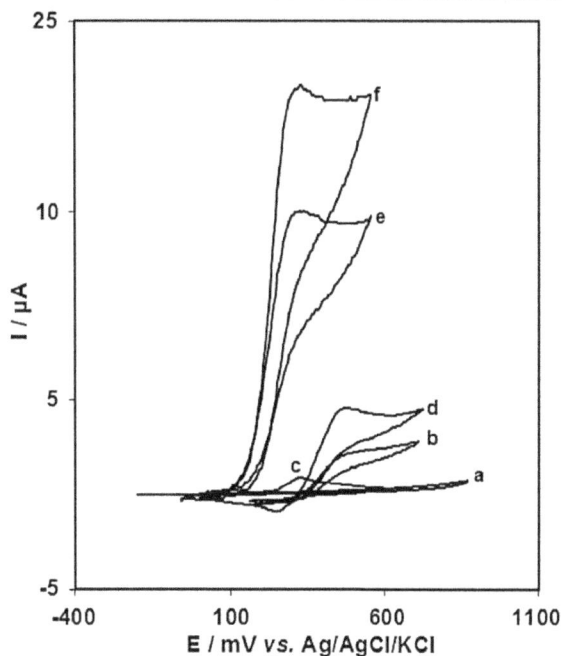

Figure 2 CV responses. (a) Unmodified CPE in 0.1 M PBS (pH 7.0) at scan rate of 10 mV s^{-1}. (b) As (a) + 0.35 mM methyldopa. (c) As (a) at the surface of 2,7-BFGPE. (d) As (b) at the surface of GPE. (e) As (b) at the surface of 2,7-BFCPE. (f) As (b) at the surface of 2,7-BFGPE.

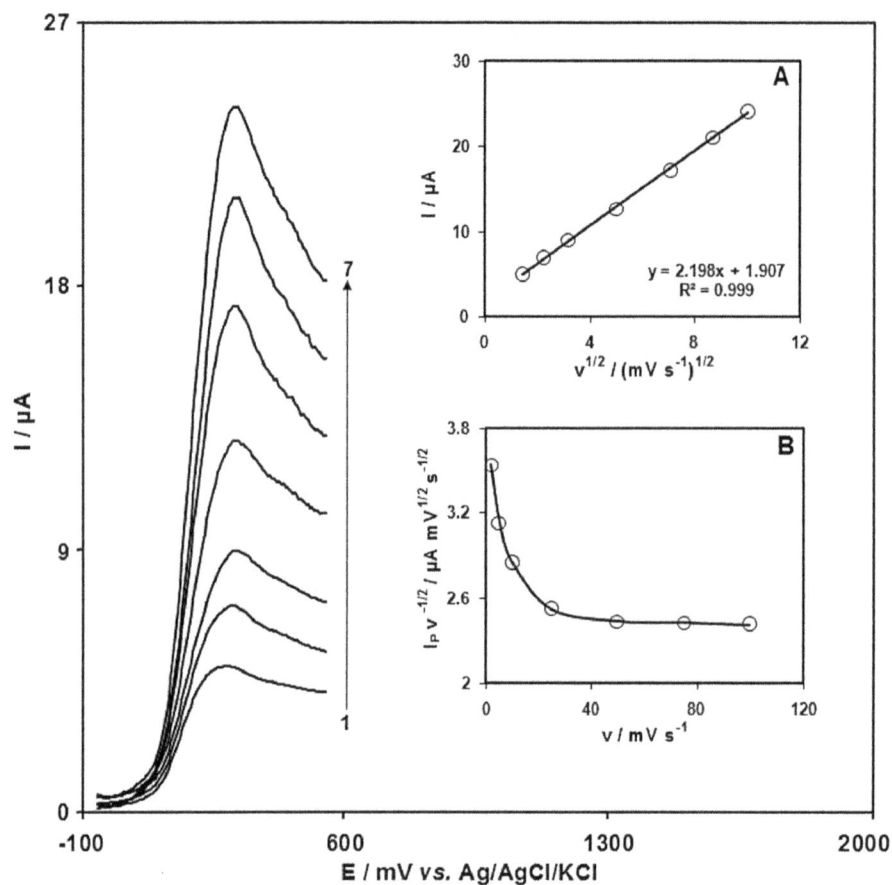

Figure 3 LSVs of 2,7-BFGPE in 0.1 M PBS (pH 7.0) containing 20.0 µM methyldopa at various scan rates. Numbers 1 to 7 correspond to 2, 5, 10, 25, 50, 75, and 100 mV s^{-1}, respectively. Insets: Variation of **(A)** anodic peak current vs. $v^{1/2}$ and **(B)** normalized current ($I_p/v^{1/2}$) vs. v.

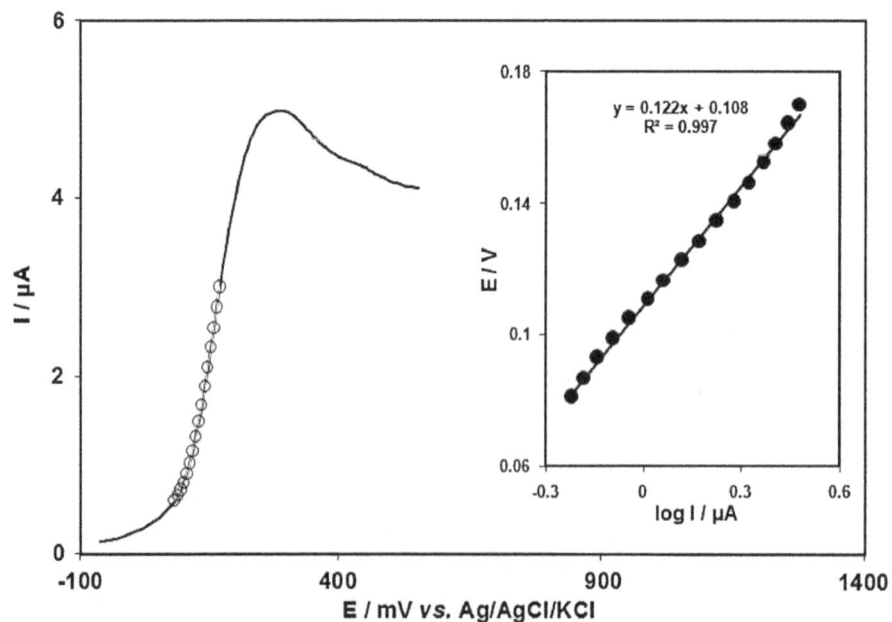

Figure 4 LSV (at 2 mV s^{-1}) of a 2,7-BFGPE in 0.1 M PBS (pH 7.0) containing 20.0 µM methyldopa. The points are the data used in the Tafel plot. The inset shows the Tafel plot derived from the LSV.

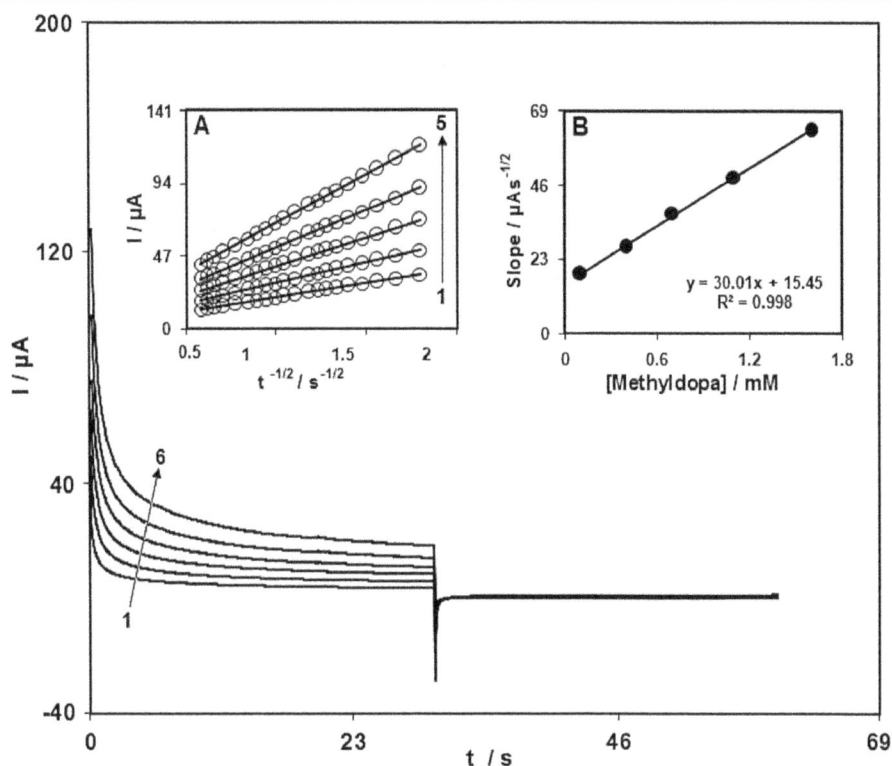

Figure 5 Chronoamperograms obtained at 2,7-BFGPE in 0.1 M PBS (pH 7.0) for different concentrations of methyldopa. Numbers 1 to 6 correspond to 0.0, 0.1, 0.4, 0.7, 1.1, and 1.6 mM of methyldopa, respectively. Insets: **(A)** Plots of I vs. $t^{-1/2}$ obtained from chronoamperograms 2 to 6. **(B)** Plot of the slope of the straight lines against methyldopa concentration.

was unchanged and the current signals showed less than 2.1% decrease relative to the initial response. The antifouling properties of the modified electrode toward methyldopa oxidation and its oxidation products were investigated by recording the cyclic voltammograms of the modified electrode before and after use in the presence of methyldopa. Cyclic voltammograms were recorded in the presence of methyldopa after having cycled the potential 20 times at a scan rate of 10 mV s^{-1}. The peak potentials were unchanged, and the currents decreased by less than 2.3%. Therefore, at the surface of 2,7-BFGPE, not only the sensitivity increased, but the fouling effect of the analyte and its oxidation product also decreased.

Influence of pH

The electrochemical behavior of methyldopa is dependent on the pH value of the aqueous solution, whereas the electrochemical properties of the 2,7-bis(ferrocenyl ethyl) fluoren-9-one/2,7-bis(ferricenium ethyl)fluoren-9-one (Fc/Fc$^+$) redox couple are independent on pH. Therefore, pH optimization of the solution seems to be necessary in order to obtain the electrocatalytic oxidation of methyldopa. Thus, the electrochemical behavior of methyldopa was studied in 0.1 M PBS in different pH values (2.0 < pH < 11.0) at the surface of 2,7-BFGPE by CV. It was found

that the electrocatalytic oxidation of methyldopa at the surface of 2,7-BFGPE was more favored under neutral conditions than in acidic or basic medium. This appears as a gradual growth in the anodic peak current and a simultaneous decrease in the cathodic peak current in the CVs of 2,7-BFGPE. Thus, pH 7.0 was chosen as the optimum pH for electrocatalysis of methyldopa oxidation at the surface of 2,7-BFGPE.

Electrocatalytic oxidation of methyldopa at a 2,7-BFGPE

Figure 2 depicts the CV responses for the electrochemical oxidation of 0.35 mM methyldopa at the unmodified CPE (curve b), GPE (curve d), 2,7-BFCPE (curve e), and 2,7-BFGPE (curve f). As it is seen, while the anodic peak potential for methyldopa oxidation at the GPE and unmodified CPE are 480 and 520 mV, respectively, the corresponding potential at 2,7-BFGPE and 2,7-BFCPE is approximately 320 mV. These results indicate that the peak potential for methyldopa oxidation at 2,7-BFGPE and 2,7-BFCPE shift by approximately 160 and 200 mV toward negative values compared to GPE and unmodified CPE, respectively. However, 2,7-BFGPE shows much higher anodic peak current for the oxidation of methyldopa compared to 2,7-BFCPE, indicating that the combination of G and the mediator (2,7-BF) has

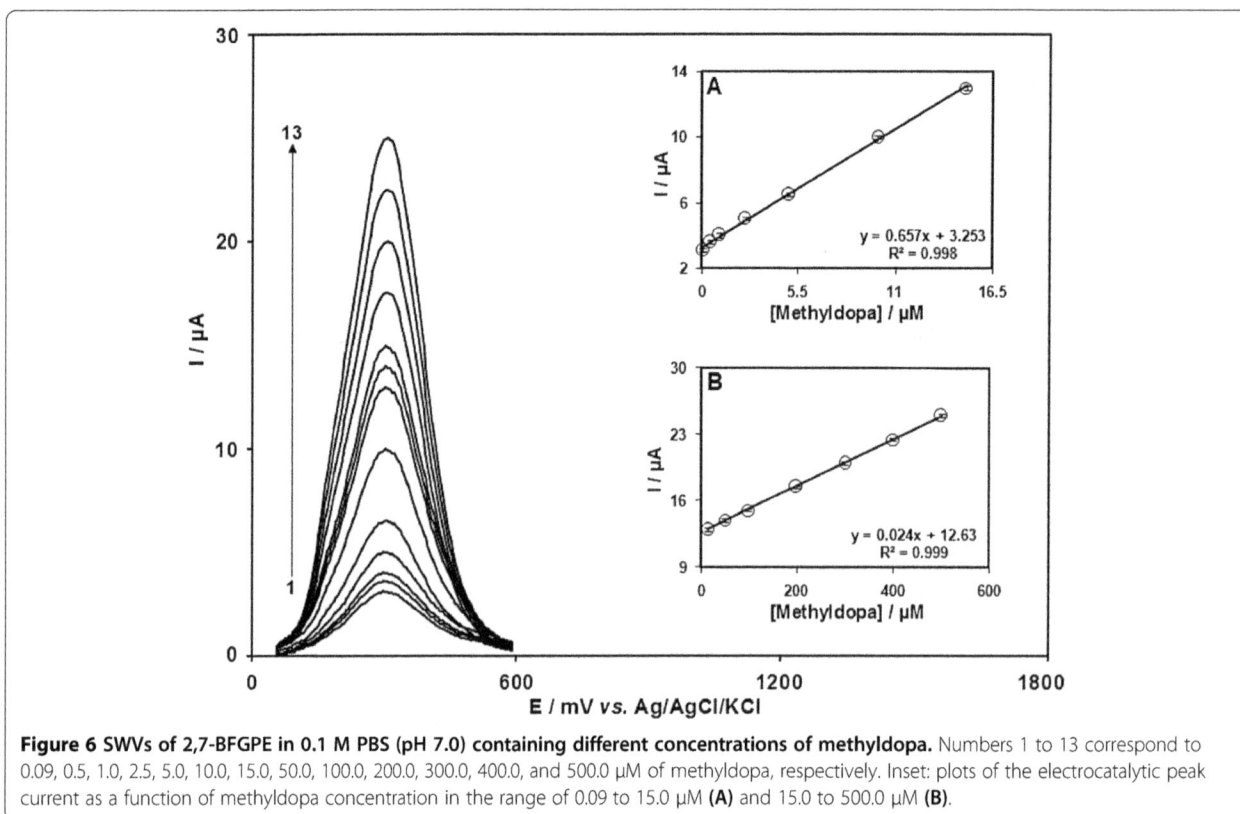

Figure 6 SWVs of 2,7-BFGPE in 0.1 M PBS (pH 7.0) containing different concentrations of methyldopa. Numbers 1 to 13 correspond to 0.09, 0.5, 1.0, 2.5, 5.0, 10.0, 15.0, 50.0, 100.0, 200.0, 300.0, 400.0, and 500.0 μM of methyldopa, respectively. Inset: plots of the electrocatalytic peak current as a function of methyldopa concentration in the range of 0.09 to 15.0 μM (**A**) and 15.0 to 500.0 μM (**B**).

significantly improved the performance of the electrode toward methyldopa oxidation. In fact, 2,7-BFGPE, in the absence of methyldopa, exhibited a well-behaved redox reaction (Figure 2, curve c) in 0.1 M PBS (pH 7.0). However, there was a drastic increase in the anodic peak current in the presence of 0.35 mM methyldopa (curve f), which can be related to the strong electrocatalytic effect of 2,7-BFGPE toward this compound (Bard and Faulkner 2001).

The effect of scan rate on the electrocatalytic oxidation of methyldopa at 2,7-BFGPE was investigated by linear sweep voltammetry (Figure 3). As can be observed in Figure 3, the oxidation peak potential shifted to more positive potentials with increasing scan rate, confirming the kinetic limitation in the electrochemical reaction. Also, a plot of peak height (I_p) vs. the square root of scan rate ($v^{1/2}$) was found to be linear in the range of 2 to 100 mV s^{-1}, suggesting that, at

sufficient overpotential, the process is diffusion- rather than surface-controlled (Figure 3A) (Bard and Faulkner 2001). A plot of the scan rate-normalized current ($I_p/v^{1/2}$) vs. scan rate (Figure 3B) exhibits the characteristic shape typical of an EC process (Bard and Faulkner 2001).

Figure 4 shows the linear sweep voltammograms (LSVs) of an 2,7-BFGPE obtained in 0.1 M PBS (pH 7.0) containing 20.0 μM methyldopa, with a sweep rate of 2 mV s^{-1}. The points show the rising part of the voltammogram (known as the Tafel region), which is affected by the electron transfer kinetics between methyldopa and 2,7-BFGPE. If deprotonation of methyldopa is a sufficiently fast step, the number of electrons involved in the rate-determining step can be estimated from the slope of the Tafel plot. The inset of Figure 4 shows a Tafel plot that was drawn from points of the Tafel region of the LSV. The Tafel slope of

Table 1 Comparison of the efficiency of some modified electrodes used in the electrocatalysis of methyldopa

Electrode	Modifier	Method	pH	Dynamic range (M)	Limit of detection (M)	Reference
Carbon paste	Ferrocene monocarboxylic acid	Voltammetry	7.0	2.0×10^{-7} to 1.0×10^{-4}	8.0×10^{-8}	Molaakbari et al. (2014)
Glassy carbon	Pt-Ru nanoparticles	Voltammetry	3.0	5.0×10^{-8} to 4.0×10^{-5}	1.0×10^{-8}	Shahrokhian and Rastgar (2011)
Carbon paste	Cellulose acetate/ionic liquids	Voltammetry	5.5	3.48×10^{-5} to 3.7×10^{-4}	5.5×10^{-6}	Moccelini et al. (2011)
Carbon nanotube paste	5AEB	Voltammetry	8.0	1.0×10^{-7} to 2.1×10^{-4}	4.8×10^{-8}	Tajik et al. (2013a)
Graphene paste	2,7-BF	Voltammetry	7.0	8.0×10^{-8} to 5.0×10^{-4}	5.0×10^{-8}	This work

Table 2 The application of 2,7-BFGPE for determination of methyldopa in methyldopa tablet and urine samples

Sample	Original content	Spiked	Found	Recovery (%)	R.S.D. (%)
Methyldopa tablet					
	15.0	0	15.3	102.0	3.5
	15.0	5.0	19.8	99.0	1.9
	15.0	1.0	24.4	97.6	2.5
	15.0	15.0	30.5	101.7	2.9
Urine					
	-	7.5	7.4	98.7	1.8
	-	12.5	12.9	103.2	3.1
	-	17.5	17.4	99.4	2.3
	-	22.5	23.1	102.7	2.6

All concentrations are in micromolar ($n = 5$).

0.122 V obtained in this case agrees well with the involvement of one electron in the rate-determining step of the electrode process, assuming a charge transfer coefficient of $\alpha = 0.52$ (Bard and Faulkner 2001).

Chronoamperometric measurements

Chronoamperometric measurements of methyldopa at 2,7-BFGPE were carried out by setting the working electrode potential at 0.4 V (at the first potential step) and at 0.1 V (at the second potential step) vs. Ag/AgCl/KCl (3.0 M) for the various concentrations of methyldopa in buffered aqueous solutions (pH 7.0) (Figure 5). For an electroactive material (methyldopa in this case) with a diffusion coefficient of D, the current observed for the electrochemical reaction at the mass transport-limited condition is described by the Cottrell equation (Bard and Faulkner 2001). Experimental plots of I vs. $t^{-1/2}$ were employed, with the best fits for different concentrations of methyldopa (Figure 5A). The slopes of the resulting straight lines were then plotted vs. the methyldopa concentration (Figure 5B). From the resulting slope and Cottrell equation, the mean value of D was found to be 9.35×10^{-6} cm^2 s^{-1}.

Calibration plot and limit of detection

The Square Wave Voltammetry (SWV) method was used to determine the concentration of methyldopa (initial potential = 0.06 V, end potential = 0.6 V, step potential = 0.001 V, amplitude = 0.02 V, frequency = 10 Hz) (Figure 6). The plot of peak current vs. methyldopa concentration consisted of two linear segments with slopes of 0.657 and 0.024 μA μM^{-1} in the concentration ranges of 0.09 to 15.0 μM and 15.0 to 500.0 μM, respectively. The decrease in sensitivity (slope) of the second linear segment is likely due to kinetic limitation (Bard and Faulkner 2001). The detection limit (3σ) of methyldopa was found to be 50.0 nM. These values are comparable with values reported by other research groups for electrocatalytic oxidation of methyldopa at the surface of chemically modified electrodes by other mediators (Table 1).

Interference studies

The influence of various substances as compounds potentially interfering with the determination of methyldopa was studied under optimum conditions. The potentially interfering substances were chosen from the group of substances commonly found with methyldopa in pharmaceuticals and/or in biological fluids. The tolerance limit was defined as the maximum concentration of the interfering substance that caused an error of less than ±5% in the determination of methyldopa. According to the results, L-lysine, glucose, NADH, acetaminophen, uric acid, L-asparagine, L-serine, L-threonine, L-proline, L-histidine, L-glycine, L-tryptophan, L-phenylalanine, lactose, saccharose, fructose, benzoic acid, methanol, ethanol, urea, caffeine, Mg^{2+}, Al^{3+}, NH$_4^+$, Fe^{2+}, Fe^{3+}, F$^-$, SO$_4^{2-}$, and S^{2-} did not show interference in the determination of methyldopa. However, levodopa, carbidopa, dopamine, and ascorbic acid with equal molar concentration make interference. Although ascorbic acid showed interference, this interference could be minimized, if necessary, by using ascorbic oxidase enzyme, which exhibits a high selectivity to the oxidation of ascorbic acid.

Real sample analysis

Determination of methyldopa in methyldopa tablet and urine samples

In order to evaluate the analytical applicability of the proposed method, it was also applied for the determination of methyldopa in methyldopa tablet (each tablet containing 250 mg methyldopa from Darou-Pakhsh, Tehran, Iran). The results for determination of methyldopa in the methyldopa tablet are given in Table 2. Satisfactory recovery of the experimental results was found for methyldopa. The reproducibility of the method was demonstrated by the mean relative standard deviation (R.S.D.).

Also, in order to evaluate the analytical applicability of the proposed method, it was applied for the determination of methyldopa in urine samples. Known amounts of methyldopa were added to the urine sample, and its concentrations were estimated with the proposed method. The urine sample was found to be free from methyldopa. Therefore, different amounts of methyldopa were spiked to the sample and analyzed by the proposed method. The results for determination of methyldopa in real samples are given in Table 2. Satisfactory recovery of the experimental results was found for methyldopa. The reproducibility of the method was demonstrated by the mean R.S.D.

Conclusions

2,7-BFGPE was prepared and used for the investigation of the electrochemical behavior of methyldopa. Two pairs of well-defined redox peaks were obtained at 2,7-BFGPE. 2,7-BFGPE showed excellent electrocatalytic activity for the redox of methyldopa. Compared with the bare electrode, the oxidation current of methyldopa increased greatly and the oxidation peak potential shifted negatively by 200 mV. This sensor showed a wide linear range (0.09 to 500.0 μM) with good detection limit (0.05 μM) for methyldopa. This sensor was successfully applied to determine methyldopa in some real samples.

Competing interests
The authors declare that they have no competing interests.

Authors' contributions
Hadi Beitollahi, Somayeh Tajik and Hossein Asadi performed the fields of experimental sections and analysis of data. Pourya Biparva synthesized the graphene nanosheets. All authors read and approved the final manuscript.

Author details
[1]Environment Department, Institute of Science and High Technology and Environmental Sciences, Graduate University of Advanced Technology, P.O. Box 76315-117, Kerman, Iran. [2]Department of Chemistry, Shahid Bahonar University of Kerman, P.O. Box 76175-133, Kerman, Iran. [3]Biotechnology Department, Institute of Science and High Technology and Environmental Sciences, Graduate University of Advanced Technology, P.O. Box 76315-117, Kerman, Iran. [4]Department of Basic Sciences, Sari Agricultural Sciences and Natural Resources University, P.O. Box 79316-217, Sari, Iran.

References
Athanasiou-Malaki EM, Koupparis MA (1984) Indirect potentiometric determination of α-amino acids with a copper-selective electrode and determination of dopa and methyldopa in pharmaceutical preparations. Anal Chim Acta 161:349

Bard AJ, Faulkner LR (2001) Electrochemical methods: fundamentals and applications, 2nd edition. Wiley, New York

Beitollahi H, Raoof JB, Hosseinzadeh R (2011a) Application of a carbon-paste electrode modified with 2,7-bis(ferrocenyl ethyl)fluoren-9-one and carbon nanotubes for voltammetric determination of levodopa in the presence of uric acid and folic acid. Electroanalysis 23:1934

Beitollahi H, Raoof JB, Hosseinzadeh R (2011b) Electroanalysis and simultaneous determination of 6-thioguanine in the presence of uric acid and folic acid using a modified carbon nanotube paste electrode. Anal Sci 27:991

Beitollahi H, Taher MA, Ahmadipour M, Hosseinzadeh R (2014c) Electrocatalytic determination of captopril using a modified carbon nanotube paste electrode: application to determination of captopril in pharmaceutical and biological samples. Measurement 47:770

Díaz C, García C, Iturriaga-Vásquez P, Jesús Aguirre M, Pablo Muena J, Contreras R, Ormazábal-Toledo R, Isaacs M (2013) Experimental and theoretical study on the oxidation mechanism of dopamine in n-octyl pyridinium based ionic liquids–carbon paste modified electrodes. Electrochimi Acta 111:846

Dönmez S, Arslan F, Sarı N, Kurnaz Yetim N, Arslan H (2014) Preparation of carbon paste electrodes including poly(styrene) attached glycine–Pt(IV) for amperometric detection of glucose. Biosens Bioelectron 54:146

Gholivand MB, Amiri M (2013) Highly sensitive and selective determination methyldopa in the presence of ascorbic acid using OPPy/TY/Au modified electrode. J Electroanal Chem 694:56

Gholivand MB, Mohammadi-Behzad L (2014) Fabrication of a highly sensitive sumatriptan sensor based on ultrasonic-electrodeposition of Pt nanoparticles on the ZrO₂ nanoparticles modified carbon paste electrode. J Electroanal Chem 712:33

Ghoreishi SM, Behpour M, Golestaneh M (2012) Simultaneous determination of Sunset yellow and Tartrazine in soft drinks using gold nanoparticles, carbon paste electrode. Food Chem 132:637

Hummers WS, Offeman RE (1958) Preparation of graphitic oxide. J Am Chem Soc 80:1339

Huo J, Shangguan E, Li Q (2013) A pre-anodized inlaying ultrathin carbon paste electrode for simultaneous determination of uric acid and folic acid. Electrochim Acta 89:600

Joon OY, Yoo JJ, Kim Y, Il YJK, Yoon HN, Kim JH, Bin Park S (2014) Oxygen functional groups and electrochemical capacitive behavior of incompletely reduced graphene oxides as a thin-film electrode of supercapacitor. Electrochim Acta 116:118

Khoobi A, Ghoreishi SM, Masoum S, Behpour M (2013) Multivariate curve resolution-alternating least squares assisted by voltammetry for simultaneous determination of betaxolol and atenolol using carbon nanotube paste electrode. Bioelectrochemistry 94:100

Kwan KC, Foltz EL, Breault GO, Baer JE, Totaro JA (1976) Pharmacokinetics of methyldopa in man. J Pharmacol Exp Ther 198:264

Li BL, WuZ L, Xiong CH, Luo HQ, Li NB (2012) Anodic stripping voltammetric measurement of trace cadmium at tin-coated carbon paste electrode. Talanta 88:707

Luo JH, Jiao XX, Li NB, Luo HQ (2013) Sensitive determination of Cd(II) by square wave anodic stripping voltammetry with in situ bismuth-modified multiwalled carbon nanotubes doped carbon paste electrodes. J Electroanal Chem 689:130

Ma J, Zhou L, Li C, Yang J, Meng T, Zhou H, Yang M, Yu F, Chen J (2014) Surfactant-free synthesis of graphene-functionalized carbon nanotube film as a catalytic counter electrode in dye-sensitized solar cells. J Power Sour 247:999

Mazloum-Ardakani M, Beitollahi H, Amini MK, Mirkhalaf F, Abdollahi-Alibeik M (2010) New strategy for simultaneous and selective voltammetric determination of norepinephrine, acetaminophen and folic acid using ZrO₂ nanoparticles-modified carbon paste electrode. Sens. Actuators B 151:243

Moccelini SK, Franzoi AC, Vieira IC, Dupont J, Scheeren CW (2011) A novel support for laccase immobilization: cellulose acetate modified with ionic liquid and application in biosensor for methyldopa detection. Biosens Bioelectron 26:3549

Mohammadi S, Beitollahi H, Mohadesi A (2013) Electrochemical behaviour of a modified carbon nanotube paste electrode and its application for simultaneous determination of epinephrine, uric acid and folic acid. Sensor Lett 11:388

Mokhtari A, Karimi-Maleh H, Ensafi AA, Beitollahi H (2012) Application of modified multiwall carbon nanotubes paste electrode for simultaneous voltammetric determination of morphine and diclofenac in biological and pharmaceutical samples. Sens Actuators B 169:96

Molaakbari E, Mostafavi A, Beitollahi H (2014) First report for voltammetric determination of methyldopa in the presence of folic acid and glycine. Mater Sci Engin C 36:168–172

Myhre E, Rugstad HE, Hansen T (1982) Clinical pharmacokinetics of methyldopa. Clin Pharmacokinet 7:221

Oliveira KM, Santos TCC, Dinelli LR, Marinho JZ, Lima RC, Bogado AL (2013) Aggregates of gold nanoparticles with complexes containing ruthenium as modifiers in carbon paste electrodes. Polyhedron 50:410

Ping J, Wang Y, Wu J, Ying Y (2014) Development of an electrochemically reduced graphene oxide modified disposable bismuth film electrode and its application for stripping analysis of heavy metals in milk. Food Chem 151:65

Raoof JB, Ojani R, Beitollahi H, Hossienzadeh R (2006a) Electrocatalytic determination of ascorbic acid at the surface of 2,7-bis(ferrocenyl ethyl) fluoren-9-one modified carbon paste electrode. Electroanalysis 18:1193

Raoof JB, Ojani R, Beitollahi H, Hosseinzadeh R (2006b) Electrocatalytic oxidation and highly selective voltammetric determination of L-cysteine at the surface of a 1-[4-(ferrocenyl ethynyl)phenyl]-1-ethanone modified carbon paste electrode. Anal Sci 22:1213

Raoof JB, Ojani R, Beitollahi H (2007) L-cysteine voltammetry at a carbon paste electrode bulk-modified with ferrocenedicarboxylic acid. Electroanalysis 19:1822

Rezaei B, Askarpour N, Ensafi AA (2013) Adsorptive stripping voltammetric determination of methyldopa on the surface of a carboxylated multiwall carbon nanotubes modified glassy carbon electrode in biological and pharmaceutical samples. Colloids Surf B 109:53

Sanghavi BJ, Mobin SM, Mathur P, Lahiri GK, Srivastava AK (2013) Biomimetic sensor for certain catecholamines employing copper(II) complex and silver nanoparticle modified glassy carbon paste electrode. Biosens Bioelectron 39:124

Shahrokhian S, Rastgar S (2011) Electrodeposition of Pt–Ru nanoparticles on multi-walled carbon nanotubes: application in sensitive voltammetric determination of methyldopa. Electrochim Acta 58:125

Silva H, Pacheco JG, Magalhães JMCS, Viswanathan S, Delerue-Matos C (2014) MIP-graphene-modified glassy carbon electrode for the determination of trimethoprim. Biosens Bioelectron 52:56–61

Sun W, Wang Y, Zhang Y, Ju X, Li G, Sun Z (2012) Poly(methylene blue) functionalized graphene modified carbon ionic liquid electrode for the electrochemical detection of dopamine. Anal Chim Acta 751:59

Tajik S, Taher MA, Beitollahi H (2013a) First report for simultaneous determination of methyldopa and hydrochlorothiazide using a nanostructured based electrochemical sensor. J Electroanal Chem 704:137

Tajik S, Taher MA, Beitollahi H (2013b) Simultaneous determination of droxidopa and carbidopa using a carbon nanotubes paste electrode. Sens Actuators B 188:923

Taleat Z, Mazloum Ardakani M, Naeimi H, Beitollahi H, Nejati M, Zare HR (2008) Electrochemical behavior of ascorbic acid at a 2,2'-[3,6-dioxa-1,8-octanediylbis (nitriloethylidyne)]-bis-hydroquinone carbon paste electrode. Anal Sci 24:1039

Thomas T, Mascarenhas RJ, Cotta F, Guha KS, Kumara Swamy BE, Martis P, Mekhalif Z (2013a) Poly(Patton and Reeder's reagent) modified carbon paste electrode for the sensitive detection of acetaminophen in biological fluid and pharmaceutical formulations. Colloids Surf B 101:91

Thomas T, Mascarenhas RJ, D'Souza OJ, Martis P, Dalhalle J, Kumara Swamy BE (2013b) Multi-walled carbon nanotube modified carbon paste electrode as a sensor for the amperometric detection of L-tryptophan in biological samples. J Colloid Interf Sci 402:223

Thomas T, Mascarenhas RJ, Kumara Swamy BE, Martis P, Mekhalif Z, Sherigara BS (2013c) Multi-walled carbon nanotube/poly(glycine) modified carbon paste electrode for the determination of dopamine in biological fluids and pharmaceuticals. Colloids Surf B 110:458

Xi F, Zhao D, Wang X, Chen P (2013) Non-enzymatic detection of hydrogen peroxide using a functionalized three-dimensional graphene electrode. Electrochem Commun 26:81

Yildiz G, Oztekin N, Orbay A, Senkal F (2014) Voltammetric determination of nitrite in meat products using polyvinylimidazole modified carbon paste electrode. Food Chem 152:245

Zhu W, Chen T, Ma X, Ma H, Chen S (2013) Highly sensitive and selective detection of dopamine based on hollow gold nanoparticles-graphene nanocomposite modified electrode. Colloids Surfaces B 111:321

22

Development and validation of RP-HPLC method for glimepiride and its application for a novel self-nanoemulsifying powder (SNEP) formulation analysis and dissolution study

Abdul Bari Mohd[1], Krishna Sanka[2], Rakesh Gullapelly[2], Prakash V Diwan[1] and Nalini Shastri[3]*

Abstract

Background: There are many analytical methods available for estimation of glimepiride in biological samples and pharmaceutical preparations. To our knowledge, there is no specific reverse-phase high-performance liquid chromatography (RP-HPLC) method for estimation of glimepiride and its dissolution study in self-nanoemulsifying powder (SNEP) formulation.

Methods: A simple method was carried out on a 5-μm particle octadesyl silane (ODS) column (250×4.6 mm) with acetonitrile: 0.2 M phosphate buffer (pH = 7.4) 40:60 *v/v* as a mobile phase at a flow rate of 1 mL/min, and quantification was achieved at 228 nm using PDA detector.

Results: The correlation coefficient (r^2) was found to be 0.999 over the concentration range of 0.2 to 2 μg/mL for glimepiride. The method was validated for linearity, accuracy, and precision. The limit of detection and limit of quantification were found to be 0.38 and 1.17 μg/mL, respectively.

Conclusions: The proposed method was found to be simple, precise, suitable, and accurate for quantification of glimepiride as an alternative to the existing methods for the routine analysis of glimepiride in pharmaceutical formulations and *in vitro* dissolution studies.

Keywords: Glimepiride; Self-nanoemulsifying powder; RP-HPLC method; PDA detector; *In vitro* dissolution studies

Background

Glimepiride (GLM), a potent first III-generation sulfonylurea derivative is widely used in the treatment of non-insulin-dependent type II diabetes mellitus as an oral hypoglycemic agent (Langtry and Balfour 1998; McCall 2001; Rosenstock et al. 1996). Chemically, it is 1-{(p-[2-(3-ethyl-4-methyl-2-oxo-3-pyrroline-1-carboxamide) ethyl] phenyl) sulfonyl}-3-(trans-4-methylcyclohexyl) urea (Figure 1).

Like other sulfonylureas, GLM acts as an insulin secretagogue (Davis 2004) lowering blood glucose by stimulating insulin secretions from functioning pancreatic beta cells and by inducing extra-pancreatic effects (increasing sensitivity of peripheral tissues to insulin) thereby

decreasing the insulin resistance. GLM potentially binds to ATP-sensitive potassium channel receptors on the pancreatic beta cell surface, dropping potassium conductance across the membrane and causing depolarization of the membrane which stimulates calcium ion influx through voltage-sensitive calcium channels. This increase in intracellular calcium ion concentration induces the secretion of insulin. It can be employed for concomitant use with metformin, thiazolidinediones, alpha-glucosidase inhibitors and insulin for the treatment of noninsulin-dependent (type II) diabetes mellitus (Bell 2004). After oral administration, it is completely absorbed from the gastrointestinal tract. Severe hypoglycemic reactions with coma, seizure, or other neurological impairment are the possible toxic effects. Other side effects of sulfonylureas include nausea and vomiting, cholestatic jaundice, agranulocytosis, aplastic and hemolytic anemias, generalized

---
* Correspondence: svcphod@yahoo.co.in
[3]Department of Pharmaceutics, National Institute of Pharmaceutical Education and Research (NIPER), Hyderabad 500 037, AP, India
Full list of author information is available at the end of the article

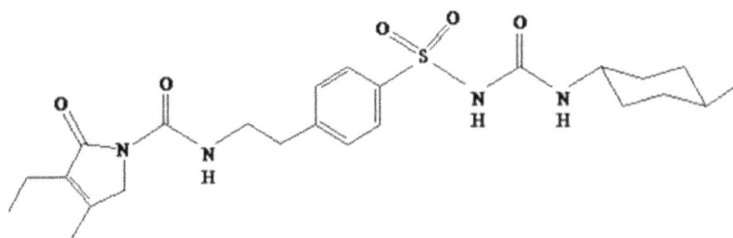

Figure 1 Structure of glimepiride.

hypersensitivity reactions, and rashes (Goodman and Gilman 2008).

Comprehensive literature survey revealed that quite a few diverse methods have been reported for qualitative and quantitative analysis of GLM in biological samples plasma/serum/urine and in pharmaceutical formulations containing single drug as well as in combination with other drugs. These include miceller electrokinetic capillary chromatography (MEEC) with diode-array detection (DAD) or ultraviolet (UV) detection (Nunez et al. 1995; Roche et al. 1997), high-performance liquid chromatography (HPLC) with DAD (Drummer et al. 1993) and UV detection (Jingar et al. 2008) and derivate UV spectrometric detection (Altinoz and Tekeli 2001), using semimicro bore high-performance liquid chromatography with column switching (Song et al. 2004), with pre-column derivatization (Lehr and Damm 1990), using monolithic column and flow program (El Deeb et al. 2006), HPLC-first derivative spectroscopy (Khan et al. 2009), reverse-phase high performance column chromatography (RP-HPLC, Sujatha et al. 2011; Wanjari and Gaikwad 2005), other HPLC methods (Kovaríkova et al. 2004; Lydia et al. 2005), liquid chromatography-electrospray ionization-tandem mass spectrometry (LC-ESI-MS, Kim et al. 2004a, b; Salem et al. 2004), liquid chromatography-mass spectroscopy (LC-MS, Chang et al. 2004; Yuzuak et al. 2007), and other liquid chromatographic techniques (Pathare et al. 2007; Sukumar et al. 2005), thin layer chromatography (TLC) (Valentina et al. 2013; Gumieniczeka et al. 2009), polarographic determination (Ma et al. 2005), square-wave voltammetric technique (Suslu and Altinoz 2011). Methods have also been developed for the estimation of GLM in combination with other drugs simultaneously in pharmaceutical formulations by RP-HPLC techniques (Deepti et al. 2008; Ravi et al. 2011; El-Enany et al. 2012). From the literature survey, it was concluded that HPLC methods have been used most extensively for analysis of GLM (Bonfilio et al. 2010).

Most of the earlier methods are not ideal since they are time-consuming, have high limits of detections, use of surplus organic solvents, strenuous sample preparation, involve expensive instrumentation and long chromatographic run times. In recent years, dissolution studies have emerged in the pharmaceutical field as a very imperative tool based on the reality that for a drug to be absorbed and available to the systemic circulation, it must previously be solubilized. Consequently, the dissolution studies are used not only to evaluate batch-to-batch consistency of drug release from solid dosage forms, but also in several crucial stages of formulation development, for screening and proper assessment of different formulations. Moreover, the information obtained from *in vitro* dissolution studies has been used for the successful characterization of the *in vivo* behavior of drugs. To our knowledge, there is no specific RP-HPLC method for quantification and assessing dissolution rate profile for GLM in self-nanoemulsifying powder (SNEP) formulation.

The main purpose of the present work was to develop and validate a simple RP-HPLC method to be applied for the quantification and dissolution studies of GLM in SNEP formulation. The developed and validated method is rapid, reproducible with simple mobile phase, trouble-free sample preparation steps, improved sensitivity and a short chromatographic run time, which therefore serves as a tool for the quality control of pharmaceutical dosage forms.

Experimental

Materials and methods

Glimepiride was a gift sample from Dr. Reddy's Laboratories Ltd, Hyderabad, India and was used without further purification. Amaryl® tablets containing 2 mg GLM as per labels claim (manufactured by Sun Pharmaceutical Industries, Mumbai, Maharashtra, India) were obtained from a local pharmacy. Methanol and acetonitrile of HPLC grade were procured from E. Merck Ltd., Mumbai, India. Sodium hydroxide, sodium dihydrogen phosphate, ortho phosphoric acid, TEA of AR grade, sesame oil, Tween® 20, PEG 400, and Aerosil® 200 were obtained from SD Fine Chemicals Ltd. Mumbai, India. Purified HPLC grade water was obtained by reverse osmosis and filtration through a Milli-Q® system (Millipore, Milford, MA, USA), and the same was used to prepare all solutions.

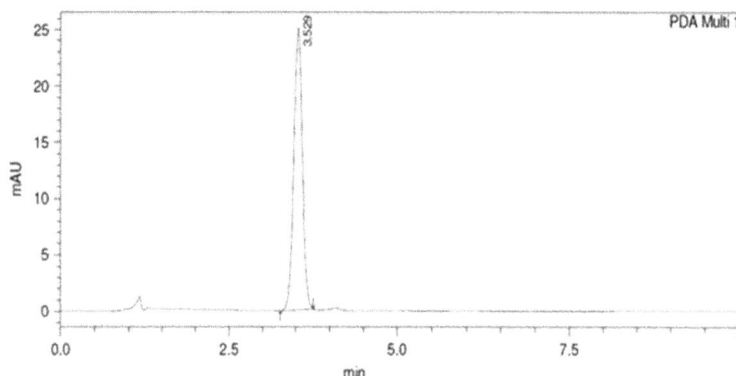

Figure 2 Typical chromatogram of GLM standard.

HPLC instrumentation and chromatographic conditions

The HPLC analysis was carried out on Shimadzu HPLC-LC-20 AD series binary gradient pump with Shimadzu SPD-M20A detector (Tokyo, Japan). The column used was Phenomenex Luna C18 (2) (250 × 4.6 mm) packed with 5 μm particles. The injection volume of sample 20 μL was used in all the experiments. In an isocratic mobile phase containing acetonitrile and 0.2 M phosphate buffer (pH 7.4), 40:60 (v/v) was pumped through the column with a flow rate of 1 mL/min and the quantification was achieved at 228 nm using PDA detector. The mobile phase was filtered through a 0.45-μm membrane filter and degassed before use.

Methods

Preparation of liquid self-nanoemulsifying drug delivery system and self-nanoemulsifying powder formulation

The vehicle (sesame oil), surfactant (Tween® 20), and co-surfactants (PEG 400) were selected for the preparation of self-nanoemulsifying drug delivery systems (SNEDDS). The formulation was prepared by dissolving GLM in the mixture of oil, surfactant, and co-surfactant accurately weighed in glass vials. Then, the components were mixed by gentle stirring and vortex mixing using vortex mixer (REMI CM 101DX, REMI Equipment, Mumbai, India) and heated at 50 °C in an isothermal water bath to obtain a homogenous isotropic mixture. The final formulation was inspected for signs of turbidity or phase separation and drug precipitation prior to self-emulsification. The formulation was stored at ambient temperature for further use. The simplest technique to convert liquid SNEDDS to SNEP is, by adsorption onto the surface of carriers. In the present study, Aerosil® 200 was used as an adsorption carrier. SNEP was prepared by mixing liquid SNEDDS containing GLM with Aerosil® 200 in 1:1 proportion. In brief, liquid SNEDDS was added drop wise over Aerosil® 200 contained in a broad porcelain dish. After each addition, mixture was homogenized using glass rod to ensure uniform distribution of formulation. Resultant damp mass was passed through sieve no. 120 and dried at ambient temperature. Then the dose-equivalent free-flow powder was filled into hard gelatin capsules and stored until further use.

Preparation of stock and standard solutions

A stock solution of 100 μg/mL was prepared by transferring 10 mg of GLM into a 100-mL volumetric flask; 30 mL of 0.1 N NaOH was added, and the mixture was sonicated to dissolve and the final volume of the solution was made up with HPLC grade methanol. The stock solution was protected from light using aluminum foil and aliquots of the standard stock solution of GLM were transferred using A-grade bulb pipettes into 10-mL volumetric flasks and the solutions were made up to volume with mobile phase to give final concentrations in the range of 0.2, 0.4, 0.8, 0.9, 1.2, 1.4, and 2 μg/mL.

Method validation

The optimized chromatographic method was completely validated according to the procedures described in ICH guidelines Q2 (R1) for the validation of analytical methods.

Table 1 Optimized chromatographic conditions

Stationary phase (column)	Phenomenex luna C1 (250 × 4.5 mm) packed with 5 μm particles
Mobile phase	Acetonitrile, 0.2 M phosphate buffer (pH 7.4) 40:60 (v/v)
Detection wave length (nm)	228
Run time (min)	10
Flow rate (mL/min)	1
Volume of injection loop (μL)	20
Column temperature	Ambient
Glimepiride R_t (min)	3.543

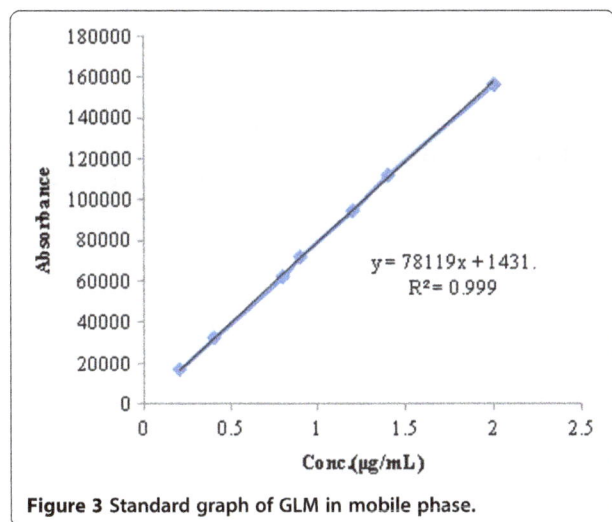

Figure 3 Standard graph of GLM in mobile phase.

The equation shown on the graph:

$$y = 78119x + 1431.$$
$$R^2 = 0.999$$

Table 3 System suitability parameters

Concentration	Injection	Area	R_t (min)
1.2 µg/mL	Inj-1	95,187	3.54
	Inj-2	95,245	3.52
	Inj-3	95,307	3.52
	Inj-4	95,377	3.53
	Inj-5	95,442	3.54
	Inj-6	95,517	3.52
	Mean	95,345.83	3.528
	SD	123.62	0.00983
Statistical analysis	%RSD	0.129	0.278
	Tailing factor	0.899	
	Plate count	1,771.634	

Linearity and range

Standard stock solution was diluted to prepare solutions containing 0.2 to 2 µg/mL of the GLM. The solutions were injected in triplicate into the HPLC column, keeping the injection volume constant (20 µL).

System suitability

Twenty microliters of the standard solution (1.2 µg/mL) was injected six times under optimized chromatographic conditions to evaluate the suitability of the system.

Precision

Three injections, of two different concentrations (1.2 and 1.4 µg/mL), were given on the same day and the values of percent relative standard deviation (%RSD) were calculated to determine intra-day precision. These studies were also repeated on different days to determine inter-day precision.

Accuracy

Accuracy was evaluated by fortifying a mixture of common excipient solutions with two known GLM reference standards. The recovery of the added drug was determined.

Specificity

To ascertain specificity, a placebo solution was prepared using the same excipients as those are present in the marketed tablet without GLM. Placebo solution was injected into the HPLC system under the optimized test conditions and the chromatogram was recorded. Responses of the peaks were noted for any possible interferences of the excipient at the retention time of the GLM.

Limit of detection and limit of quantification

The limit of detection (LOD) is the lowest amount of analyte that can be detected in a sample, but not necessarily quantified, under the stated experimental conditions. The limit of quantification (LOQ) was identified as the lowest plasma concentration of the standard curve that could be quantified with acceptable accuracy, precision, and variability. They are determined by the signal-to-noise method.

Assay

For the analysis of marketed formulation Amaryl®, 20 tablets were accurately weighed and powdered. The powder equivalent to 1.0 mg of GLM was weighed accurately and transferred to a 10-mL volumetric flask containing 1.0 mL of 0.1 N NaOH. The mixture was sonicated to dissolve, made up the volume with methanol and filtered through a 0.45-µm membrane filter. Aliquots of

Table 2 Linearity parameter for glimepiride

Conc. (µg/mL)	Area
0.2	17,055.22
0.4	32,679
0.8	62,567.25
0.9	72,346.5
1.2	95,187
1.4	112,383
2.0	156,821

Table 4 Reproducibility and precision data evaluated through intra-day and inter-day studies

Conc. (µg/mL)	Intra-day ($n = 3$)		Inter-day ($n = 3$)	
	Mean peak area ± SD ($n = 3$)	%RSD	Mean peak area ± SD ($n = 3$)	%RSD
1.2	95,187 ± 605	0.63	96,391 ± 426	0.44
1.4	112,849 ± 1,077	0.95	115,782 ± 1,121	0.96
2.0	165,844 ± 1,317	0.79	169,267 ± 541	0.319

Table 5 Recovery studies

Actual conc. (μg/mL)	Calculated conc. (μg/mL) ± SD ($n = 3$)	%RSD	%Recovery
1.2	1.1983 ± 0.00153	0.127	99.87
1.4	1.403 ± 0.01058	0.754	100.3

this standard solution were transferred using A-grade bulb pipettes into 10-mL volumetric flasks, and the solutions were made up to volume with mobile phase to give final concentration of 10 μg/mL. The above solution was then analyzed for the content of GLM using the proposed method.

Dissolution release study of pure drug, marketed and SNEPS formulation

The dissolution studies of GLM-loaded SNEP formulation was performed in a USP-II dissolution test apparatus (DS 8000, LABINDIA, Mumbai, India). The dissolution

studies were conducted according to the dissolution procedure recommended for single-entity products in 900 mL of 0.1 N HCl (75 rpm). The temperature of the cell was maintained at 37 ± 0.5 °C by using a thermostatic bath. At predetermined time intervals (0, 5, 10, 15, 30, 60, 90, and 120 min) an aliquot (5 mL) of the sample was withdrawn from each vessel and immediately replaced with an equal volume of fresh medium to maintain sink conditions. The samples collected were filtered through a membrane filter (0.45 μm) and further analyzed by HPLC. In order to obtain the dissolution profile, the cumulative percentage of drug released was plotted against time (min).

Results and discussion
Method development

Development of new HPLC methods are often useful in regular quality control assessment of pharmaceuticals which may convey relevant information in establishing

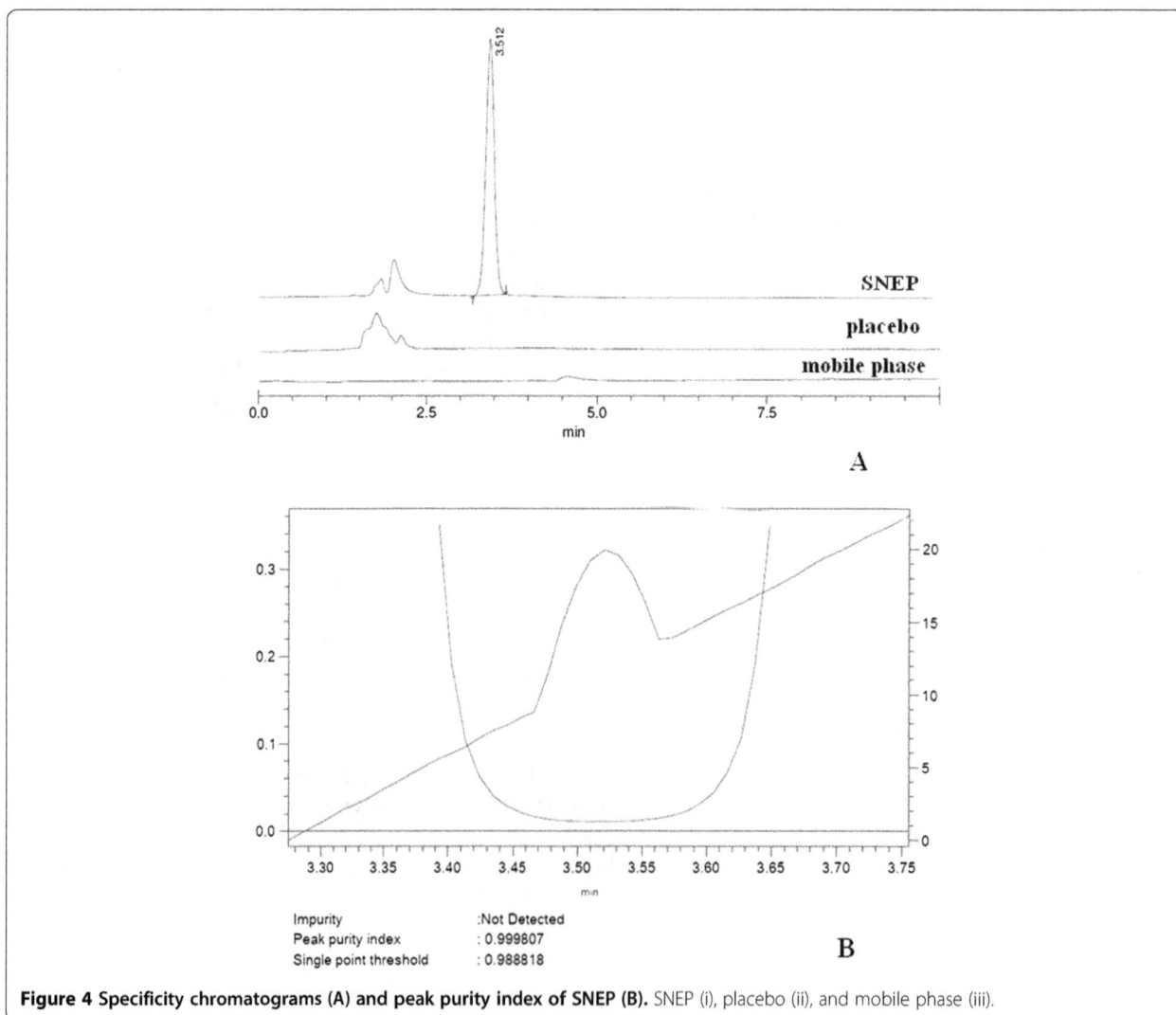

Figure 4 Specificity chromatograms (A) and peak purity index of SNEP (B). SNEP (i), placebo (ii), and mobile phase (iii).

optimal experimental conditions for the better usage of drugs. In this study, a simple, specific, selective, and accurate RP-HPLC method to quantify and to study drug release profile of GLM was developed and validated according to ICH guidelines. Acetonitrile and 0.2 M phosphate buffer (pH 7.4) in different proportions were tried, and finally, a ratio of acetonitrile - 0.2 M phosphate buffer (pH 7.4) (40:60) - was selected as an appropriate combination which gave good resolution and acceptable system suitability parameters. The chromatogram of working standard of GLM solution was shown in Figure 2. Optimized chromatographic conditions were given in Table 1. The mobile phase was filtered through a 0.45-μm membrane filter before use. The contents were finally transferred to solvent reservoir of the LC20AD pump and purged the solvent line with 30 mL of fresh mobile phase.

Linearity

The required test samples were prepared freshly using the stock solution in the range of 0.2 to 2 μg/mL (GLM). Triplicate 20-μL injections were made for each

concentration and were analyzed under the conditions optimized chromatographic conditions. A calibration curve was obtained by plotting the response (peak area) versus concentration of drug and represented in Figure 3. Linearity parameter for GLM was given in Table 2.

System suitability

System suitability tests were carried out on freshly prepared standard stock solutions of GLM and it was calculated by determining the standard deviation of GLM standards by injecting in six replicates at short time intervals and the peak areas were recorded and represented in Table 3.

Precision

The precision of the method was demonstrated by inter-day and intra-day variation studies. In the intra-day studies, solutions of the standard and the sample were repeated thrice in a day, and %RSD for the response factor was calculated; the results were tabulated in Table 4. The %RSD values in the two cases were <2%, which indicates that the method was sufficiently precise.

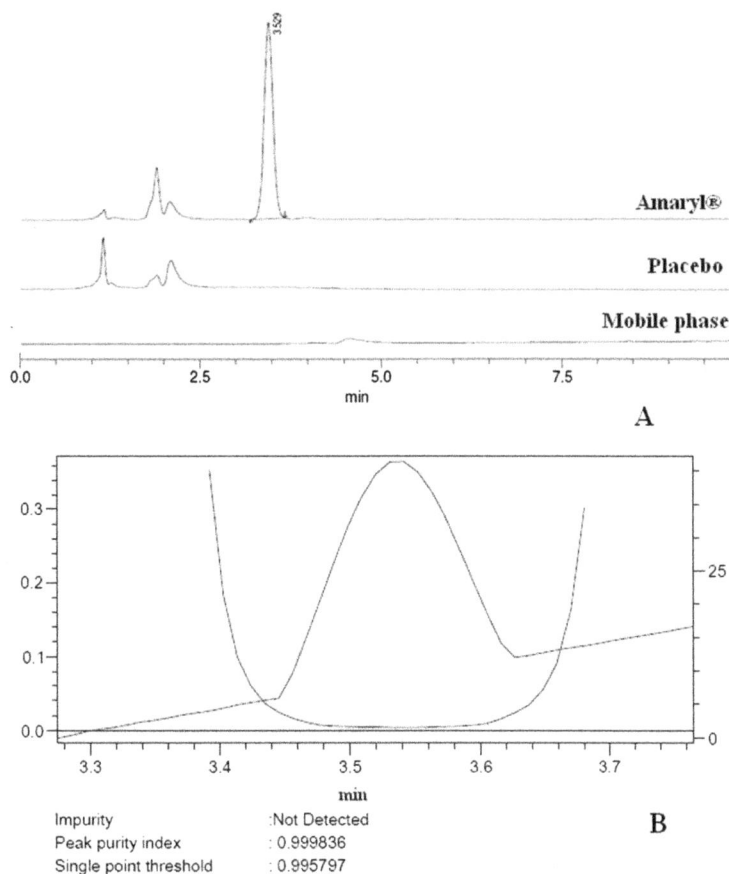

Figure 5 Specificity chromatograms (A) and peak purity index of Amaryl® (B). Amaryl® (i), Placebo (ii), and Mobile phase (iii).

Accuracy

The accuracy of the method was determined by recovery experiments. The recovery studies were performed by using standard addition method. GLM reference standards were accurately weighed and added to the fixed concentration of self-nanoemulsifying powder at different concentration levels (1.2 and 1.4 µg/mL). Percent recovery was calculated by comparing the area before and after the addition of reference standard. The recovery studies were performed in triplicate. Percent recovery was within the range of 99.8% to 100.3% as shown in Table 5 for GLM which indicates that the method was accurate.

Specificity and selectivity

Specificity was tested against standard compounds and possible interference peaks in the presence of placebo under optimized test conditions. The comparison of the chromatograms of the placebo mixture and the spiked drug solution revealed that there were no additional peaks co-eluting with the peaks of GLM in the sample solution. No interference from the placebo was observed at the retention time of the GLM (Figure 4A and Figure 5A). Therefore, it was concluded that the method is specific and can assess unequivocally the analyte of the interest in the presence of possible interferences. Peak purity indices for SNEP and Amaryl® are shown in Figures 4B in 5B.

Limit of detection and limit of quantification

Standard stock solutions of GLM (1 mg/mL) were prepared. Standard solutions of GLM (0.2, 0.4, 0.8, 0.9, 1.2, 1.4, and 2 µg/mL) were prepared by diluting the standard stock solutions with mobile phase. The LOD and LOQ GLM under the present chromatographic conditions were estimated at a signal-to-noise ratio (S/N) of 3:1 and 10:1 respectively, by injecting a series of diluted solutions with known concentrations. The LOD and

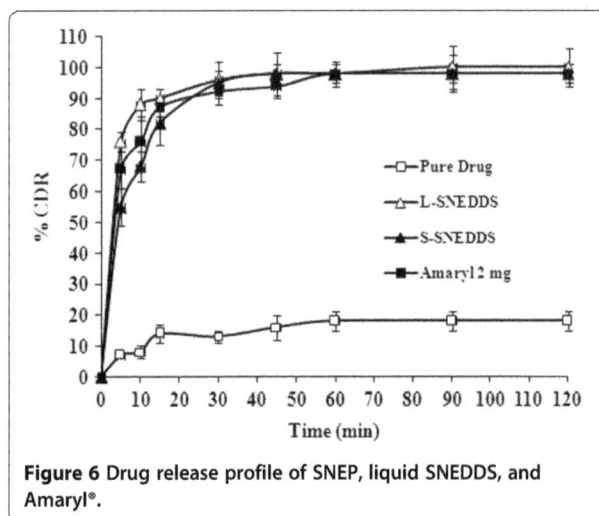

Figure 6 Drug release profile of SNEP, liquid SNEDDS, and Amaryl®.

Table 6 Robustness study

System suitability parameters (variations)		%RSD peak area ($n = 6$)	Mean tailing factor ($n = 6$)	Mean R_t (min) ($n = 6$)
Varied pH (±0.2%)	7.2	1.354	0.875	0.321
	7.6	1.371	0.858	0.336
Mobile phase ratio (±20 v/v)	60:40	1.362	0.891	0.338
	20:80	1.348	0.915	0.346

LOQ for GLM were found to be 0.38 and 1.17 µg/mL, respectively.

Robustness

Robustness of the method was checked by making slight changes in chromatographic conditions like mobile phase ratio, pH of buffer, flow rate. It was observed that there were no noticeable changes in chromatograms, which demonstrated that the developed RP-HPLC method is robust and is represented in Table 6.

Assay of marketed tablets

The results of assay of marketed tablets Amaryl® as described earlier showed good conformity with the label claim and the assay values are represented in Table 7.

In vitro dissolution study

A dissolution release study was carried out for liquid SNEDDS, SNEP of GLM, and marketed formulation Amaryl®. As evident from the drug release profiles, the % CDR of pure drug, liquid SNEDDS, SNEP and Amaryl® were 14.68 ± 3.88, 90.36 ± 3.74, 82.22 ± 7.32, and 87.3 ± 2.84, respectively at the 15th min. The results indicate instantaneous and remarkably higher and faster dissolution rate of GLM from SNEP, liquid SNEDDS, and marketed formulation compared to pure drug. The % CDR profile for liquid SNEDDS, SNEP of GLM, and Amaryl® are shown in Figure 6.

Conclusion

The proposed method was rapid, accurate, precise, and sensitive for the quantification of GLM from its pharmaceutical dosage forms. The method relies on the use of simple working procedure; hence, this method can be routinely employed in quality control for analysis of GLM in pharmaceutical dosage forms and dissolution studies.

Table 7 Assay of GLM marketed tablets Amaryl® ($n = 3$)

Label claim (mg/tab)	Mean estimated amt (mg)	%Label claim ± SD	%RSD
2	1.995	99.75 ± 0.4712	0.4723
2	2.0048	100.24 ± 0.5234	0.5221
2	2.0064	100.32 ± 0.4372	0.4358

Competing interests
The authors declare that they have no competing interests.

Acknowledgements
The authors greatly acknowledge the receipt of pure GLM from Dr. Reddy's Laboratories Ltd, Hyderabad, India and are also thankful to Dr. P. Rajeshwar Reddy, Chairman, School of Pharmacy (Anurag Group of Institutions) Hyderabad for providing research facilities throughout the project work.

Author details
[1]Department of Pharmaceutics, School of Pharmacy, Nalla Narasimha Reddy Educational Society's Group of Institutions, Hyderabad -500088, AP, India. [2]Department of Pharmaceutics, School of Pharmacy, Anurag Group of Institutions, Hyderabad -500088, AP, India. [3]Department of Pharmaceutics, National Institute of Pharmaceutical Education and Research (NIPER), Hyderabad 500 037, AP, India.

References

Altinoz S, Tekeli D (2001) Analysis of glimepiride by using derivative UV spectrophotometric method. J Pharm Biomed Anal 24(3):507–515

Bell DS (2004) Practical Considerations and Guidelines for Dosing Sulfonylureas in Monotherapy or Combination Therapy. Clin Ther 26(11):1714–1727

Bonfilio Rudy MD, Araújo D, Benjamim M, Regina Nunes SH (2010) A Review of Analytical Techniques for Determination of Glimepiride: Present and Perspectives. Ther Drug Monit 32(5):550–559

Davis SN (2004) The Role of Glimepiride in the Effective Management of Type 2 Diabetes. J Diabetes Complicat 18(6):367–376

Deepti J, Surendra J, Deepak J, Maulik A (2008) Simultaneous Estimation of Metformin Hydrochloride, Pioglitazone Hydrochloride, and Glimepiride by RP-HPLC in Tablet Formulation. J Chromatogr Sci 46:501–504

Drummer OH, Kotsos A, McIntyre IM (1993) J Anal Toxicol 17:225–229

El Deeb S, Schepers U, Watzig H (2006) Fast HPLC method for the determination of glimepiride, glibenclamide, and related substances using monolithic column and flow program. J Sep Sci 29(11):1571–7

El-Enany NM, Abdelal AA, Belal FF, Itoh YI, Nakamura MN (2012) Development and validation of a reversed phase-HPLC method for simultaneous determination of rosiglitazone and glimepiride in combined dosage forms and human plasma. Chem Cent J 6(9):1–10

Goodman & Gilman (2008) Manual of Pharmacology and Therapeutics. Mc Graw Hill, New York, pp 1037–1058

Gumieniczeka A, Hopkałab H, Bereckab A (2009) Ant diabetic Drugs: HPLC/TLC Determination. Encyclopedia of Chromatography, 3 [rd] edn. vol II.

Jingar JN, Rajput SJ, Dasandi B, Rathnam S (2008) Development and Validation of LC-UV for Simultaneous Estimation of Rosiglitazone and Glimepiride in Human Plasma. Chromatographia 67(11–12):951–955

Khan IU, Aslam F, Ashfaq M, Asghar MN (2009) Determination of Glimepiride in Pharmaceutical Formulations Using High-Performance Liquid Chromatography and First-Derivative Spectrophotometric Methods. J Anal Chem 64(2):171–175

Kim H, Chang KY, Lee HJ, Han SB (2004a) Determination of Glimepiride in Human Plasma by Liquid Chromatography-Electro spray Ionization Tandem Mass Spectrometry. Bull Korean Chem Soc 25(1):109–114

Kim H, Chang KY, Park CH, Jang MS, Lee JA, Lee HJ, Lee KR (2004b) Determination of Glimepiride in Human Plasma by LC-MS-MS and Comparison of Sample Preparation Methods for Glimepiride. Chromatographia 60(1–2):93–98

Kovaríkova P, Klimes J, Dohnal J, Tisovska L (2004) HPLC study of glimepiride under hydrolytic stress conditions. J Pharm Biomed Anal 36(1):205–9

Langtry HD, Balfour JA (1998) Glimepiride: A review of its use in the management of type 2 diabetics. Drugs 55:563–84

Lehr KH, Damm P (1990) Simultaneous Determination of the Sulphonylurea Glimepiride and Its Metabolites in Human Serum and Urine by High-Performance Liquid Chromatography after Pre-Column Derivatization. J Chromatogr B 526(1):497–505

Lydia RK, Rita AD, Dolla KS, Chawki A, Antoine Z (2005) A Simple and Sensitive Method for Determination of Glimepiride in Human Serum by HPLC. J of Liq Chromatogr R T 28(20):3255–3263

Ma HL, Xu MT, Qu P, Ma XH (2005) Polarographic behavior and determination of glimepiride. Acta Pharmaceut Se 40(8):750–3

McCall AL (2001) Clinical Review of Glimepiride. Expert Opinion on Pharmacotherapy 2(4):699–713

Nunez M, Ferguson JE, Machacek D, Jacob G, Oda RP, Lawson GM, Landers JP (1995) Anal Chem 67:3668–3675

Pathare DB, Jadhav AS, Shingare MS (2007) RP-LC Determination of the Cis-Isomer of Glimepiride in a Bulk Drug Substance. Chromatographia 66(7–8):639–641

Ravi S, Gagan S, Darpan C, Jain PK (2011) Analytical Method Development And Validation For The Simultaneous Estimation Of Pioglitazone And Glimepiride In Tablet Dosage Form By RP-HPLC. Int J Pharm Sci Res 2(3):637–642

Roche ME, Oda RP, Lawson GM, Landers JP (1997) Capillary Electrophoretic Detection of Metabolites in the Urine of Patients Receiving Hypoglycemic Drug Therapy. Electrophoresis 18(10):1865–1874

Rosenstock J, Samols E, Muchmore DB, Schneider J (1996) Glimepiride, a New Once-Daily Sulfonylurea: A Double-Blind Placebo-Controlled Study of NIDDM Patients. Diabetes Care 19(11):1194–1199

Salem II, Idrees J, Al Tamimi JI (2004) Determination of Glimepiride in Human Plasma by Liquid Chromatography-Electro spray Ionization Tandem Mass Spectrometry. J Chromatogr B Analyt Technol Biomed Life Sci 799(1):103–9

Song YK, Maeng JE, Hwang HR, Park JS, Kim BC, Kim JK, Kim CK (2004) Determination of glimepiride in human plasma using semi-micro bore high performance liquid chromatography with column-switching. J Chromatogr B 810(1):143–149

Sujatha S, Sandhya RT, Veeresham C (2011) Determination of Glimepiride in Rat Serum by RP-HPLC Method. Am J Anal Chem 2:152–157

Suslu I, Altinoz S (2011) Determination of Glimepiride in Pharmaceutical Formulations by Square-Wave Voltammetric Method. Curr Anal Chem 7(4):333–340

Valentina T, Slavica F, Gordana P, Katarina N, Danica A (2013) TLC Determination Of Glimepiride And Its Main Impurities In Pharmaceuticals. J of Liq Chromatogr R T 36(17):2422–2430

Wanjari DB, Gaikwad NJ (2005) Reversed Phase HPLC Method for Determination of Glimepride in Tablet Dosage Form. Indian J Pharm sci 2(67):253–255

Yuzuak N, Ozden T, Eren S, Ozilhan S (2007) Determination of Glimepiride in Human Plasma by LC-MS-MS. Chromatographia 66(1):165–168

23

Neural substrates associated with humor processing

Jihye Noh[1], Ji-woo Seok[2], Suk-Hee Kim[3], Chaejoon Cheong[1] and Jin-Hun Sohn[2*]

Abstract

Background: Humor is composed of a cognitive element related to the detection of humor and an affective element related to the appreciation of humor. To investigate activated areas of the brain related to the two components of humor and to identify neural substrates associated with the degree of humor intensity, 13 participants were scanned while watching cartoons.

Findings: While watching humorous scenes, various areas of the brain were activated, including (1) the inferior gyrus, an area involved in reconciling ambiguous semantic content with stored knowledge, and (2) the temporal gyrus and fusiform gyrus, brain regions associated with the feeling of mirth. Further, humor intensity was positively correlated with BOLD signal magnitude in the nucleus accumbens, a region known to be involved in psychologically and psychopharmacologically driven rewards.

Conclusions: Our findings demonstrate a two-component neural circuit model of humor processing and a key region important in pleasurable feelings accompanied by humor.

Keywords: Emotion; Humor; Detection; Appreciation; Event-related fMRI

Findings

Humor plays a central and unique role in human life. Without humor, life would undeniably be less exhilarating. Humor provides an effective means of communicating ideas, attracting partners, boosting mood, and even coping in times of trauma and stress (Brownell and Gardner 1988; Dixon 1980; Garilovic et al. 2003; Martin 2001; Mobbs et al. 2003; Neuhoff and Schaefer 2002; Nezlek and Derks 2001).

Humor involves both cognitive and affective elements (Gardner et al. 1975). The cognitive element refers to 'getting the joke' which includes moments during which the perceiver attempts to comprehend disparities between a punch line and prior experience (Brownell et al. 1983). The affective element refers to 'enjoying a joke'; these are moments during which the perceiver experiences pure visceral, emotional responses depending on the hilarity of the experience (Shammi and Stuss 2003).

Studies have been conducted to identify biological neural systems related to humor. Gardner et al. (1975) examined patients with brain injury. They found that the left hemisphere of the brain is related to the integration of information that is required for understanding humor and that the right hemisphere is associated with the emotional processing of humor. In another study, patients with an injury in the right hemisphere showed a low physical reaction and emotional response to humor (Shammi and Stuss 1999).

Studies comparing activated areas of the brain responsible for the affective element and the cognitive element have also been conducted. Moran et al. (2004) examined a brain region that is activated during humor detection (cognitive element) and humor appreciation (affective element). The inferior frontal gyrus and posterior middle temporal gyrus were found to be activated during humor detection condition, while the insula and amygdala were activated during humor appreciation condition.

While numerous studies have focused on block-designed functional magnetic resonance imaging (fMRI) related to humor, few studies have explored event-related fMRI. Whether emotion-inducing stimuli should be presented in a block-designed paradigm or event-related paradigm

* Correspondence: jhsohn@cun.ac.kr
[2]Department of Psychology, Brain Research Institute, Chungnam National University, Daejeon, South Korea
Full list of author information is available at the end of the article

during fMRI remains controversial. Block-designed paradigms are often used because of their easy implementation and because randomization, jittering, and spacing of different stimulus categories is not necessary (Josephs et al. 1997). In blocked designs, stimulus presentation is lengthened and consecutive stimuli in a block are predictable (Zarahn et al. 1997). Prolonged exposure of stimuli may decrease emotional involvement and hence alter underlying brain activation. In emotion research, presentation duration is particularly important, not only from a methodological point of view but also in respect of differences in information processing (Buhler et al. 2008). Event-related designs are superior in terms of rapid estimation of the hemodynamic response function to a short stimulus and are useful for emotion experiments, in part because of their ability to avoid the effects of confounding factors, such as habituation and anticipation (Rosen et al. 1998). In this study, we examined differences in brain activation associated with the two elements of humor, the cognitive element and the affective element, and identified brain areas positively correlated with the rating of funniness using an event-related fMRI paradigm.

Availability and requirements
Participants
Thirteen healthy, right-handed subjects participated in the experiment (mean age 24.8 ± 3.8 years, range 23–33 years, four men and nine women). No participant had a history of psychiatric or neurological disorders. The subjects were instructed to watch cartoons without laughing and to not move their heads.

Stimuli
Five cartoons were used in this study. All images were selected from a pilot study. The cartoons consisted of 7, 8, 9, 11, or 13 scenes. For fMRI study, cartoons were displayed on a monitor and presented to the subject through a 45° angled mirror positioned above the head coil.

Experimental design
Stimuli were presented by showing five cartoons selected from a pilot experiment. Stimuli were presented according to an event-related fMRI paradigm with each cartoon being presented for 32 to 46 s. The subjects were instructed to press a button on a keypad immediately if they found the cartoon to be funny. The interval between the cartoons was 4 s. Following the scan, each subject was instructed to assess humor intensity. The subjects were asked to state whether they found the cartoon funny. If they did find it funny, they were asked to rate their perceived humor intensity on a scale of 1 to 7

(1 least funny, 7 most funny). The subjects were then asked to explain the meaning of the cartoons (Figure 1).

Image acquisition
fMRI experiments were conducted using an ISOL 3 T Forte scanner (ISOL Technology, Gyeonggi, Korea). During the presentation of visual stimuli, fMRI scanning was performed with the single shot Echo Planar Imaging sequence (repetition time (TR), 2,000 ms; echo time (TE), 28 ms; flip angle, 80°; field of view (FOV), 240 mm; matrix size, 64×64; slice thickness, 5 mm, no gap; and in-plane resolution, 3.75 mm, three dummy scans). Anatomical T1-weighted images were obtained with a 3-D FLAIR sequence (TR 280, TE 14, FA 60, FOV 240, matrix 256×256, 4-mm slice thickness).

Data analysis
Functional images were analyzed using SPM99 (http://www.fil.ion.ucl.ac.uk/spm/software/spm99/). Data including head motion artifacts that could not be corrected were excluded from analysis. All functional images were realigned with six movement parameters (translation; x, y, z and rotation; pitch, roll, yaw) to correct head motion. Echo-planar imaging (EPI) and T1-weighted images were coregistered and spatially normalized to the Montreal Neurological Institute template (MNI template) using an automated spatial transformation. Normalized images were smoothed using a 7-mm isotropic Gaussian kernel.

Following preprocessing, statistical analysis was performed. fMRI data were analyzed for each subject individually in the context of the general linear model (GLM) and theory of Gaussian random fields. Using subtraction and correlation procedures, activated areas in the brain while observing different pictures were color-coded by T-score.

Results and discussion
Behavioral results
After fMRI experiments, all participants rated the intensity of humor. The number of subjects who experienced humor while watching each cartoon was 9 for cartoon #1, 11 for cartoon #2, 8 for cartoon #3, 13 for cartoon #4, and 8 for cartoon #5 (Figure 2, upper image). Participants who recognized the cartoons as funny reported an average of 3.5 points for cartoon #1, 3.2 points for cartoon #2, 2.5 points for cartoon #3, 5.2 points for cartoon #4, and 1.9 points for cartoon #5, respectively (Figure 2, lower image).

fMRI results
While viewing humorous scenes, significant activation was observed in the bilateral middle temporal gyrus, left superior temporal gyrus, right fusiform gyrus, right parahippocampal gyrus, left uncus, left inferior frontal gyrus,

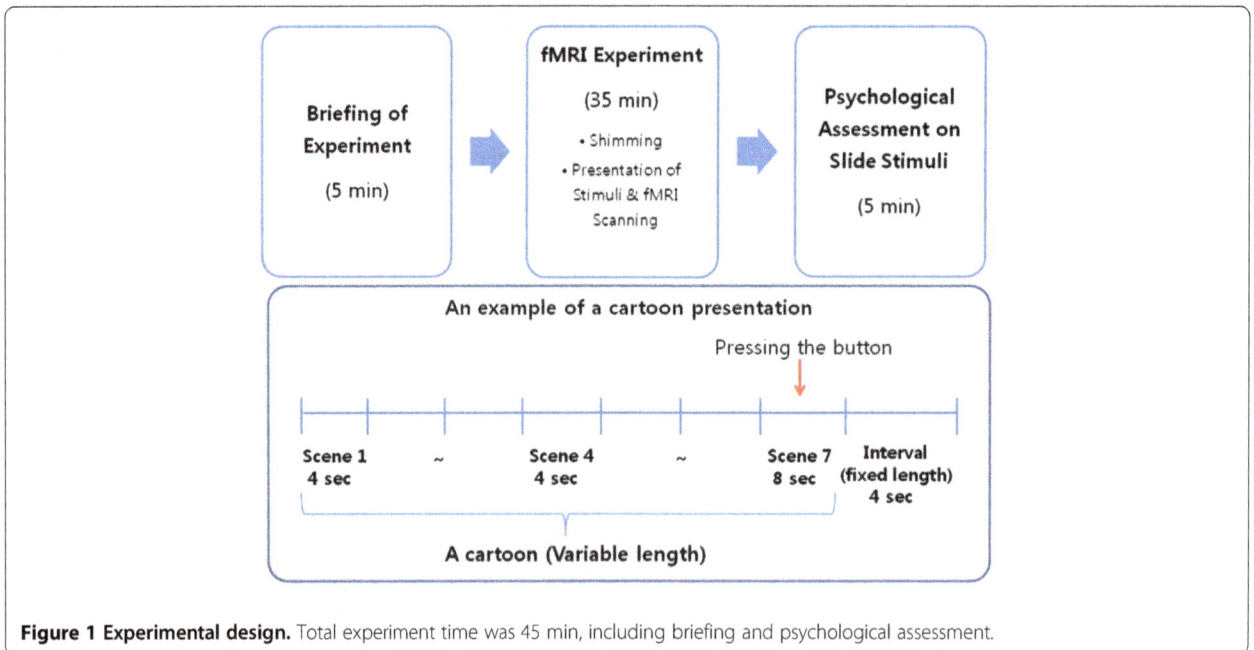

Figure 1 Experimental design. Total experiment time was 45 min, including briefing and psychological assessment.

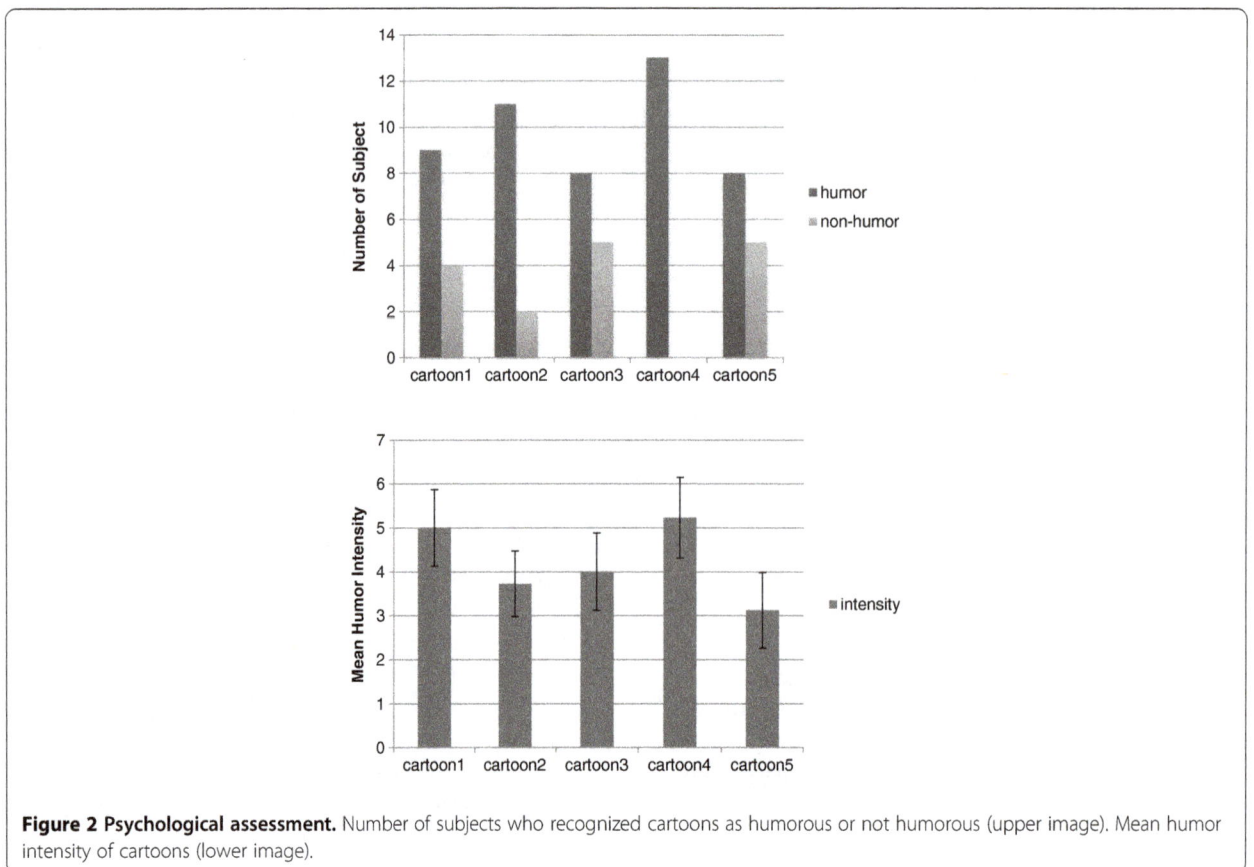

Figure 2 Psychological assessment. Number of subjects who recognized cartoons as humorous or not humorous (upper image). Mean humor intensity of cartoons (lower image).

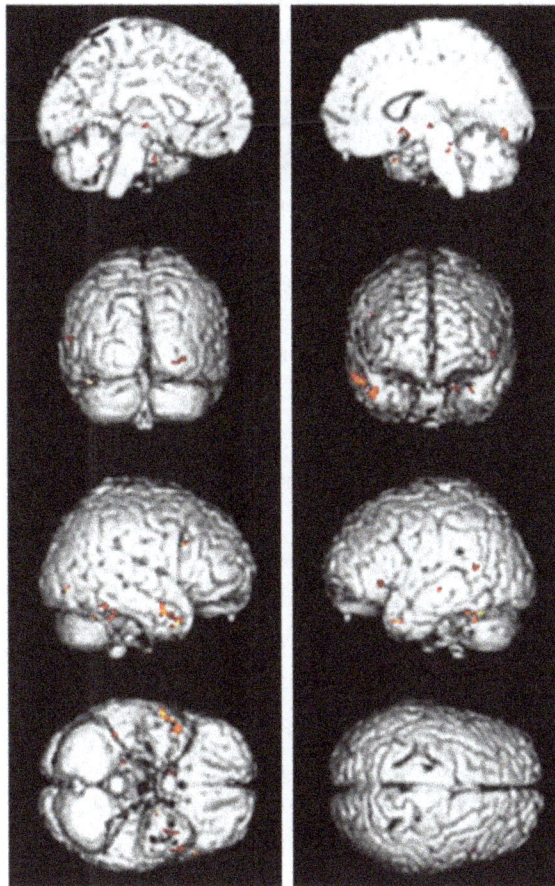

Figure 3 Areas of the brain activated by humorous scenes. Bilateral middle temporal gyrus, left superior temporal gyrus, right fusiform gyrus, right parahippocampal gyrus, left uncus, left inferior frontal gyrus, and right middle frontal gyrus were activated while experiencing humor.

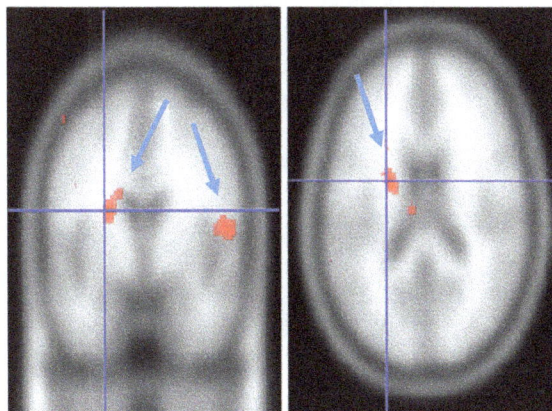

Figure 4 Areas of the brain activated during cartoon scenes with different degrees of humor intensity. Activation in the left nucleus accumbens and right middle temporal gyrus is correlated with humor intensity.

and right middle frontal gyrus ($p < 0.001$, uncorrected; Figure 3).

Humor detection is critically dependent upon resolving incongruities between punch lines and expectations shaped by the storyline (Sul 1972). Consistent with this notion, frontal regions engaged during humor detection have been implicated in language tasks that encourage the retrieval and appraisal of relevant semantic knowledge (Binder et al. 1997, Price et al. 1999). Recent studies have indicated further specialization within the left inferior frontal cortex for reconciling ambiguous semantic content with stored knowledge (Gold and Buckner 2002, Thompson-Schill et al. 1997). Inferior frontal regions may resolve ambiguities between these expectations and punch lines.

Regression analysis was used to examine the association between humor intensity (i.e., the degree of funniness as rated by each subject) and BOLD signal magnitude. This analysis revealed that humor intensity was associated with increased activation in the left nucleus accumbens and right middle temporal gyrus ($p < 0.001$, uncorrected; Figure 4).

Activation of the fusiform gyrus and anterior temporal region caused by electrical stimulation induced laughter accompanied by a feeling of mirth (i.e., positive emotion; Arroyo et al. 1993). The temporal area, including the temporoparietal junction, is involved in the integration of multisensory information and coherence building and inferring knowledge (Ferstl and von Cramon 2002; Goel et al. 1995). Additionally, the temporal lobe may contribute to generating, testing, and correcting internal prediction regarding external sensory events, which is crucial for resolving incongruity in humor processing (Samson et al. 2009). These regions may be involved in the incongruent or surprising (Brownell et al. 1983) elements of a joke and thus may play a pivotal role in the early stages of the humor network.

The nucleus accumbens has been implicated in psychologically and psychopharmacologically driven rewards in various studies (Breiter et al. 2001; Knutson et al. 2001). Activation of the nucleus accumbens elicited by humor converges with findings from fMRI studies across a number of psychologically rewarding tasks, suggesting that this structure is involved in processing a diverse number of stimuli with rewarding characteristics (Aharon et al. 2001; Breiter et al. 2001; Erk et al. 2002; Rilling et al. 2002). Additionally, electrical stimulation of the nucleus accumbens results in laughter and giddiness (Okun et al. 2004). Although we cannot exclude other intervening factors (e.g., novelty), given the results of prior fMRI and physiological studies implicating the nucleus accumbens modulation in self-reported happiness (Knutson et al. 2001) and cocaine/amphetamine-induced euphoria in humans (Brieter et al. 2001; Drevets et al. 2001), it is reasonable to conclude that nucleus accumbens activation

observed in this study reflects the hedonic feeling accompanying humor.

Conclusions

In this study, using event-related fMRI, we identified areas of the brain that were activated during humor processing. We have presented evidence for differential systems underlying the cognitive and affective processes of humor and the brain region correlated with the degree of humor intensity.

Competing interests
The authors declare that they have no competing interests.

Authors' contributions
JN, JWS, JHS, and CC carried out fMRI experiments and analysis. JN and SHK drafted the manuscript. All authors read and approved the final manuscript.

Acknowledgements
This research has been supported by the Converging Research Center Program funded by the Ministry of Education, Science and Technology (2013K000332), the Korea Science and Engineering Foundation (No. 20120006577), and the Korea Basic Science Institute (T33408).

Author details
[1]Division of Magnetic Resonance Research, Korea Basic Science Institute, Ochang, Chungbuk, South Korea. [2]Department of Psychology, Brain Research Institute, Chungnam National University, Daejeon, South Korea. [3]Department of Professional Counseling and Psychotherapy, Graduate School of Health and Complementary Medicine, Wonkwang University, Iksan, Cheonbuk 570-749, South Korea.

References
Aharon I, Etcoff N, Ariely D, Chabris CF, O'Connor E, Breiter HC (2001) Beautiful faces have variable reward value: fMRI and behavioral evidence. Neuron 32(3):537–551
Arroyo S, Lesser RP, Gordon B, Uematsu S, Hart H, Schwerdt P, Andeasson K, Fisher RS (1993) Mirth, laughter and gelastic seizures. Brain 116(4):757–780
Binder JR, Frost JA, Hammeke TA, Cox RW, Rao SM, Prieto T (1997) Human brain language areas identified by functional magnetic resonance imaging. J Neurosci 17(1):353–362
Breiter HC, Aharon I, Kahneman D, Dale A, Shizgal P (2001) Functional imaging of neural responses to expectancy and experience of monetary gains and losses. Neuron 30:619–639
Brownell HH, Gardner H (1988) Neuropsychological insights into humour. In: Durant J, Miller J (eds) Laughing matters: a serious look at humour. Longman Scientific and Technia, Harlow, UK
Brownell HH, Michel D, Powelson J, Gardner H (1983) Surprise but not coherence: sensitivity to verbal humor in right-hemisphere patients. Brain Language 18:20–27
Buhler M, Klein SV, Klemen J, Smolka MN (2008) Does erotic stimulus presentation design affect brain activation patterns? Event-related vs. blocked fMRI designs. Behav Brain Funct 4(1):30
Dixon NF (1980) Humor: A cognitive alternative to stress. In Spielberger CD, Sarason IG (eds) Anxiety and stress, Hemisphere, Washington DC
Drevets WC, Gautier C, Price JC, Kupfer DJ, Kinahan PE, Grace AA, Price JL, Mathis CA (2001) Amphetamine-induced dopamine release in human ventral striatum correlates with euphoria. Society of Biological Psychiatry 49:81–96
Erk S, Spitzer J, Wunderlich AP, Galley L, Walter H (2002) Cultural objects modulate reward circuitry. Neuroreport 13:2499–2503
Ferstl EC, von Cramon DY (2002) What does the frontomedian cortex contribute to language processing: coherence or theory of mind? Neuroimage 17:1599–1612
Gardner H, Ling PK, Flamm L, Silverman J (1975) Comprehension and appreciation of humorous material following brain damage. Brain 98:399–412

Gavrilobic J, Lecic-Tosevski D, Dimic S, Pejovic-Milovancevic M, Knezevic G, Priebe S (2003) Coping strategies in civilians during air attacks. Soc Psychiatry Psychiatr Epidemiol 38(3):128–133

Goel V, Grafman JNS, Sadato N, Hallett M (1995) Modeling other minds. Neuroreport 6:1741–1746

Gold BT, Buckner RL (2002) Common prefrontal regions coactivate with dissociable posterior regions during controlled semantic and phonological task. Neuron 35(4):803–812

Josephs O, Turner R, Friston K (1997) Event-related fMRI. Hum Brain Mapp 5:243–248

Knutson B, Adams CM, Fong GW, Hommer D (2001) Anticipation of increasing monetary reward selectively recruits nucleus accumbens. J Neurosci 21:RC159

Martin RA (2001) Humor, laughter, and physical health: methodological issues and research findings. Psychol Bull 127(4):504–519

Mobbs D, Grecius MD, Abdel-Azim E, Menon V, Reiss AL (2003) Humor modulates the mesolimbic reward centers. Neuron 40:1041–1048

Moran JM, Wig GS, Adams RB, Janata P, Kelley WM (2004) Neural correlates of humor detection and appreciation. Neuroimage 21(3):1055–1060

Netzlek JB, Derks P (2001) Use of humor as a copying mechanism, psychological adjustment, and social interaction. Humor International Journal of Humor Research 14:395–413

Neuhoff CC, Scahaefer C (2002) Effects of laughing, smiling, and howling on mood. Psychol Rep 91:1079–1080

Okun MS, Bowers D, Springer U, Shapira NA, Malone D, Rezai AR, Nuttin B, Heilman KM, Morecraft RJ, Rasmussen SA, Greenberg BD, Foote KD, Goodman WK (2004) What's in a smile? Intra-operative observation of contralateral smiles induced by deep brain stimulation. Neurocase 10(4):271–279

Price CJ, Green DW, von Studnitz RA (1999) Functional imaging study of translation and language switching. Brain 122(12):2221–2235

Rilling JK, Gutman DA, Zeh TR, Pagnoni G, Berns GS, Kilts CD (2002) A neural basis for social cooperation. Neuron 35(2):395–405

Rosen BR, Buckner RL, Dale AM (1998) Event-related functional MRI: past, present and future. PNAS Proc Natl Acad Sci U S A 95(3):773–780

Samson AC, Hempelmann CF, Huber O, Zysset S (2009) Neural substrates of incongruity-resolution and nonsense humor. Neuropsychologia 47:1023–1033

Shammi P, Stuss DT (1999) Humour appreciation: a role of the right frontal lobe. Brain 122:657–666

Shammi P, Stuss DT (2003) The effects of normal aging on humor appreciation. J Int Neuropsychol Soc 9:855–863

Suls J (1972) A two-stage model for the appreciation of jokes and cartoons. In: Goldstein PE, McGhee JH (eds) The psychology of humor: theoretical perspectives and empirical issue. Thieme Medical Publishers, New York, pp 81–100

Thompson-Schill SL, E'Esposito M, Aguirre GK, Farah M (1997) Role of left inferior prefrontal cortex in retrieval of semantic knowledge: a reevaluation. PNAS 94(26):14792–14797

Zarahn E, Aguirre G, D'Esposito M (1997) A trial-based experimental design for fMRI. Neuroimage 6:122–138

24

A selective and sensitive LC-MS/MS method for the simultaneous determination of two potential genotoxic impurities in celecoxib

Ambavaram Vijaya Bhaskar Reddy, Nandigam Venugopal and Gajulapalle Madhavi[*]

Abstract

Background: Impurity profiling is now receiving critical attention from regulatory authorities. For trace level quantification of potential genotoxic impurities (PGIs), conventional analytical techniques like high-performance liquid chromatography (HPLC) and gas chromatography (GC) are inadequate; consequently, there is a great need to apply hyphenated analytical techniques to develop sensitive analytical methods for the analysis of pharmaceuticals.

Methods: A selective and sensitive liquid chromatography-tandem mass spectrometry (LC-MS/MS) method was developed for the simultaneous determination of (4-sulfamoylphenyl)hydrazine hydrochloride (SHH) and (4-methyl-acetophenone)*para*-sulfonamide phenylhydrazine hydrochloride (MAP) PGIs in celecoxib active pharmaceutical ingredient (API). The LC-MS/MS analysis of SHH and MAP PGIs was done on Symmetry C18 (150 mm × 4.6 mm, 3.5 μm) analytical column, and the mobile phase used was 5.0 mM ammonium acetate-acetonitrile in the ratio of 30:70 (*v/v*). The flow rate used was 0.7 mL/min. Triple quadrupole mass detector coupled to positive electrospray ionization operated in multiple reaction monitoring (MRM) mode was used for the quantification of SHH and MAP PGIs. The method was validated as per International Conference on Harmonization (ICH) guidelines and was able to quantitate both SHH and MAP PGIs at 1.0 ppm with respect to 10 mg/mL of celecoxib.

Results: The proposed method was specific, linear, accurate, precise, and robust. The calibration curves show good linearity between the concentration range of 0.06 and 7.5 ppm for both SHH and MAP PGIs. The correlation coefficient obtained was >0.9998 in each case. The method has very low limit of detection (LOD) and limit of quantification (LOQ). The obtained LOD and LOQ values were 0.02 and 0.06 ppm, respectively, for both SHH and MAP PGIs. For both the PGIs, excellent recoveries of 95.0% to 104.0% were obtained at a concentration range of 0.06 to 3.0 ppm. The developed method was also applied to determine the SHH and MAP PGIs in three formulation batches of celecoxib.

Conclusions: The proposed method is simple and accurate and is a good quality control tool for the simultaneous quantitative determination of SHH and MAP PGIs at very low levels in celecoxib during its manufacturing.

Keywords: LC-MS/MS; Method validation; Genotoxicity; Ionization; Quantification

Background

The presence of potential genotoxic impurities (PGIs) even in smaller quantities may affect the efficacy and safety of pharmaceutical products. Impurity profiling is now receiving critical attention from regulatory authorities. The different pharmacopoeias such as BP (British pharmacopoeias), USP (United States pharmacopoeias), IP (Indian pharmacopoeias), and so on, are slowly incorporating limits to the allowable levels of impurities present in the active pharmaceutical ingredients (APIs). Celecoxib is one of the most popular non-steroidal anti-inflammatory drug (NSAID) and a selective cyclooxygenase-2 (COX-2) inhibitor used to treat osteoarthritis, rheumatoid arthritis, acute pain, painful menstruation, and menstrual symptoms (Dembo et al. 2005). Celecoxib also reduces the number of colon and rectum polyps in patients with familial adenomatous polyposis (Clemett and Goa 2000; Silverstein et al. 2000). It is chemically named as 4-[5-(4-methylphenyl)-3-(trifluoromethyl)

* Correspondence: gmchem01@gmail.com
Department of Chemistry, Sri Venkateswara University, Tirupati 517502, India

pyrazol-1-yl]benzene sulfonamide, and the chemical structure of celecoxib is shown in Figure 1. (4-Sulfamoylphenyl) hydrazine hydrochloride (SHH) and (4-methyl-acetophenone)*para*-sulfonamide phenylhydrazine hydrochloride (MAP) are the two important key intermediates used in the synthesis of celecoxib, which are identified as PGIs in finished pharmaceutical substances due to their electrophilic functional groups (Ashby and Tennant 1988; Muller et al. 2006). Several analytical methods have been used to determine celecoxib concentrations in human plasma with various analytical techniques such as high-performance liquid chromatography-UV (HPLC-UV), liquid chromatography-mass spectrometry (LC-MS), and liquid chromatography-tandem mass spectrometry (LC-MS/MS) (Jalalizadeh et al. 2004; Zarghi et al. 2006; Emami et al. 2006; Chow et al. 2004; Stormer et al. 2003; Abdel-Hamid et al. 2001; Werner et al. 2002; Bräutigam et al. 2001), and few methods have been reported for the determination of impurities in celecoxib using HPLC and LC-MS/MS (Satyanarayana et al. 2004; Rao et al. 2006; Jadhav and Shinqare 2005). Ideally, many conventional analytical instruments in pharmaceutical industry such as HPLC with UV detection and GC with flame ionization detector (FID) detection should be employed as the standards in the first attempt for PGIs analysis. However, there are some drawbacks with the abovementioned techniques because HPLC retention times can vary, and some methods are needed to characterize the impurities on line when the

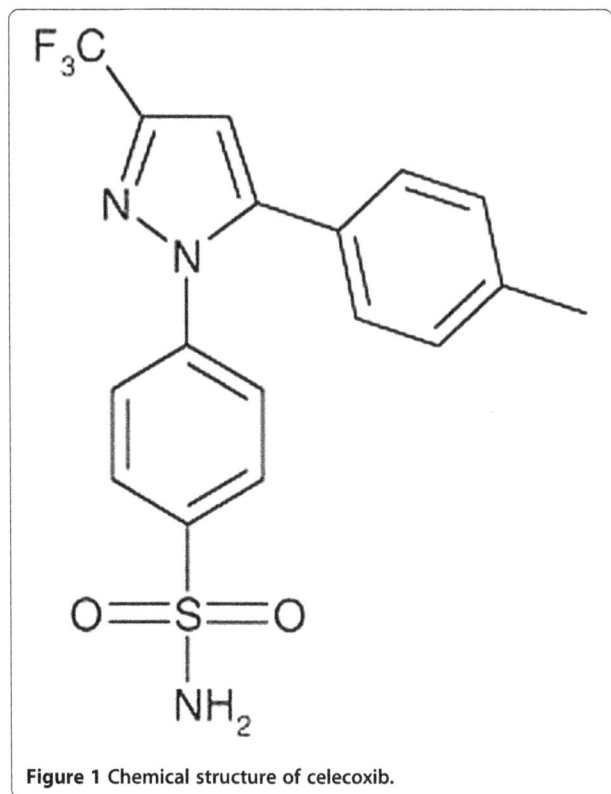

Figure 1 Chemical structure of celecoxib.

impurity standards are not available (Hsieh and Korfmacher 2006; Lee and Kems 1999). Therefore, for accurate determination of PGIs at trace levels, the abovementioned techniques are inadequate; consequently, there is a great need to develop better analytical methods for the analysis of such PGIs in pharmaceutical industries. As a result, various kinds of hyphenated chromatographic techniques and methodologies have been explored as useful approaches.

Based on the threshold of toxicological concern (TTC) of 1.5 µg/person/day, the impurity concentration in celecoxib must not exceed 7.5 ppm considering the worst case scenario where 200-mg daily dose of celecoxib is applied. To the best of our knowledge, no analytical method for the simultaneous determination of SHH and MAP PGIs in celecoxib has been reported in the literature. Therefore, in the present study, we have developed a simple LC-MS/MS method that can quantify two PGIs in celecoxib at permitted levels. The method was validated as per ICH guidelines in terms of limit of detection (LOD), limit of quantification (LOQ), linearity, precision, accuracy, specificity, robustness, and solution stability. The developed method was also applied to determine SHH and MAP PGIs in three formulation batches of celecoxib.

Methods

Chemicals and reagents

All chemicals and solvents were of analytical grade. HPLC grade acetonitrile and ammonium acetate were purchased from Merck (Mumbai, India). Formic acid, trifluoroacetic acid, and methanol were obtained in their highest grade from SD fine chemicals limited (Mumbai, India). Reference substances of SHH, MAP, and celecoxib with the highest purity (>99.0) were obtained from Sigma-Aldrich (St. Louis, MA, USA). High-purity Milli-Q water was used with the help of Millipore Milli-Q plus purification system (Bedford, MA, USA).

Preparation of stock and standard solutions

A stock solution of celecoxib (10 mg/mL) was prepared by dissolving appropriate amount in the methanol. A stock solution of mixture of PGIs (SHH and MAP) at 1.0 mg/mL was also prepared in methanol. The diluted stock solution (0.01 mg/mL) was prepared by diluting 1.0 mL of the 1.0 mg/mL solutions to 100 mL with methanol. Then, 0.1 µg/mL diluted stock solution was prepared by diluting 1.0 mL of 0.01 mg/mL diluted stock solution to 100 mL with methanol. The working standard solution was prepared by weighing accurately 100 mg of celecoxib into 10-mL volumetric flask and made the solution up to the graduation mark after adding 10 µL of 0.1 µg/mL diluted stock solution to give 10 ng/mL and 10 mg/mL of PGIs with respect to celecoxib which corresponds to 1.0 ppm of PGI contamination relative to the drug substance. The PGI samples for validation at 0.06-, 0.5-, 1.0-, 3.0-, 5.0-, and 7.5-ppm concentrations relative to the drug substance were prepared in the same manner using 0.5 µg/mL of diluted stock solution. The concentration of the standard solutions and samples was optimized to achieve a desired signal-to-noise ratio (S/N) and good peak shape. All the standards were sonicated well and filtered through 0.22-µm membrane filters before the analysis.

Chromatographic conditions

All chromatographic experiments were carried out on a HPLC consisting of LC-20AD binary gradient pump, SPD-10AVP UV detector, SIL-10HTC autosampler, and a column oven CTO-10ASVP (Shimadzu, Switzerland) system coupled with MS/MS (Applied Biosystems Sciex API 4000 model, Rotkreuz, Switzerland). The analytical column used was Symmetry C18 (150 mm × 4.6 mm, 3.5 µm). The mobile phase flow operated in isocratic mode using 5.0 mM ammonium acetate-acetonitrile in the ratio of 30:70 (*v/v*). The flow rate of the mobile phase was set at 0.7 mL/min, and the column oven temperature was maintained at 40°C. The injection volume was 10 µL. All the solutions were filtered through 0.22-µm nylon filter before the analysis.

Mass spectrometer

The MS/MS system used was an Applied Biosystems Sciex API 4000 triple quadrupole mass spectrometer with electrospray ionization (ESI) probe operated in positive polarity. Multiple reaction monitoring (MRM) mode was selected for the quantification of SHH and MAP PGIs, and the data acquisition and processing were conducted using the Analyst 1.5.1 software. Typical operating conditions were as follows: ion spray voltage 5,500 V, source temperature 410°C, declustering potential (50 and 55 V), entrance potential (10 and 10 V), collision energy (25 and 20 V), respectively, for both SHH and MAP PGIs. The curtain gas flow, ion source gas 1, and ion source gas 2 nebulization pressure were maintained as 25, 30, and 35 psi, respectively. Electrospray ionization in positive MRM mode was used for the quantification of SHH and MAP PGIs at their transition ion pairs of m/z 188.2→99.2 (protonated) and m/z 304.2→209.2 (protonated), respectively. Celecoxib was monitored with its transition ion pair m/z 382.2→214.1 (protonated).

Method validation

To demonstrate the feasibility of the newly developed method, validation was performed in relation to specificity, linearity, LOQ, LOD, accuracy, precision, robustness, and solution stability. These parameters were validated in agreement with the ICH guidelines.

The linearity was performed by diluting the impurity stock solution to the required concentrations. The solutions were prepared at six concentration levels between 0.06 to 7.5 ppm for both SHH and MAP PGIs and were subjected to linear regression analysis with the least squares method. Calibration equation obtained from regression analysis was used to calculate the corresponding predicted responses. System precision of the mass spectrometric response was established by injecting six individual preparations of the standard solution. The method precision was evaluated by spiking each analyte and determining the percent relative standard deviation (%RSD). LOD and LOQ were evaluated by considering the impurity concentration that would yield S/N ratios of 3:1 and 10:1, respectively. The precision of LOD and LOQ values were experimentally verified by six injections of standard solutions of the compounds at the determined concentrations. Recoveries of SHH and MAP PGIs in spiked samples were studied at three different concentration levels, viz. 0.06, 1.5, and 3.0 ppm. At each concentration level, three independent sample preparations were injected, and the percentage recoveries were determined by comparing the concentration of the spiked sample obtained with the concentration of the spiking standard. The robustness of the method was evaluated by changing mobile phase flow and column temperature, and the stability of the impurities in the sample solution was evaluated by analyzing spiked sample solution at different time intervals at room temperature.

Results and discussion
Optimization of sample preparation

Sample preparation is an important part in the pharmaceutical impurity analysis, because matrix effects in trace analysis were enlarged, causing loss of sensitivity, abnormal recovery, and analyte instability. Different diluents were evaluated with respect to chromatographic efficiency. Solubility of both celecoxib and impurities were good in methanol. Good response and proper peak shapes were obtained for both the impurities when methanol was used as the diluent. Good recoveries (95.0% to 104.0%) were also observed for both SHH and MAP PGIs when methanol was used as a diluent. Therefore, methanol was employed as the diluent throughout the analysis.

Column selection and separation

The present method was developed by testing different stationary phases to achieve good separation of the impurity peaks from drug substance peak. It is important to achieve proper separation among the two PGIs and celecoxib, because of similar chemical structure of two PGIs and celecoxib. In order to obtain a short analysis time, various analytical columns like Kromasil C18 150 mm × 4.6 mm, 3.5 µm (Altmann Analytik, Munich, Germany), Hypersil BDS C8 150 mm × 4.6 mm, 3.5 µm

(Altmann Analytik), Symmetry C18 150 mm × 4.6 mm, 3.5 μm (Waters, Milford, MA, USA), and Zorbax Rx C8 150 mm × 4.6 mm, 3.5 μm (Agilent Technologies, Inc., Santa Clara, CA, USA) were evaluated. The tested columns were checked under the same conditions; with the Kromasil C18 and Zorbax Rx C8 columns, the peaks of impurities were overlapped with celecoxib peak. The resolution between celecoxib and impurities were poor with Hypersil BDS C8 column. On Symmetry C18 column (150 mm × 4.6 mm, 3.5 μm), the separation and responses for both the impurities and celecoxib were found good. On this column, the analytes were well retained and separated from each other and from the drug substance. This separation is achieved due to polar group technology that 'shields' the silica residual silanol surface from highly basic analytes; this reduced silanol activity for the symmetry column significantly improved the peak shape and resolution. Different compositions of mobile phases using 10 mM ammonium acetate and 5.0 mM ammonium acetate with acetonitrile were tested; finally, good separation and response were observed at a ratio of 5.0 mM ammonium acetate-acetonitrile (30:70, v/v). Both isocratic and gradient elution modes were evaluated. Isocratic elution was observed to be more efficient in achieving optimum separation of impurities from each other with respect to drug substance peak. The column was thermostated at 40°C to avoid any shift in retention time. Retention times of SHH and MAP PGIs were observed at 3.08 and 4.02 min, respectively. Peaks were well separated from the drug substance peak (5.79 min).

Table 1 The precision at LOD and LOQ concentrations of SHH and MAP PGIs

Injection ID	SHH		MAP	
	LOD (peak area)	LOQ (peak area)	LOD (peak area)	LOQ (peak area)
1	2,196	6,280	2,496	7,109
2	2,094	6,300	2,344	7,350
3	2,173	6,351	2,342	6,973
4	2,085	6,240	2,349	7,300
5	2,210	6,190	2,488	7,246
6	2,090	6,250	2,371	6,920
Mean	2,141.33	6,268.50	2,398.66	7,149.66
Standard deviation	57.88	55.22	73.58	177.52
%RSD	2.70	0.88	2.94	2.48
Concentration	0.02 ppm	0.06 ppm	0.02 ppm	0.06 ppm

Optimization of MS-MS parameters

Selection of a detection method is also the most important part of pharmaceutical impurity analysis. From the instrument simplicity and availability, first, we have evaluated with HPLC-UV and GC-FID. However, on these techniques sufficient sensitivity for the trace level analysis of SHH and MAP PGIs was not achieved. In view of this, a sensitive and specific mass LC-MS/MS technique in MRM mode was evaluated for the quantification of SHH and MAP PGIs in celecoxib drug substance. Then, the possibility of using electrospray ionization (ESI) source under positive ion detection mode was evaluated during the early stage of

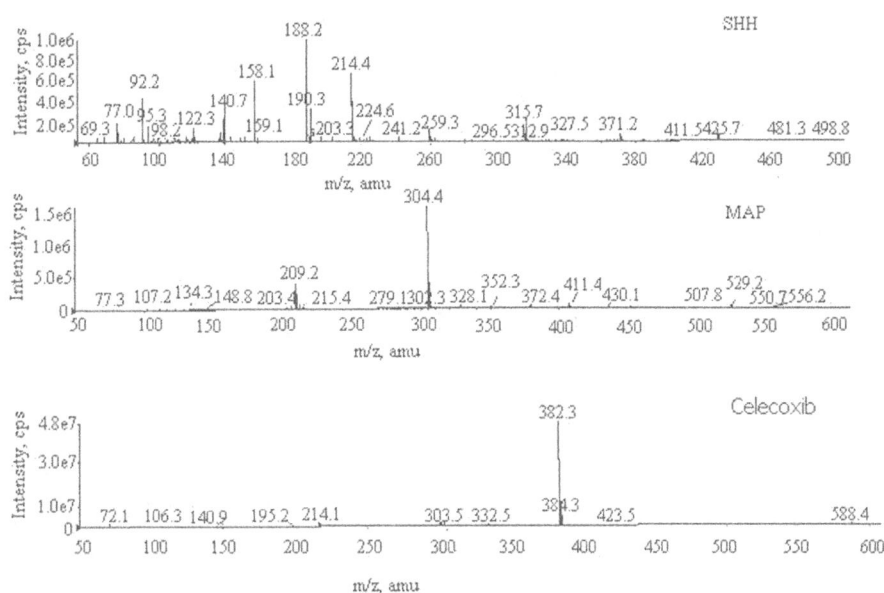

Figure 2 Representative mass spectra of SHH, MAP PGIs, and celecoxib.

method development. The signal intensity in positive mode was much higher than that in negative mode. Further, the method development was carried out with ESI source operated in positive polarity mode. The ion source parameters were optimized to get proper response. The representative mass spectra of SHH, MAP, and celecoxib are shown in Figure 2.

Method validation

In order to prove that the method is capable of its intended use, the newly developed method for the quantification of SHH and MAP PGIs in celecoxib drug substance was validated according to the international guidelines (Vijaya Bhaskar Reddy et al. 2013; ICH 2005).

Limit of detection and limit of quantification

The method validation was started by injecting 1.0-ppm concentration of individual solutions of SHH and MAP PGIs of each with respect to the drug substance concentration of 10 mg/mL and determining their S/N ratios. Now, to evaluate LOD and LOQ values, their concentrations were reduced sequentially such that they yield S/N ratios as 3:1 and 10:1, respectively. Each predicted concentration was verified for their precision by preparing the solutions at predicted concentrations and injected each solution six times for analyses. The LOD and LOQ values calculated form S/N ratio was found to be 0.02 and 0.06 ppm, respectively. It is noteworthy that the LOD values for both the impurities were below the required concentration limit (7.5 ppm) for PGIs in celecoxib (Table 1).

Linearity

By MRM, the linearity of SHH and MAP PGIs was satisfactorily demonstrated with a six-point calibration graph between 0.06 and 7.5 ppm with respect to a sample concentration of 10 mg/mL. The calibration curves were produced by plotting the average of triplicate PGI

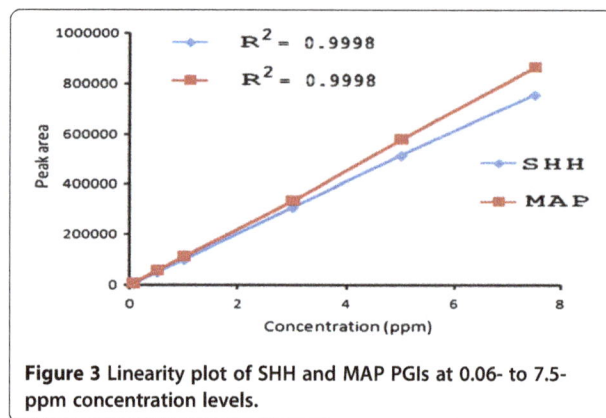

Figure 3 Linearity plot of SHH and MAP PGIs at 0.06- to 7.5-ppm concentration levels.

injections against the concentration expressed in percentage. The slope, intercept, and correlation coefficient values were derived from linear least squares regression analysis. The correlation coefficient obtained in each case was >0.9998. The corresponding linearity data is presented in Figure 3. The results indicated that an excellent correlation existed between the peak areas and the concentrations of impurities.

Precision

The precision of the method was evaluated at two levels, viz. repeatability and intermediate precision. Repeatability was checked by calculating the %RSD of six replicate determinations by injecting six freshly prepared solutions containing 1.0 ppm each of the mixture of impurities on the same day. The same experiments were done on six different days to evaluate the intermediate precision.

Table 2 Intra-day and inter-day precision of SHH and MAP PGIs at 1.0-ppm concentration

Injection ID	SHH (peak area)		MAP (peak area)	
	Intra-day	Inter-day	Intra-day	Inter-day
1	101,680	101,680	113,540	113,540
2	104,534	102,641	113,471	108,618
3	103,820	101,950	109,346	116,864
4	99,495	102,700	108,510	112,951
5	102,350	102,681	114,570	113,470
6	103,554	103,987	109,500	108,650
Standard deviation	1,826.69	801.93	252.78	3,194.58
%RSD	1.78	0.78	2.37	2.84

Table 3 The recovery data of SHH and MAP PGIs at three different concentrations

Parameter	SHH	MAP
Accuracy at LOQ level ($n = 3$)		
Amount added (ppm)	0.06	0.06
Amount recovered (ppm)	0.057	0.059
%recovery	95.3	98.6
%RSD	1.95	1.84
Accuracy at 100% level ($n = 3$)		
Amount added (ppm)	1.5	1.5
Amount recovered (ppm)	1.479	1.521
%recovery	98.6	101.4
%RSD	1.95	1.84
Accuracy at 150% level ($n = 3$)		
Amount added (ppm)	3.0	3.0
Amount recovered (ppm)	3.102	3.108
%recovery	103.4	103.6
%RSD	1.21	1.44

n, number of determinations.

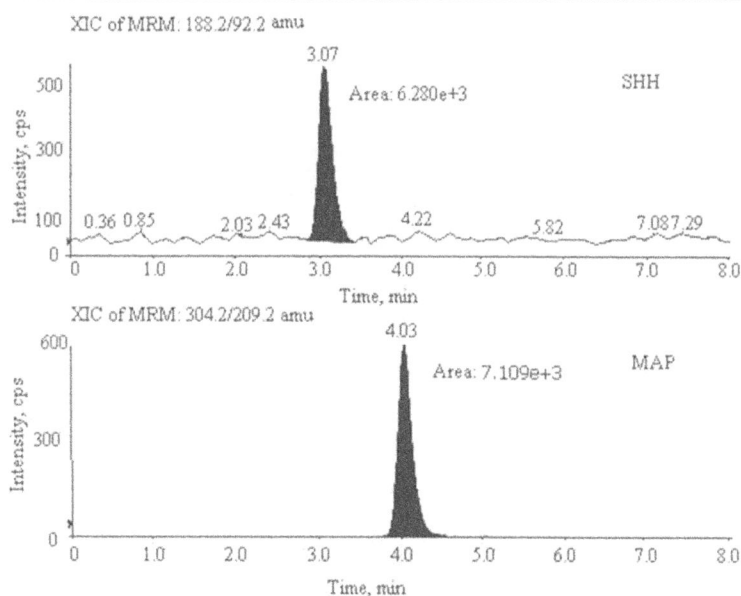

Figure 4 Recovery chromatogram of SHH and MAP PGIs at LOQ concentration.

As reported in Table 2, %RSD values were lower than 3.0% for both the impurities; this confirmed an adequate precision of the developed method.

Accuracy and specificity studies
When three pure and formulation sample solutions of 10 mg/mL of celecoxib were injected, impurities were not at all detected in them. Hence, recovery studies by the standard addition method were performed to evaluate accuracy and specificity. Accordingly, the accuracy of the method was determined by spiking at (LOQ) 0.06-, 1.5-, and 3.0-ppm concentrations separately to three batches of pure and formulation solutions of celecoxib (10 mg/mL). Each determination was carried out three times. The recovery data is presented in Table 3, and the corresponding chromatogram is shown in Figure 4. Satisfactory recoveries of 95.3% to 98.6% for 0.06 ppm, 98.6% to 101.4% for 1.5 ppm, and 103.4% to 103.6% for

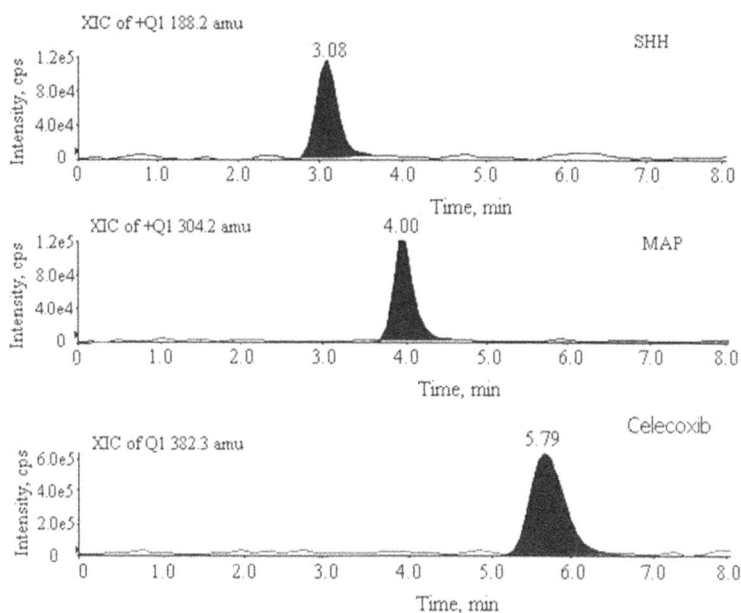

Figure 5 Specificity chromatogram of celecoxib spiked with SHH and MAP PGIs.

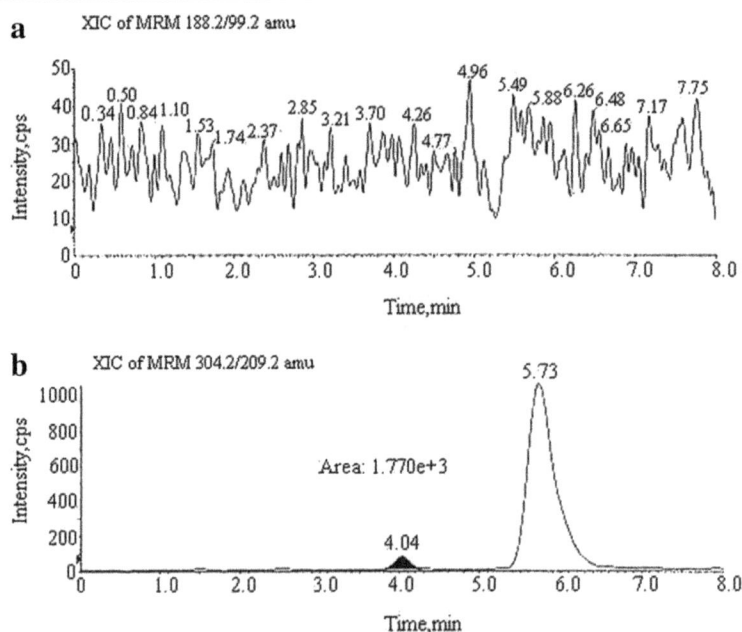

Figure 6 Representative chromatograms of (a) blank and (b) formulation sample of celecoxib.

3.0 ppm were obtained. At such low concentrations, these recoveries and %RSDs were satisfactory. The specificity of the method was established by injecting blank celecoxib (tablet) solution and celecoxib spiked with two PGIs. It was observed that the common excipients used in the tablets were not interfered at the retention times of any PGIs and drug substance. The corresponding specificity chromatogram is shown in Figure 5. The developed method was also successfully applied for the determination of SHH and MAP PGIs in three different batches of celecoxib. In two batches, the PGIs were not detected. In one of the batches of celecoxib, only MAP was observed; however, its concentration was below the specification. The corresponding chromatogram is shown in Figure 6.

Robustness

The robustness of the method was studied with deliberate modifications in the flow rate of the mobile phase and the column temperature. The optimized flow rate of the mobile phase was 0.7 mL/min, and the same was altered by 10% of its flow, i.e., from 0.63 to 0.77 mL/min. The effect of column temperature on resolution was studied at 38°C and 42°C (altered by 2°C). However, the mobile phase components were held constant as described above. As reported in Table 4, the %RSD in both the cases does not exceeded 3.0%, which demonstrates the robustness of the method.

Solution stability

Stability of SHH and MAP PGIs in methanol was checked by keeping them in an autosampler and observing the variations in their peak areas. From the stability results, we found that SHH and MAP were stable up to 48 h. The corresponding data is presented in Table 5.

Table 4 Robustness data of SHH and MAP PGIs at LOD and LOQ concentrations

Parameter	Actual	Low	High
Flow variation	0.7	0.63	0.77
Column oven temperature (°C)	40	38	42
SHH			
%RSD at LOD	1.37	1.34	1.76
%RSD at LOQ	1.42	1.78	2.04
MAP			
%RSD at LOD	0.68	1.42	0.74
%RSD at LOQ	2.14	1.63	1.91

Table 5 Solution stability data of SHH and MAP PGIs at LOQ concentration

Parameter	SHH	MAP
Solution stability		
Theoretical concentration (ppm)	0.06	0.06
Percent recovery (n = 3)		
At 0 h	98.2 ± 0.94	96.2 ± 1.24
At 12 h	101.4 ± 1.13	95.6 ± 0.91
At 24 h	102.6 ± 0.82	96.4 ± 0.88
At 48 h	99.8 ± 1.45	100.4 ± 1.36

n, number of determinations.

Conclusions

The proposed method is a direct LC-MS/MS method for the separation and quantification of SHH and MAP PGIs in celecoxib drug substance. The method utilized MRM mode for the quantitation, which provided the better sensitivity. The method was fully validated and presents good linearity, specificity, accuracy, precision, and robustness, and it is also found to be simple, sensitive, selective, cost effective, and stability indicating. The LOD and LOQ of the method were found very low, as 0.02 and 0.06 ppm for both SHH and MAP impurities. The proposed method was successfully applied for the determination of the two PGIs in three formulation batches of celecoxib. The method presented here could be very useful to monitor SHH and MAP PGIs in celecoxib during its manufacturing.

Competing interests
The author declares no competing interests.

Authors' contributions
VBR designed the experiment, carried out the experiment, and contributed in framing the article. V assisted during the method development and analysis using LC-MS/MS. M assisted during the analysis and contributed in framing the article. All authors read and approved the final manuscript

Acknowledgements
One of the authors Dr. A. Vijaya Bhaskar Reddy is highly grateful to the UGC (BSR), Government of India, New Delhi for financial assistance in the form of an award of Meritorious Research Fellowship (RFSMS), and the authors are also thankful to Sipra Labs Limited, Hyderabad for supporting this work.

References

Abdel-Hamid M, Novotny L, Hamza H (2001) Liquid chromatographic-mass spectrometric determination of celecoxib in plasma using single-ion monitoring and its use in clinical pharmacokinetics. J Chrom B 753:401–408

Ashby J, Tennant RW (1988) Chemical structure, Salmonella mutagenicity and extent of carcinogenicity as indicators of genotoxic carcinogenesis among 222 chemicals tested in rodents by the U.S. NCI/NTP. Mutat Res 204:17–115

Bräutigam L, Vetter G, Tegeder I, Heinkele G, Geisslinger G (2001) Determination of celecoxib in human plasma and rat microdialysis samples by liquid chromatography tandem mass spectrometry. J Chrom B 761(2):203–212

Chow HS, Anavy N, Salazar D, Frank DH, Alberts DS (2004) Determination of celecoxib in human plasma using solid-phase extraction and high-performance liquid chromatography. J Pharma Biomed Anal 34:167–174

Clemett D, Goa KL (2000) Celecoxib: a review of its use in osteoarthritis, rheumatoid arthritis and acute pain. Drugs 59(4):957–980

Dembo G, Park SB, Kharasch ED (2005) Central nervous system concentrations of cyclooxygenase-2 inhibitors in humans. Anesthesia 102(2):409–415

Emami J, Fallah R, Ajami A (2006) A rapid and sensitive HPLC method for the analysis of celecoxib in human plasma: application to pharmacokinetic studies. J Pharma Sci 16(4):211–217

ICH (2005) Validation of analytical procedures: test and methodology. Q2 (R1). ICH, Geneva

Hsieh Y, Korfmacher WA (2006) Increasing speed and throughput when using HPLC-MS/MS systems for drug metabolism and pharmacokinetic screening. Curr Drug Metabol 7:479–489

Jadhav AS, Shingare MS (2005) A new stability-indicating RP-HPLC method to determine assay and known impurity of celecoxib API. Drug Dev Indust Pharm 31(8):779–783

Jalalizadeh H, Amini M, Ziaee V, Safa A, Farsam H, Shafiee A (2004) Determination of celecoxib in human plasma by high performance liquid chromatography. J Pharma Biomed Anal 35:665–670

Lee MS, Kems EH (1999) LC/MS applications in drug development. Mass Spec Rev 18:187–279

Muller L, Mauthe RJ, Riley CM, Andino MM, De Antonis D, Beels C, De George J, De Knaep AGM, Ellison D, Fagerland JA (2006) A rationale for determining, testing and controlling specific impurities in pharmaceuticals that possess potential for genotoxicity. Regul Toxicol Pharmacol 44:198–211

Rao RN, Meena S, Nagaraju D, Rao AR, Ravikanth S (2006) Liquid-chromatographic separation and determination of process-related impurities, including a regio-specific isomer of celecoxib on reversed-phase C18 column dynamically coated with hexamethyldisilazane. Anal Sci 22:157–1260

Satyanarayana U, Sreenivas Rao D, Ravindra Kumar Y, Moses Babu J, Rajender Kumar P, Tirupathi Reddy J (2004) Isolation, synthesis and characterization of impurities in celecoxib, a COX-2 inhibitor. J Pharma Biomed Anal 35:951–957

Silverstein FE, Faich G, Goldstein JL, Simon LS, Pincus T, Whelton A, Makuch R, Eisen G, Agrawal NM, Stenson WF, Burr AM, Zhao WW, Kent JD, Lefkowith JB, Verburg KM, Geis GS (2000) Gastrointestinal toxicity with celecoxib vs nonsteroidal anti-inflammatory drugs for osteoarthritis and rheumatoid arthritis: the CLASS study: a randomized controlled trial. Celecoxib Long-term Arthritis Safety Study. Amer Med Assoc 284(10):1247–1255

Stormer E, Bauer S, Kirchheiner J, Brockmoller J, Roots I (2003) Simultaneous determination of celecoxib, hydroxycelecoxib, and carboxycelecoxib in human plasma using gradient reversed-phase liquid chromatography with ultraviolet absorbance detection. J Chrom B 783(1):207–212

Vijaya Bhaskar Reddy A, Venugopal N, Madhavi G, Gangadhara Reddy K, Madhavi V (2013) A selective and sensitive UPLC-MS/MS approach for trace level quantification of four potential genotoxic impurities in zolmitriptan drug substance. J Pharma Biomed Anal 84:84–89

Werner U, Werner D, Pahl A, Mundkowski R, Gillich M, Brune K (2002) Investigation of the pharmacokinetics of celecoxib by liquid chromatography-mass spectrometry. Biomed Chrom 16(1):56–60

Zarghi A, Shafaati A, Foroutan SM, Khoddam A (2006) Simple and rapid high performance liquid chromatographic method for determination of celecoxib in plasma using UV detection: application in pharmacokinetic studies. J Chroma B 835(1–2):100–104

25

Rapid ultra-performance liquid chromatography assay of losartan potassium in bulk and formulations

Tarab J Ahmad[4*], Amruth Raj[1], Rayapura T Radhika[2], Sannaiah Ananda[3], Netkal M Gowda[4] and Bellale M Venkatesha[1*]

Abstract

Background: Losartan potassium is a non-peptide AT1 receptor drug used in the treatment of hypertension.

Methods: A simple, rapid, sensitive, and validated isocratic reverse-phase ultra-performance liquid chromatographic (RP-UPLC) method was developed and validated for the determination of losartan potassium (LOS) in bulk drug and tablets. The assay was developed using Waters Acquity BEH C18 (100 mm × 2.1 mm), 1.7-μm column with a mobile phase consisting of a mixture of phosphate buffer (pH 3.2) and acetonitrile (50:50 v/v).

Results: An assay with a total run time of only 5 min was developed. The method monitored at 245 nm exhibited linearity over a concentration range of 2.0 to 15.0 μg mL^{-1} LOS. The limits of detection and quantification (signal-to-noise ratio (S/N) = 10) were found be 0.018 and 0.054 μg mL^{-1}, respectively. The intraday and interday RSDs were less than 1.0%. The method was validated by the determination of LOS levels in tablets where the percentage on the label claim was 100 ± 2. The accuracy of the method was further ascertained by recovery studies via the standard addition procedure, which yielded satisfactory results.

Conclusion: A rapid UPLC assay of LOS in bulk drug and tablets was developed and validated.

Keywords: Losartan potassium; Ultra-performance liquid chromatography; Assay; Pharmaceutical; C-18 column

Background

Losartan potassium, a monopotassium salt of 2-butyl-4-chloro-1-[p-(o-1H-tetrazol-5-ylphenyl)benzyl] imidazole-5-methanol or (2-butyl-4-chloro-1-{[2'-(1H-tetrazol-5-yl) biphenyl-4-yl]methyl}-1H-imidazol-5-yl)methanol (Figure 1), is a non-peptide AT1 receptor antagonist used for the treatment of hypertension (Conlin 2001). Losartan potassium was the first angiotensin II receptor antagonist to be marketed. Currently, it is marketed by Merck and Co. Inc. under the trade name, Cozaar. Several analytical techniques have been reported for the determination of losartan potassium (LOS) in different pharmaceutical formulations and in biological fluids. Most of these methods employ high-performance liquid chromatography (HPLC) with UV detection (Seburg et al. 2006; Pedroso et al. 2009). The drug LOS is determined by HPLC in the presence of other drugs

such as hydrochlorothiazide (Carlucci et al. 2000; Erk 2001). The LC-MS-MS method works for LOS in the presence of its degradation products and in plasma (Yeung et al. 2000; Gonzalez et al. 2002).

The separation science plays a key role in pharmaceutical industry ranging from impurity profiling to the final assay for monitoring the finished products. The batch assay of the pharmaceuticals in a quality control setup needs to be rapid, accurate, and sensitive. The fast quality monitoring of the products using ultra-performance liquid chromatography (UPLC) is gaining pronounced interest. Known for its advanced technology, UPLC is based on the principles of liquid chromatography, which utilizes 1.7-μm column particles. This enhances the separation process without affecting the resolutions. Due to small particle size, the system entails the use of high pressure of the order 15,000 psi to pump the mobile phase. The elevated mobile phase linear velocity results in high resolution, sensitivity, and shorter analysis time. Owing to its speed and sensitivity, this technique is gaining considerable attention

* Correspondence: tj-ahmad@wiu.edu; venkichem123@rediffmail.com
[4]Department of Chemistry, Western Illinois University, Macomb, IL 61455, USA
[1]Department of Chemistry, Yuvaraja's College, University of Mysore, Mysore-570005, India
Full list of author information is available at the end of the article

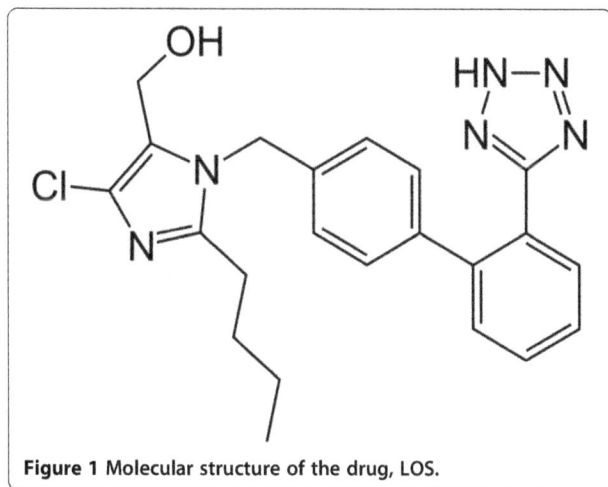

Figure 1 Molecular structure of the drug, LOS.

in recent years in different fields of pharmaceutical and biomedical analysis (Krishnaiah et al. 2010; Waren and Tchlitcheff 2006). The literature survey shows that, despite these advantages, the UPLC has not been applied for the assay of the drug, LOS.

The aim of this study is to develop and validate, according to the current ICH guidelines, a fast, accurate, precise, and sensitive UPLC method for the analysis of LOS in tablets without the interference from inactive ingredients.

Methods
Materials and reagents
The pure active ingredient sample of LOS was given as a gift by Jubilant Life Sciences, Mysore, India. Tablet formulations, *viz.* Cosart from Cipla, and Covance from Ranbaxy, were purchased from local commercial sources. Solvents such as methanol and acetonitrile (HPLC grade), potassium dihydrogen orthophosphate, and orthophosphoric acid (Qualigens, Mumbai, India) were purchased from Merck & Co., Inc., Whitehouse Station, NJ, USA. Double-distilled water was used throughout the investigation.

Chromatographic conditions and equipment
Analyses were carried out on a Waters Acquity UPLC (LabX, Midland, ON, Canada) with a tunable UV detector. The output signal was monitored and processed using an Empower software. The chromatographic column used was Waters Acquity UPLC BEH C18 (100 mm × 2.1 mm with 1.7-µm particle size). The isocratic elution process was adopted throughout the analysis.

Mobile phase preparation
An aqueous phosphate buffer solution was prepared by dissolving 2.000 g of potassium dihydrogen orthophosphate in approximately 400 mL of water. The pH of this solution was adjusted to 3.2 with 10% phosphoric acid before diluting to a final volume of 500.0 mL. A mixture of 500.0 mL phosphate buffer and 500.0 mL acetonitrile

was stirred and filtered using a 0.22-µm nylon membrane filter. This solution was also used as the solvent in all the subsequent preparations of analyte samples.

Instrumental parameters
The isocratic flow rate of the mobile phase was maintained at 0.20 mL min^{-1}. The column temperature was adjusted to 40°C. The injection volume was 4.0 µL. The elution was monitored at 220 nm and the total run time was 5.0 min.

Preparation of stock solution
A standard stock solution of LOS (100 µg mL^{-1}) was prepared by dissolving an accurately weighed amount (5.0 mg) of the drug in the solvent to a final volume of 50.0 mL in a volumetric flask.

Procedures
Procedure for calibration curve
Working standard solutions containing 2.0 to 15.0 µg mL^{-1} of LOS were prepared by serial dilutions of the stock solution (100 µg mL^{-1}). Aliquots of 4.0 µL were injected (six injections) and eluted with the mobile phase under the reported chromatographic conditions. The average peak area vs. concentration of LOS (in µg mL^{-1}) was plotted to obtain the standard curve for determining the unknown concentrations of the analyte. Alternatively, the corresponding regression equation was derived using mean peak area-concentration data, and the concentration of the unknown analyte can be computed from the regression equation.

Preparation of tablet extracts and assay procedure
Ten tablets (approximately 25-mg LOS each) were weighed and ground to a fine powder. A quantity equivalent to a tablet was weighed and transferred into a 100-mL flask, dissolved in 60 mL of the mobile phase, sonicated for 20 min, and then diluted to the final volume with the same mobile phase to yield a concentration of 250 µg mL^{-1}. The solution was passed through a 0.22-µm nylon membrane filter. Appropriate volumes of the filtered solution were diluted with the mobile phase to obtain the desired concentrations such as 5.0 ppm.

Procedure for method validation
Accuracy and precision To determine the accuracy and intraday precision, pure LOS solutions of three different concentrations were analyzed in six replicates each during the same day. Mobile phase was injected as the blank solution before the sample injection, and the relative standard deviation (%RSD) values of the peak area and retention time were determined.

Limits of detection and quantification The limit of detection (LOD) and limit of quantification (LOQ) were determined by the signal-to-noise (S/N) ratio method.

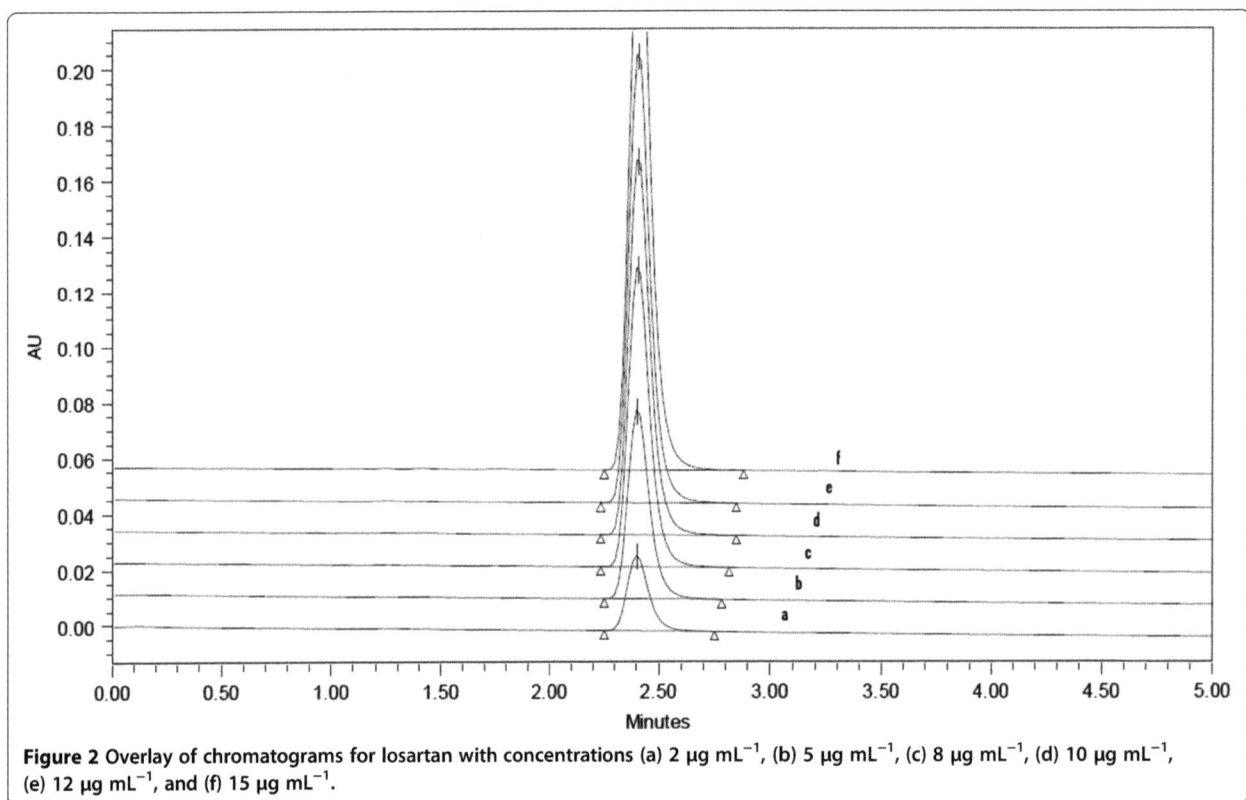

Figure 2 Overlay of chromatograms for losartan with concentrations (a) 2 µg mL^{-1}, (b) 5 µg mL^{-1}, (c) 8 µg mL^{-1}, (d) 10 µg mL^{-1}, (e) 12 µg mL^{-1}, and (f) 15 µg mL^{-1}.

These were obtained by a series of dilutions of the LOS stock solution. Precision study was performed at the LOQ level also. LOQ solution was injected six times (n = 6) and the %RSD values for the obtained peak area and retention time were calculated.

Solution and mobile phase stability The stability of the LOS solution was tested by injecting the sample into the C-18 column. The peak area was recorded at time intervals of 0, 3, 6, 8, 12, and 15 h, and the RSD and time values were calculated. The mobile phase stability was studied by injecting a freshly prepared sample solution at

the same time periods, and the RSD values of the peak areas were calculated. The RSD values of both studies were found to be less than 3.0% exhibiting compatibility of the diluent and the stability of the mobile phase.

Results and discussion
Method development
The drug LOS is a basic due to the presence of imidazole and tetrazole moieties in the molecule (Figure 1). The log P value of LOS was found to be 2.25 by ChemDraw Ultra Version 7.0 indicating a high lipophilicity. Acidic mobile phase with a buffer of pH 3.2 was chosen to protonate nitrogen atoms for a fast elution. In order to achieve better efficiency of the chromatographic system, the experimental conditions such as composition and pH of the mobile phase, detection wavelength, nature of column, and column temperature were optimized by varying one parameter at a time while keeping the other conditions constant. Several proportions of buffer, water-acetonitrile mixture, and methanol were evaluated to obtain suitable composition of the mobile phase. Parameters such as the retention time, peak shape, theoretical plates, and run time were the major tasks while developing the method. Several combinations of gradient methods were also performed. Isocratic method was found to be better for the assay. Finally, at the mobile phase composition described under the 'Methods' section, the method gave the lowest peak tailing factor and the highest theoretical plate count.

Table 1 Regression and sensitivity parameters for UPLC analysis of LOS

Parameter	Value
Linearity range, µg mL^{-1}	2.0 to 15.0
Slope (b)	95,938
Intercept (a)	−3,271.6
Standard deviation of intercept (S$_a$)	±5,726.3
Standard deviation of slope (S$_b$)	±591.7
Correlation co-efficient (r)	0.9999
Limit of detection (LOD), µg mL^{-1}	0.0543
Limit of quantification (LOQ), µg mL^{-1}	0.018
$\pm t S_a / \sqrt{n}$	4,581.7
$\pm t S_b / \sqrt{n}$	473.4

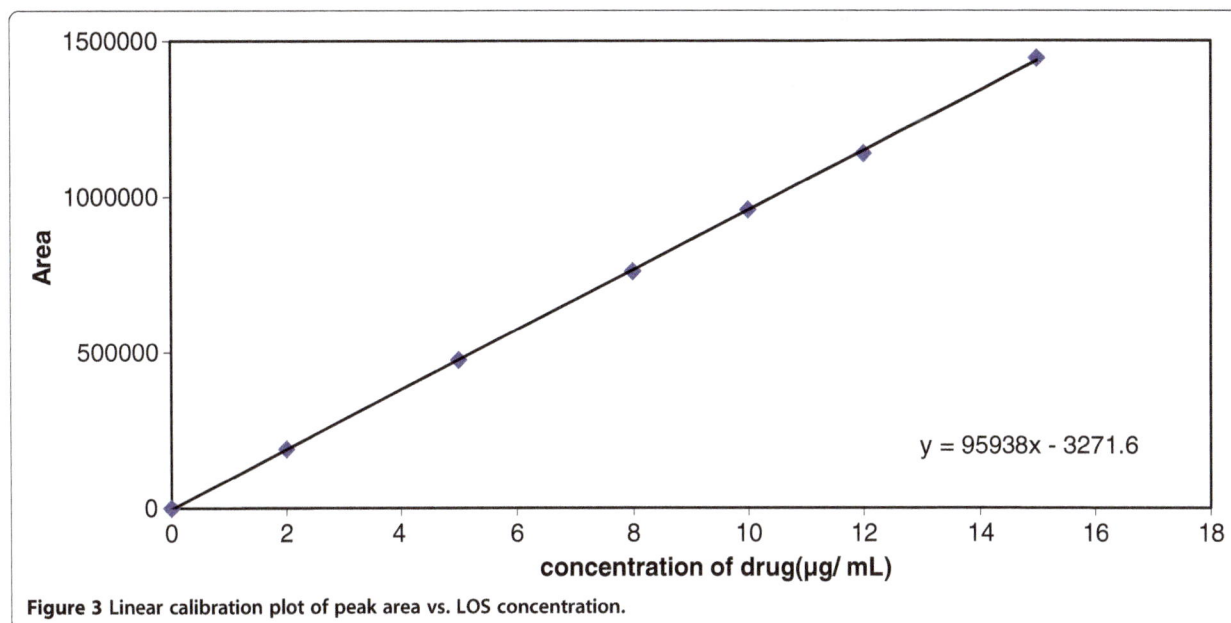

Figure 3 Linear calibration plot of peak area vs. LOS concentration.

The equation shown on the plot: $y = 95938x - 3271.6$

Validation of the method

The described method for the assay of LOS has been validated as per the current ICH Q2 (R1) guidelines.

Analytical parameters

Figure 2 shows an overlay of the chromatographic peaks for LOS at different concentrations. A linear correlation was obtained between the peak area and the concentrations in the range 2.00 to 15.0 $\mu g\ mL^{-1}$ LOS, from which the linear regression equation was computed to be $A = 96{,}192.3C - 3{,}271.6$ ($r = 0.9999$), where A is the peak area and C is the concentration of LOS (in $\mu g\ mL^{-1}$). The LOD and LOQ values, slope, y-intercept, and their standard deviations evaluated are presented in Table 1 and Figure 3. These results confirm the existence of a linear relationship between the concentrations of LOS and the peak areas along with the sensitivity of the method.

Accuracy and precision

Table 2 shows the data for three concentration levels of the analyte LOS in tablets determined with and without the standard addition of an equal amount of the pure LOS. The data include method accuracy and precision represented by the relative error (RE) and RSD, respectively, for six determinations at each concentration level. Both RE and RSD decrease with the increase in the sample size showing the lowest values for the 8 $\mu g\ mL^{-1}$ sample size. However, the relatively low %RSDs indicate the high precision of the method.

Robustness of the method and stability of the solution

The robustness of an analytical procedure is a measure of its capacity to remain unaffected by small but deliberate variations made in method parameters. It provides an indication of its reliability during normal usage. At varied chromatographic conditions (flow rate, temperature, and

Table 2 Results of determination of LOS in tablets and in standard samples

Tablet brand name[a]	Nominal amount (mg)	LOS in tablet ($\mu g\ mL^{-1}$)	Pure LOS added ($\mu g\ mL^{-1}$)	Total area	%RE	%RSD
Covance	25.0	2.0	2.0	380,159	−22.0	0.078
				380,892		
				380,532		
		5.0	5.0	663,598	−9.14	0.033
				663,259		
				663,124		
		8.0	8.0	949,892	−2.60	0.022
				950,129		
				950,321		

Mean value of six determinations. [a]Marketed by Covance from Ranbaxy, Mumbai, India.

Table 3 Robustness of the analytical method

	Value				
Column temperature, 15-ppm LOS	39°C, area	40°C, area	41°C, area	%RE	%RSD
	1,672,455	1,675,725	1,674,952	−0.097 for 39°C −0.095 for 41°C	0.13 for 39°C 0.12 for 41°C
	1,671,846	1,672,374	1,671,854		
	1,674,985	1,671,377	1,671,853		
	1,673,917	1,671,377	1,670,988		
	1,674,992	1,671,377	1,669,852		
	1,677,866	1,669,455	1,673,479		
Wavelength, 15-ppm LOS	243 nm, area	245 nm, area	247 nm, area	%RE	%RSD
	1,672,379	1,675,725	1,672,874	−0.093 for 241 nm −0.090 for 245 nm	0.13 for 241 nm 0.06 for 245 nm
	1,671,895	1,672,374	1,671,893		
	1,674,813	1,671,377	1,671,623		
	1,673,739	1,671,898	1,672,098		
	1,674,385	1,670,491	1,671,254		
	1,677,930	1,669,455	1,669,695		

mobile phase composition, absorption wavelength of the detector, etc.), the analyte peak %RSD, tailing factor, and theoretical plate count should remain close to the actual values. The RSD values ranging from 0.06% to 0.13% represent the robustness of the proposed system. Results of RE and RSD determined for the variation of temperature and absorption wavelength are presented in Table 3. At a specified time interval, values of %RSD for the peak areas obtained for the stabilities of the drug solution and the mobile phase were within 1%. This shows that there is no

significant change in the elution of the peak and its system suitability criteria (%RSD, tailing factor, theoretical plate count). The results also confirm that the standard drug solution in the mobile phase was stable at least for 15 h during the assay performance. The constant peak area for different time intervals is shown in Figure 4.

Selectivity

Selectivity of the method was evaluated by injecting the mobile phase, standard drug solution, and tablet extract.

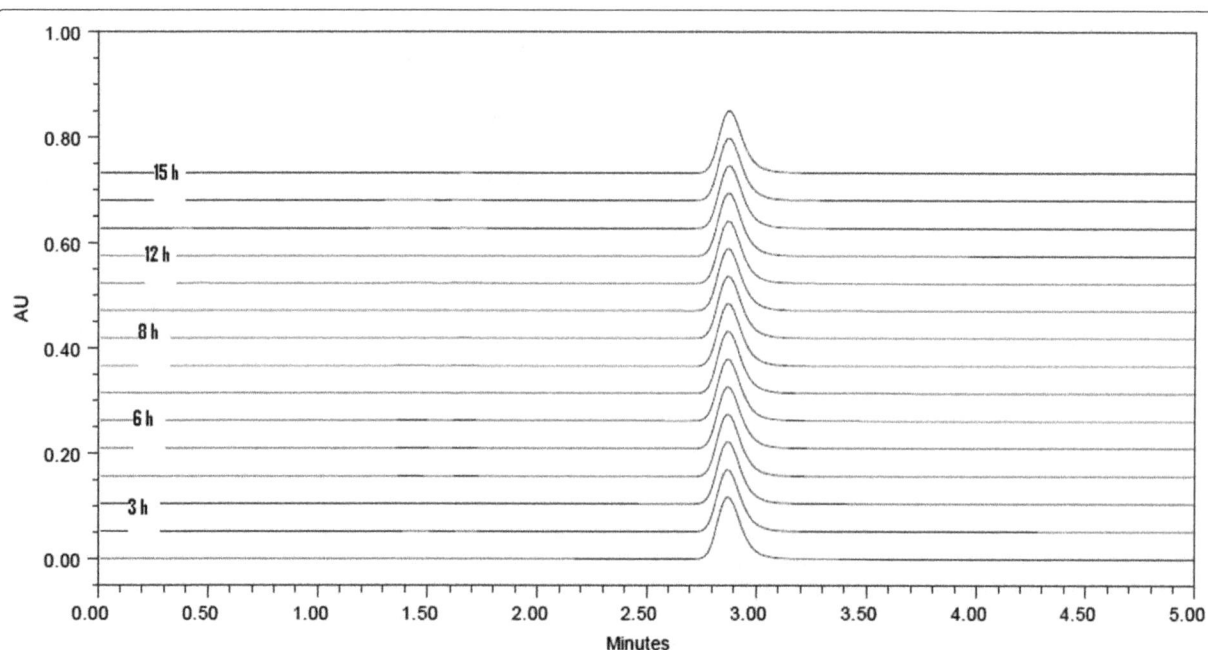

Figure 4 Chromatograms for LOS solution stability for periods of 3, 6, 8, 12, and 15 h in triplicate.

Under the experimental conditions, there was only a single peak for the drug (LOS) elusion, which showed a high selectivity of the method.

Application to tablet

Aliquots containing 250 µg mL^{-1} of LOS in extract and the pure drug solution were separately injected in triplicate to the UPLC system. The mean peak area of the tablets was found to be equivalent to that of the pure drug used as a positive control at the same concentration level.

Recovery study

A standard addition procedure was used to evaluate the accuracy and precision of the method. The solutions were prepared by spiking the pure LOS solution into a pre-analyzed LOS tablet extract at three different concentration levels followed by injection into the chromatographic column. The relatively low values of %RE and %RSD show high accuracy and precision of the developed UPLC method for the drug, LOS.

Conclusions

A rapid, isocratic reverse-phase ultra-performance liquid chromatographic (RP-UPLC) method was developed for the quantitative analysis of the drug, losartan potassium or LOS, in pharmaceutical dosage formulations. This method is precise, accurate, robust, and specific. Satisfactory results were obtained from the validation of the method. The short retention time obtained (2.40 min) enables rapid determination of LOS, which is important for its routine analysis in quality control. The method exhibits an excellent performance in terms of sensitivity and speed. Each experiment was repeated three times. Recovery of known amounts of the added analyte was calculated and is presented in Table 2. The reported values of the recovery are the average of three experiments.

Competing interests
The author declares no competing interests.

Author details
[1]Department of Chemistry, Yuvaraja's College, University of Mysore, Mysore-570005, India. [2]Department of Chemistry, Government First Grade College, K.R. Nagar, Mysore, India. [3]Department of studies in Chemistry, University of Mysore, Manasagangothri, Mysore, India. [4]Department of Chemistry, Western Illinois University, Macomb, IL 61455, USA.

References
Carlucci G, Palumbo G, Mazzeo P, Quaglia MG (2000) Simultaneous determination of losartan and hydrochlorothiazide in tablets by high-performance liquid chromatography. J Pharm Biomed Anal 23:185–189
Conlin PR (2001) Efficacy and safety of angiotensin receptor blockers: a review of losartan in essential hypertension. Curr Ther Res Clin Exp 62:673–673
Erk N (2001) Analysis of binary mixtures of losartan potassium and hydrochlorothiazide by using high performance liquid chromatography, ratio derivative spectrophotometric and compensation technique. J Pharm Biomed Anal 24:603–611
Gonzalez L, Lopez JA, Alonso RM, Jimenez RM (2002) Fast screening method for the determination of angiotensin II receptor antagonists in human plasma by high-performance liquid chromatography with fluorimetric detection. J Chromatogr A 949:49–60
Krishnaiah C, Reddy AR, Kumar R, Mukkanti K (2010) Stability-indicating UPLC method for determination of Valsartan and their degradation products in active pharmaceutical ingredient and pharmaceutical dosage forms. J Pharm Biomed Anal 53:483–489
Pedroso CF, de Oliveira JG, Campos FR, Gonzalves AG, Trindade CLB, Pontarolo R (2009) A Validated RP–LC Method for Simultaneous Determination of Losartan Potassium and Amlodipine Besilate in Pharmaceutical Preparations. Chromatographia 69:S201–S206
Seburg RA, Ballard JM, Hwang TL, Sullivan CM (2006) Photosensitized degradation of losartan potassium in an extemporaneous suspension formulation. J Pharm Biomed Anal 42:411–422
Waren SAC, Tchlitcheff P (2006) Use of ultra-performance liquid chromatography in pharmaceutical development. J Chromatogr A 1119:140–146
Yeung PK, Jamieson A, Smith GJ, Fice D, Pollak PT (2000) Determination of plasma concentrations of losartan in patients by HPLC using solid phase extraction and UV detection. Int J Pharm 204:17–22

Permissions

List of Contributors

Min Seok Choi
Division of Earth and Environmental Sciences, Korea Basic Science Institute, Chungbuk 363-883, South Korea

Chang-Sik Cheong
Division of Earth and Environmental Sciences, Korea Basic Science Institute, Chungbuk 363-883, South Korea

Jeongmin Kim
Division of Earth and Environmental Sciences, Korea Basic Science Institute, Chungbuk 363-883, South Korea

Hyung Seon Shin
Division of Earth and Environmental Sciences, Korea Basic Science Institute, Chungbuk 363-883, South Korea

Mahmoud A Omar
Analytical Chemistry Department, Faculty of pharmacy, Minia University, Minia 61519, Egypt

Osama H Abdelmageed
Pharmaceutical Chemistry Department, Faculty of Pharmacy, King Abdulaziz University, Jeddah, Kingdom of Saudi Arabia

Sayed M Derayea
Analytical Chemistry Department, Faculty of pharmacy, Minia University, Minia 61519, Egypt

Tadayuki Uno
Graduate School of Pharmaceutical Sciences, Osaka University, 1-6 Yamadaoka, Suita, Osaka 565-0871, Japan

Tamer Z Atia
Analytical Chemistry Department, Faculty of pharmacy, Minia University, Minia 61519, Egypt
Graduate School of Pharmaceutical Sciences, Osaka University, 1-6 Yamadaoka, Suita, Osaka 565-0871, Japan

Kannissery Pramod
Department of Pharmaceutics, Faculty of Pharmacy, Jamia Hamdard, Hamdard Nagar, New Delhi – 110 062, India

Ura Kottil Ilyas
Department of Pharmacognosy & Phytochemistry, Faculty of Pharmacy, Jamia Hamdard, Hamdard Nagar, New Delhi – 110 062, India

Yoonuskunju Thajudeenkoya Kamal
Department of Pharmacognosy & Phytochemistry, Faculty of Pharmacy, Jamia Hamdard, Hamdard Nagar, New Delhi – 110 062, India

Sayeed Ahmad
Department of Pharmacognosy & Phytochemistry, Faculty of Pharmacy, Jamia Hamdard, Hamdard Nagar, New Delhi – 110 062, India

Shahid Hussain Ansari
Department of Pharmacognosy & Phytochemistry, Faculty of Pharmacy, Jamia Hamdard, Hamdard Nagar, New Delhi – 110 062, India

Javed Ali
Department of Pharmaceutics, Faculty of Pharmacy, Jamia Hamdard, Hamdard Nagar, New Delhi – 110 062, India

Mohd Idris
Chemistry Division, Central Forensic Science Laboratory, Hyderabad, India

Cijo John
Chemistry Division, Central Forensic Science Laboratory, Hyderabad, India

Priyankar Ghosh
Chemistry Division, Central Forensic Science Laboratory, Hyderabad, India

Sudhir Kumar Shukla
Chemistry Division, Central Forensic Science Laboratory, Chandigarh, India

Tulsidas Ramachandra Rao Baggi
Forensic Science Institute, Osmania University, Hyderabad, India

M H Sanad
Labeled Compounds Department, Radioisotopes Production and Radioactive Sources Division, Hot Laboratories Center, Atomic Energy Authority, P.O. Box 13759, Cairo, Egypt

Swarali S Hingse
Food Engineering and Technology Department, Institute of Chemical Technology, Nathalal Parekh Marg, Matunga, Mumbai - 400019, India

Shraddha B Digole
Food Engineering and Technology Department, Institute of Chemical Technology, Nathalal Parekh Marg, Matunga, Mumbai - 400019, India

Uday S Annapure
Food Engineering and Technology Department, Institute of Chemical Technology, Nathalal Parekh Marg, Matunga, Mumbai - 400019, India

Amany Abd AL-Azem Gaber
Ceramic Department, National Research Centre, Cairo, Egypt

Doreya Mohamed Ibrahim
Ceramic Department, National Research Centre, Cairo, Egypt

Fawzia Fahm Abd-AImohsen
Polymers Department, National Research Centre, Cairo, Egypt

Elham Mohamed El-Zanati
Chemical Engineering Department, National Research Centre, Cairo, Egypt

Farhan Ahmed Siddiqui
Faculty of Pharmacy, Federal Urdu University Arts, Science and Technology, Karachi 75300, Pakistan

Nawab Sher
Department of Chemistry, University of Karachi, Karachi 75270, Pakistan

Nighat Shafi
Faculty of Pharmacy, Federal Urdu University Arts, Science and Technology, Karachi 75300, Pakistan

Hina Shamshad
Research Institute of Pharmaceutical Sciences, Faculty of Pharmacy, University of Karachi, Karachi 75270, Pakistan

Arif Zubair
Department of Environmental Sciences, Federal Urdu University Arts, Science and Technology, Karachi 75300, Pakistan

Chang-sik Cheong
Division of Earth and Environmental Sciences, Korea Basic Science Institute, Ochang, Chungbuk 363-883, Republic of Korea

Youn-Joong Jeong
Division of Earth and Environmental Sciences, Korea Basic Science Institute, Ochang, Chungbuk 363-883, Republic of Korea

Sung-Tack Kwon
Department of Earth System Sciences, Yonsei University, Seoul 120-749, Republic of Korea

Hina Shamshad
Research Institute of Pharmaceutical Sciences, Department of Pharmaceutical Chemistry, Faculty of Pharmacy, University of Karachi, Karachi 75270, Pakistan

M Saeed Arayne
Research Institute of Pharmaceutical Sciences, Department of Pharmaceutical Chemistry, Faculty of Pharmacy, University of Karachi, Karachi 75270, Pakistan

Najma Sultana
Department of Chemistry, University of Karachi, Karachi 75270, Pakistan

Hadi M Marwani
Department of Chemistry, Faculty of Science, King Abdulaziz University, P.O. Box 80203, Jeddah 21589, Saudi Arabia
Center of Excellence for Advanced Materials Research (CEAMR), King Abdulaziz University, P.O. Box 80203, Jeddah 21589, Saudi Arabia

Amjad E Alsafrani
Department of Chemistry, Faculty of Science, King Abdulaziz University, P.O. Box 80203, Jeddah 21589, Saudi Arabia

Amir Alhaj Sakur
Department of Analytical Chemistry, Faculty of Pharmacy, University of Aleppo, Aleppo, Syria

Tamim Chalati
Department of Pharmaceutics, Faculty of Pharmacy, University of Aleppo, Aleppo, Syria

Hanan Fael
Department of Analytical Chemistry, Faculty of Pharmacy, University of Aleppo, Aleppo, Syria

Stanislav Vrtnik
Jožef Stefan Institute, Jamova 39, SI-1000 Ljubljana, Slovenia
Faculty of Mathematics and Physics, University of Ljubljana, Jadranska 19, SI-1000 Ljubljana, Slovenia

Magdalena Wencka
Institute of Molecular Physics, Polish Academy of Sciences, Smoluchowskiego 17, PL-60-179 Poznań, Poland

Andreja Jelen
Jožef Stefan Institute, Jamova 39, SI-1000 Ljubljana, Slovenia
Faculty of Mathematics and Physics, University of Ljubljana, Jadranska 19, SI-1000
Ljubljana, Slovenia

Hae Jin Kim
Division of Materials Science, Korea Basic Science Institute, Daejeon 305-333, Republic of Korea

Janez Dolinšek
Jožef Stefan Institute, Jamova 39, SI-1000 Ljubljana, Slovenia
Faculty of Mathematics and Physics, University of Ljubljana, Jadranska 19, SI-1000
Ljubljana, Slovenia

Srinivasa Babu Puttagunta
Vignan Colllege of pharmacy, Vadlamudi, Guntur, Andhra Pradesh 522213, India

Rihana Parveen Shaik
Vignan Colllege of pharmacy, Vadlamudi, Guntur, Andhra Pradesh 522213, India
Jawaharlal Nehru Technological University, Anantapur, Andhra Pradesh 515002, India

Chandrasekhar Kothapalli Bannoth
Jawaharlal Nehru Technological University, Anantapur, Andhra Pradesh 515002, India
Bala Sekhara Reddy Challa
Vaagdevi College of Pharmacy, Gurazala, Guntur, Andhra Pradesh 522415, India

Bahlul Zayed Sh Awen
Faculty of Pharmacy, Tripoli University, Tripoli 13610, Libya

Jamie Whelan
Department of Chemical Engineering, The Petroleum Institute, P.O. Box 2533, Abu Dhabi, United Arab Emirates

Department of Chemistry, New York University Abu Dhabi, P.O. Box 129188, Abu Dhabi, UAE

Ionut Banu
Department of Chemical and Biochemical Engineering, University Politehnica of Bucharest,
313 Spl. Independentei, sector 6, 060042, Bucharest, Romania

Gisha E Luckachan
Department of Chemical Engineering, The Petroleum Institute, P.O. Box 2533, Abu Dhabi, United Arab Emirates

Nicoleta Doriana Banu
Department of Chemical Engineering, The Petroleum Institute, P.O. Box 2533, Abu Dhabi, United Arab Emirates
Center for Organic Chemistry "C.D. Nenitzescu", 060023 Bucharest, Romania

Samuel Stephen
Department of Chemical Engineering, The Petroleum Institute, P.O. Box 2533, Abu Dhabi, United Arab Emirates

Anjana Tharalekshmy
Department of Chemical Engineering, The Petroleum Institute, P.O. Box 2533, Abu Dhabi, United Arab Emirates

Saleh Al Hashimi
Department of Chemical Engineering, The Petroleum Institute, P.O. Box 2533, Abu Dhabi, United Arab Emirates

Radu V Vladea
Department of Chemical Engineering, The Petroleum Institute, P.O. Box 2533, Abu Dhabi, United Arab Emirates

Marios S Katsiotis
Department of Chemical Engineering, The Petroleum Institute, P.O. Box 2533, Abu Dhabi, United Arab Emirates

Saeed M Alhassan
Department of Chemical Engineering, The Petroleum Institute, P.O. Box 2533, Abu Dhabi, United Arab Emirates

Eun Hye Lee
Division of Magnetic Resonance Research, Korea Basic Science Institute, Ochang, Chungbuk, Korea
Division of Biotechnology, College of Life Sciences and Biotechnology, Korea University, Seoul, Korea

Hae-Kap Cheong
Division of Magnetic Resonance Research, Korea Basic Science Institute, Ochang, Chungbuk, Korea

Hye-Yeon Kim
Division of Magnetic Resonance Research, Korea Basic Science Institute, Ochang, Chungbuk, Korea

Jong-Sik Ryu
Division of Earth and Environmental Sciences, Korea Basic Science Institute, Chungbuk 363-883, South Korea

Min Seok Choi
Division of Earth and Environmental Sciences, Korea Basic Science Institute, Chungbuk 363-883, South Korea

Youn-Joong Jeong
Division of Earth and Environmental Sciences, Korea Basic Science Institute, Chungbuk 363-883, South Korea

Chang-sik Cheong
Division of Earth and Environmental Sciences, Korea Basic Science Institute, Chungbuk 363-883, South Korea

Pawan K Basniwal
School of Pharmaceutical Sciences, Rajiv Gandhi Technological University, Bhopal, Madhya Pradesh 462 033, India
LBS College of Pharmacy, Jaipur, Rajasthan 302 004, India

Deepti Jain
School of Pharmaceutical Sciences, Rajiv Gandhi Technological University, Bhopal, Madhya Pradesh 462 033, India

Raafia Najam
PG Department of Chemistry, University of Kashmir, Srinagar, Jammu and Kashmir 190006, India

Gh Mohd Shah
PG Department of Chemistry, University of Kashmir, Srinagar, Jammu and Kashmir 190006, India

S Muzaffar Ali Andrabi
University Science Instrumentation Centre, University of Kashmir, Srinagar, Jammu and Kashmir 190006, India

Deepti Jain
School of Pharmaceutical Sciences, Rajiv Gandhi Technological University, Bhopal, Madhya Pradesh 462033, India

Pawan K Basniwal
School of Pharmaceutical Sciences, Rajiv Gandhi Technological University, Bhopal, Madhya Pradesh 462033, India
LBS College of Pharmacy, Jaipur, Rajasthan 302004, India

Hadi Beitollahi
Environment Department, Institute of Science and High Technology and Environmental Sciences, Graduate University of Advanced Technology, P.O. Box 76315-117, Kerman, Iran.

Somayeh Tajik
Department of Chemistry, Shahid Bahonar University of Kerman, P.O. Box 76175-133, Kerman, Iran

Malek Hossein Asadi
Biotechnology Department, Institute of Science and High Technology and Environmental
Sciences, Graduate University of Advanced Technology, P.O. Box 76315-117, Kerman, Iran

Pourya Biparva
Department of Basic Sciences, Sari Agricultural Sciences and Natural Resources University, P.O. Box 79316-217, Sari, Iran

Abdul Bari Mohd
Department of Pharmaceutics, School of Pharmacy, Nalla Narasimha Reddy Educational Society's Group of Institutions, Hyderabad -500088, AP, India

Krishna Sanka
Department of Pharmaceutics, School of Pharmacy, Anurag Group of Institutions, Hyderabad -500088, AP, India

Rakesh Gullapelly
Department of Pharmaceutics, School of Pharmacy, Anurag Group of Institutions, Hyderabad -500088, AP, India

Prakash V Diwan
Department of Pharmaceutics, School of Pharmacy, Nalla Narasimha Reddy Educational Society's Group of Institutions, Hyderabad -500088, AP, India

Nalini Shastri
Department of Pharmaceutics, National Institute of Pharmaceutical Education and Research (NIPER), Hyderabad 500 037, AP, India

Jihye Noh
Division of Magnetic Resonance Research, Korea Basic Science Institute, Ochang, Chungbuk, South Korea

Ji-woo Seok
Department of Psychology, Brain Research Institute, Chungnam National University, Daejeon, South Korea

Suk-Hee Kim
Department of Professional Counseling and Psychotherapy, Graduate School of Health and Complementary Medicine, Wonkwang University, Iksan, Cheonbuk 570-749, South Korea

Chaejoon Cheong
Division of Magnetic Resonance Research, Korea Basic Science Institute, Ochang, Chungbuk, South Korea

Jin-Hun Sohn
Department of Psychology, Brain Research Institute, Chungnam National University, Daejeon, South Korea

Ambavaram Vijaya Bhaskar Reddy
Department of Chemistry, Sri Venkateswara University, Tirupati 517502, India

Nandigam Venugopal
Department of Chemistry, Sri Venkateswara University, Tirupati 517502, India

Gajulapalle Madhavi
Department of Chemistry, Sri Venkateswara University, Tirupati 517502, India

Tarab J Ahmad
Department of Chemistry, Western Illinois University, Macomb, IL 61455, USA

Amruth Raj
Department of Chemistry, Yuvaraja's College, University of Mysore, Mysore-570005, India

Rayapura T Radhika
Department of Chemistry, Government First Grade College, K.R. Nagar, Mysore, India

Sannaiah Ananda
Department of studies in Chemistry, University of Mysore, Manasagangothri, Mysore, India

Netkal M Gowda
Department of Chemistry, Western Illinois University, Macomb, IL 61455, USA

Bellale M Venkatesha
Department of Chemistry, Yuvaraja's

www.ingramcontent.com/pod-product-compliance
Lightning Source LLC
Chambersburg PA
CBHW080656200326

41458CB00013B/4871